MDR and XDR Tuberculosis

MDR and XDR Tuberculosis

Rajendra Prasad
MD DTCD FAMS FCCP (USA)
FNCCP FCAI FIAB FIMSA DSC (Honoris Causa)

Director
Vallabhbhai Patel Chest Institute
University of Delhi
New Delhi, India

Formerly
Professor and Head
Department of Pulmonary Medicine
King George's Medical University
Lucknow, Uttar Pradesh, India

Co-author
Nikhil Gupta MD
Assistant Professor
Department of Medicine
Era's Lucknow Medical College
Lucknow, Uttar Pradesh, India

Foreword
KC Mohanty

JAYPEE *The Health Sciences Publisher*

New Delhi | London | Philadelphia | Panama

JAYPEE **Jaypee Brothers Medical Publishers (P) Ltd**

Headquarters

Jaypee Brothers Medical Publishers (P) Ltd
4838/24, Ansari Road, Daryaganj
New Delhi 110 002, India
Phone: +91-11-43574357
Fax: +91-11-43574314
Email: jaypee@jaypeebrothers.com

Overseas Offices

J.P. Medical Ltd
83, Victoria Street, London
SW1H 0HW (UK)
Phone: +44 20 3170 8910
Fax: +44 (0)20 3008 6180
Email: info@jpmedpub.com

Jaypee-Highlights Medical Publishers Inc
City of Knowledge, Bld. 237, Clayton
Panama City, Panama
Phone: +1 507-301-0496
Fax: +1 507-301-0499
Email: cservice@jphmedical.com

Jaypee Medical Inc
The Bourse
111 South Independence Mall East
Suite 835, Philadelphia, PA 19106, USA
Phone: +1 267-519-9789
Email: jpmed.us@gmail.com

Jaypee Brothers Medical Publishers (P) Ltd
17/1-B Babar Road, Block-B, Shaymali
Mohammadpur, Dhaka-1207
Bangladesh
Mobile: +08801912003485
Email: jaypeedhaka@gmail.com

Jaypee Brothers Medical Publishers (P) Ltd
Bhotahity, Kathmandu
Nepal
Phone: +977-9741283608
Email: kathmandu@jaypeebrothers.com

Website: www.jaypeebrothers.com

Website: www.jaypeedigital.com

Inquiries for bulk sales may be solicited at: jaypee@jaypeebrothers.com

MDR and XDR Tuberculosis

First Edition: **2015**

ISBN 978-93-5152-220-1

Printed at Rajkamal Electric Press, Plot No. 2, Phase-IV, Kundli, Haryana.

Dedicated to

My teachers for their guidance, wisdom and inspiration
My parents, wife and children for their love and patience

Foreword

Professor Rajendra Prasad is a nationally-acclaimed chest physician and tuberculosis expert, possessing over 3 decades' illustrious teaching, research and administrative experience with proven excellence in quality patient care. Apart from being a clinician par excellence, he is also a very popular medical teacher in pulmonary medicine. He is currently the Director of Vallabhbhai Patel Chest Institute, New Delhi. He has earlier served as Professor and Head, Department of Pulmonary Medicine, King George's Medical University, Lucknow, Uttar Pradesh, India and Director, UP Rural Institute of Medical Sciences and Research, Saifai, Etawah, Uttar Pradesh, India. He has devoted all his energy in promoting medical education, patient care and research. Professor Prasad's contribution in the field of tuberculosis and multidrug-resistant tuberculosis (MDR-TB) are widely acclaimed. He took keen interest in Revised National Tuberculosis Control Program (RNTCP) since its inception. His dynamic leadership in academic and administrative areas has earned him a large number of awards from various international and national scientific societies.

Tuberculosis is a multisystemic disease with varied clinical presentations. Despite being a 100% curable disease, it still continues to be the world's most important infectious cause of morbidity and mortality. Globally, 1.4 million people die every year with tuberculosis, of which 0.3 million die in India. Drug-resistant tuberculosis has been reported since the early days of introduction of anti-TB chemotherapy but multidrug-resistant tuberculosis (MDR-TB) and more recently extensively drug-resistant tuberculosis (XDR-TB) has been an area of growing concern and is posing threat to global efforts to control tuberculosis.

Against this backdrop, the publication of the book *MDR and XDR Tuberculosis* by Professor Rajendra Prasad is a timely and exclusive addition to the existing literature on drug-resistant tuberculosis. The book has summarized the current status of knowledge on drug-resistant tuberculosis and also discusses the latest practical approach to various diagnostic and treatment modalities for drug-resistant tuberculosis, multidrug-resistant tuberculosis (MDR-TB) and extensively drug-resistant tuberculosis (XDR-TB). The book has been divided into 27 chapters covering all the aspects of drug-resistant tuberculosis ranging from detailed epidemiology, practical approach to diagnosis and treatment of MDR and XDR tuberculosis including HIV and drug-resistant tuberculosis. Special chapters on case-based approach to treatment of MDR-TB and XDR-TB, drug-resistant tuberculosis in children and extrapulmonary tuberculosis, fluoroquinolone resistance, infection control in drug-resistant tuberculosis and newer antituberculosis drugs are also included. The chapters in the book have been arranged in a systemic sequence for easy understanding. The chapters have been written on the basis of vast and rich clinical experience gained by the author from day-to-day patient management over the last many years.

Professor Rajendra Prasad's endeavor for elaborating the management of drug-resistant, multidrug-resistant (MDR) and extensively drug-resistant (XDR) tuberculosis in this book is very informative and is a plethora of knowledge. I am sure it will be extremely helpful to all the clinicians, undergraduate and postgraduate medical students, and all medical and healthcare professionals who are managing and who will be managing tuberculosis. This book deserves a place in the library of every medical college and healthcare providing institute.

KC Mohanty
MBBS MD (Bom) MAMS (Ind)
TDD (Bom) FCCP (USA) FICCD
FISCD FMSGE FIAMS
MIPHA FSASMS FAPI DSc
Former Professor and Head
Department of Tuberculosis and Chest Disease
Grant Medical College and Sir JJ Group of Hospitals
KJ Somaiya Medical College
Mumbai, Maharashtra, India

Preface

I look upon tuberculosis as a 100% curable disease throughout the 40 years of my clinical practice in pulmonary medicine, provided adequate regimen is prescribed by doctor and taken by patients. Practically, there should be no relapse, drug resistance and death. However, tuberculosis still continues to be the world's most important infectious cause of morbidity and mortality. Globally, nearly 9 million people develop tuberculosis disease every year and 1.4 million die every year with tuberculosis. In India, nearly 2 million people develop tuberculosis and 0.3 million people are dying every year. It is a cause for concern as India stands first in terms of absolute number of cases closely followed by China. Drug-resistant tuberculosis has been reported since the early days of introduction of anti-TB chemotherapy but multidrug-resistant tuberculosis (MDR-TB) and more recently extensively drug-resistant tuberculosis (XDR-TB) has been an area of growing concern and is posing threat to global efforts of eradication of tuberculosis.

This book was written with the aim of defining a practical approach to every aspect of drug-resistant tuberculosis, especially multidrug-resistant tuberculosis (MDR-TB) and extensively drug-resistant tuberculosis (XDR-TB). In total, there are 27 chapters in the book. Chapters practically cover all the aspects of drug-resistant tuberculosis including MDR and XDR-TB, ranging from epidemiology, diagnosis and practical approach to the treatment of MDR and XDR-TB including HIV and DR-TB. Special chapters on case-based approach to treatment of MDR-TB have also been included. Chapter on DR-TB in children, DR-TB in extrapulmonary tuberculosis, fluoroquinolone resistance, infection control in DR-TB and newer antituberculosis drugs are also included. Chapters have been written in the background of current literature and practical experience gained from day-to-day dealing with different patients suffering from drug-resistant tuberculosis. Advances up to 2013 have been included, making all the chapters well referenced with the latest references.

This book will be useful to both undergraduate and postgraduate medical students, practitioners and program managers of TB control. In toto, this book will serve as a very useful practical guide regarding all aspects of drug-resistant tuberculosis, especially MDR and XDR-TB.

Rajendra Prasad

Acknowledgments

I wish to acknowledge my indebtedness to a number of people who significantly contributed to the publication of this book. The individual to whom I would like to acknowledge first is Professor BK Khanna, who, as a Head of the Department of Tuberculosis at the King George's Medical College, Lucknow, Uttar Pradesh, India, while I was a postgraduate student in that department, markedly stimulated my interest in tuberculosis. Professor BK Khanna's own tremendous knowledge and wisdom in the field of tuberculosis, especially drug-resistant tuberculosis, set an example of thoughtfulness and meticulousness, which I have always tried to emulate. I am also indebted to Professor PK Mukherjee, Dr J Nath, Late Dr MS Agnihotri and Late Dr Jafar Jameel, for their great inspiration as a teacher during my postgraduate days. I am greatly indebted to the many postgraduate students who have been trained with me in the department at King George's Medical College, Lucknow, Uttar Pradesh, India and Vallabhbhai Patel Chest Institute, New Delhi, especially Dr Sanjay Verma, Dr Kiran Vishnu Narayan, Dr Suneesh C Anand, Dr Giridhar BH, Dr Abhijeet, Dr Jabeed P, Dr Saheer S, Dr Abhishek Agrawal, Dr Shailendra Singh, Dr Mandeep Singh, Dr Pawan Gupta. The efforts of these students are in part responsible for generating much of the data that can be incorporated in making the chapters in the book more evidence-based.

I also wish to express my appreciation to Dr Nikhil Gupta, the co-author of this book, for helping me in preparing and correcting the manuscript. I also wish to express my thanks to Mr PP Sharma and Mr Ashish Yadav, for their invaluable help in the preparation and typing of the manuscript. I am also thankful to all my patients who gave me experience in the field of tuberculosis, especially MDR and XDR-TB.

I am especially thankful to Shri Jitendar P Vij (Group Chairman), Mr Ankit Vij (Group President), Mr Tarun Duneja (Director–Publishing) and Ms Samina Khan (Executive Assistant to Director–Publishing) and all the members of M/s Jaypee Brothers Medical Publishers (P) Ltd, New Delhi, India, for all the help and cooperation they have extended to me.

Contents

Chapter 1

Case Definitions in Drug-resistant Tuberculosis

Drug-resistant tuberculosis is defined as a case of tuberculosis excreting bacilli resistant to one or more anti-tubercular drugs. DR-TB is confirmed through laboratory tests that show that the infecting isolates of *Mycobacterium tuberculosis* grow in vitro in the presence of one or more antituberculosis drugs. The following different categories of drug resistance have been established:[1]

- **Primary drug resistance:** Drug resistance in a patient who has not received any antitubercular treatment in the past.
- **Acquired drug resistance:** Drug resistance that develops in a patient who has received prior chemotherapy.
- **Combined resistance:** Defined as the sum of primary and acquired drug resistance.
- **Initial resistance:** When one is not sure whether the resistance is primary or acquired due to concealed history of previous treatment or unawareness of treatment taken before, it is known as initial drug resistance. Thus, initial resistance is primary resistance plus some undisclosed acquired resistance.
- **Monoresistance:** Resistance to one antituberculosis drug.
- **Polyresistance:** Resistance to more than one antituberculosis drug, other than both isoniazid and rifampicin.
- **MDR-TB or Multidrug-resistant TB**: Resistant to isoniazid (H) and rifampicin (R) with or without resistance to other drugs.
- **MDR-TB suspect:** A TB patient who fails an RNTCP Category I or III treatment regimen and any RNTCP Category II patient, who is sputum smear positive at the end of the fourth month of treatment or later. Recently, criteria for defining a MDR-TB suspect has been divided into three groups under programmatic management of drug-resistant tuberculosis, 2012. The program uses a strategy that screens patients with initially a very high risk of MDR-TB using DST. As laboratory and treatment capacity builds, the program will scale up to achieve universal access to quality-assured DST. The MDR suspects have been divided into three criteria based on the risk of MDR-TB. Criteria A includes all failures of new TB cases, smear positive previously treated cases who remain smear positive at fourth month onwards, all pulmonary TB cases who are contacts of the known MDR-TB case. Criteria B includes,

in addition to criteria A, all smear positive previously treated pulmonary TB cases at diagnosis, any smear positive follow-up result in new or previously treated cases. Criteria C includes, in addition to Criteria B, all smear negative previously treated pulmonary TB cases at diagnosis, HIV TB coinfected cases at diagnosis. Initially, DST will be performed in those patients fulfilling Criteria A and, as capacity builds up, it will progress to criteria B and then to criteria C.[2,3]

- **Confirmed MDR-TB case:** A TB patient whose sputum is culture positive for Mycobacterium tuberculosis and is resistant in vitro to isoniazid and rifampicin with or without other antitubercular drugs based on DST results from an RNTCP-certified Culture and DST Laboratory. An 'MDR-TB suspect' confirmed by an RNTCP-certified Culture and DST Laboratory to have MDR-TB, or any rifampicin resistance, will be treated with the RNTCP Regimen for MDR-TB.[2,3]
- **XDR-TB or Extensively Drug-resistant TB**: The term 'Extensively drug-resistant TB (XDR-TB)' is a new term which was provisionally defined as those persons with TB whose isolates were resistant to Isoniazid and Rifampicin and atleast three of the six main classes of Second Line Drugs (SLDs) (Aminoglycosides, Polypeptides, Fluoroquinolones, Thioamides, Cycloserine and Para-aminosalicylic Acid). But, in October 2006, the World Health Organization (WHO) revised the case definition of XDR-TB as TB with resistance to at least isoniazid and rifampicin as well as further resistance to a fluroquinolone and a second line injectable agent (kanamycin, amikacin or capreomycin).[4,5]
- **XDR-TB suspect**: If the sixth month follow-up culture of MDR patients under DOTS-PLUS treatment is found to be positive, then, at this time, culture isolate should to be sent for second-line DST.
- **XXDR-TB or Extremely Drug-resistant TB or Total drug-resistant TB (TDR-TB):** The term 'extremely drug-resistant XXDR-TB or TDR-TB' has been proposed for cases resistant to all available first- and second-line drugs.[5-8] The term 'totally drug-resistant' tuberculosis is not yet recognized by the WHO. For now, these cases are defined as extensively drug-resistant tuberculosis (XDR-TB), according to WHO definitions.[9]

Treatment Outcomes in DOTS-PLUS

Standardized treatment outcome definitions are to be used following treatment of an MDR-TB case, and these are as follows:

- **Cure:** An MDR-TB patient, who has completed treatment and has been consistently culture negative (with at least five consecutive negative results in the last 12–15 months). If one follow-up positive culture is reported during the last three quarters, the patient will still be considered cured, provided this positive culture is followed by at least three consecutive negative cultures, taken at least 30 days apart, provided that there is clinical evidence of improvement.
- **Treatment completed:** An MDR-TB patient who has completed treatment according to guidelines but does not meet the definition for cure or treatment failure due to lack of bacteriological results.

- **Death:** An MDR-TB patient who dies for any reason during the course of MDR-TB treatment.
- **Treatment failure:** Treatment will be considered to have failed if two or more of the five cultures recorded in the final 12 to 15 months are positive, or if any of the final three cultures are positive.
- **Treatment default:** An MDR-TB patient whose MDR-TB treatment was interrupted for two or more consecutive months for any reasons.
- **Transfer out:** An MDR-TB patient who has been transferred to another reporting unit and for whom the treatment outcome is not known.
- **Treatment stopped due to adverse drug reactions:** A patient on MDR-TB treatment who develops severe adverse reactions and could not continue the MDR-TB treatment in spite of the management of the adverse reactions as per the defined protocols and decision has been taken by the DOTS-Plus site committee to stop treatment.
- **Treatment stopped due to other reasons:** A patient on MDR-TB treatment who could not continue the MDR-TB treatment for any other medical reason (other than adverse drug reactions), and a decision has been taken by the DOTS-Plus site committee to stop treatment.
- **Still on treatment:** An MDR-TB patient who, for any reason, is still receiving his RNTCP CAT IV treatment at the time of the submission of the RNTCP DOTS-Plus Treatment Outcome Report.

References

1. Guidelines for the programmatic management of drug-resistant tuberculosis; emergency update 2008. Geneva, WHO 2008 (WHO/HTM/TB/2008.402).
2. Guidelines on Programmatic Management of Drug-resistant TB (PMDT) in India 2012. Central TB Division, Directorate General of Health Services, Ministry of Health & Family Welfare, Nirman Bhavan, NewDelhi.
3. Centers for Disease Control and Prevention (CDC). Emergence of *Mycobacterium tuberculosis* with extensive resistance to second-line drugs—Worldwide, 2000–2004. MMWR Morb Mortal Wkly Rep. 2006;55:301-5.
4. Centers for Disease Control and Prevention (CDC). Notice to readers: Revised definition of extensively drug-resistant tuberculosis. MMWR Morb Mortal Wkly Rep. 2006;55:1176.
5. Migliori GB, Loddenkemper R, Blasi F, Raviglione MC. 125 years after Robert Koch's discovery of the tubercle bacillus: the new XDR-TB threat: is "science" enough to tackle the epidemic? Eur Respir J. 2007;29:423-7.
6. Joshi JM. Preventing extremely drug-resistant tuberculosis: directly observed treatment is the only answer. Editorial. Indian J Chest Dis Allied Sci. 2008;50:183-5.
7. Velayati AA, Masjedi MR, Farnia P, et al. Emergence of new forms of totally drug-resistant tuberculosis bacilli: super-extensively drug-resistant tuberculosis or totally drug-resistant strains in Iran. Chest 2009;136:420-5.
8. Udwadia ZF, Amale RA, Ajbani KK, Rodriguez C. Totally drug-resistant tuberculosis in India. Clin Infect Dis. 2012;54:579-81.
9. WHO Stop TB Department Drug-resistant Tuberculosis—Frequently Asked Questions. Updated 24th January, 2012. Available at: http://www.who.int/tb/challenges/mdr/TDRFAQs160112.

Chapter 2

Antitubercular Drugs Used in Previously Treated Patients of Tuberculosis and Their Adverse Effects

Kanamycin

Drug Class: Aminoglycoside

Activity against TB, Mechanism of Action and Metabolism: Bactericidal, aminoglycosides: It is used as reserve drugs in MDR tuberculosis not responding to primary antitubercular drugs.[1] It was second systemically used aminoglycoside, after streptomycin, in tuberculosis.[2,3] Inhibit protein synthesis by irreversibly binding to 30S ribosomal subunit; aminoglycosides are not metabolized in the liver, they are excreted unchanged in the urine. Most strains of tuberculosis is inhibited in vitro at the concentrations of 10 μg/mL.[4]

Distribution: 0.2–0.4 L/kg; distributed in extracellular fluid, abscesses, ascitic fluid, pericardial fluid, pleural fluid, synovial fluid, lymphatic fluid and peritoneal fluid. Not well distributed into bile, aqueous humour, bronchial secretions, sputum and CSF.

Preparation and dose: Kanamycin sulfate, sterile powder for intramuscular injection in sealed vials. The powder needs to be dissolved in 2 mL of 0.9% sodium chloride or water for injections before use. The optimal dose is 15 (12–18) mg/kg body weight, usually 750 mg to 1 g given daily or 5–6 days per week, by deep intramuscular injection. Rotation of injection sites avoids local discomfort. When necessary, it is possible to give the drug at the same total dose 2 or 3 times weekly during the continuation phase, under close monitoring for adverse effects.

Storage: Powder stable at room temperature (15–25°C), diluted solution should be used the same day.

Oral absorption: There is no significant oral absorption.

CSF penetration: Penetrates inflamed meninges only.

Special Circumstances

- **Pregnancy/breastfeeding:** Safety class D. Eighth cranial nerve damage has been reported following in utero exposure to kanamycin. Excreted in breast milk. The American Academy of Paediatrics considers kanamycin to be compatible with breastfeeding.

- **Renal disease:** Use with caution. Levels should be monitored for patients with impaired renal function. Interval adjustment (12–15 mg/kg—2 or 3 times per week) is recommended for creatinine clearance < 30 mL/min. or hemodialysis.
- **Hepatic disease:** Drug levels not affected by hepatic disease (except a larger volume of distribution for alcoholic cirrhotic patients with ascites). Presumed to be safe in severe liver disease; however, use with caution—some patients with severe liver disease may progress rapidly to hepatorenal syndrome.

Adverse Effects (Table 2.1)

Frequent

- Pain at injection site
- Renal failure (usually reversible).

TABLE 2.1: Adverse effects of antitubercular drugs used in retreatment cases

Drug	*Frequent*	*Occassional*	*Rare*
Amikacin	Pain injection site Proteinuria Electrolyte disturbances (hypokalemia and hypomagnesemia)	Cochlear ototoxicity Vestibular toxicity Nephrotoxicity Peripheral neuropathy Rash Eosinophilia	Fever
Capreomycin	Nephotoxicity Tubular dysfunction Urticaria Maculopapular rash	Cochlear ototoxicity Vestibular toxicity Electrolyte disturbances (hypokalemia, hypomagnesemia and hypocalcemia) Pain at injection site, induration and sterile abscesses at site of injection Neurotoxicity	Rash
Clofazimine	Ichthyosis Dry skin Pink to brown black discolouration of skin, cornea, retina and urine Anorexia Abdominal pain	Hepatitis Hypersensitivity Nephrotoxicity Acneform eruption	Phototoxicity
Cycloserine	Neurological disturbances (headache and tremors) Psychiatric disturbances (sleep disturbances, anxiety, depression, irritability, confusion, drowsiness) Inflammation of gums Pale skin	Visual changes and eye pain Skin rash Jaundice (hepatitis) Burning, tingling and numbness in hands and feet	Seizures Suicidal thoughts Imaired hearing in fetus Hypersensitivity

Contd...

Contd...

Drug	*Frequent*	*Occassional*	*Rare*
Ethinonamide and prothionamide	Severe gastrointestinal Intolerance (including nausea, vomiting, diarrhea, abdominal pain, excessive salivation metallic taste)-dose related Headache Anorexia and weight loss Stomatitis	Neurological disturbances Psychiatric disturbances (depression, restlessness, drowsiness) Allergic reactions Postural hypotension Reversible hepatitis (transient increase in serum bilirubin) Hypothyroidism (especially when combined with PAS) Menstrual irregularity Gynecomastia Arthralgias Leukopenia	Peripheral neuritis Optic neuritis Pellagra-like syndrome Rash Photosensitivity Thrombocytopenia Alopecia Impotence Purpura
Kanamycin	Pain at injection site Renal damage (usually reversible)	Cochlear and vestibular otoxicity (usually irreversible) Peripheral neuropathy Rash Nephrotoxicity (dose related to cumulative and peak concenteration, often irreversible)	Fever
Levofloxacin	Generally well tolerated	Gastrointestinal intolerance (diarrhea) Neurological disturbances (insomnia, restlessness, dizziness) Allergic reactions Photosensitivity	QT interval prolongation Peripheral neuropathy Tendon rupture Rash
Moxifloxacin	Generally well-tolerated	Gastrointestinal intolerance (diarrhea) Neurological disturbances (insomnia, restlessness, dizziness) Allergic reactions Photosensitivity	QT internal prolongation (in isolated cases) Rash
Ofloxacin	Generally well-tolerated	Gastrointestinal intolerance (diarrhea) Neurological disturbances (headache, insomnia, restlessness)	Allergic reactions Photosensitivity Peripheral neuropathy Tendon rupture Increased liver function tests
P-aminosalicylic Acid (PAS)	Gastrointestinal intolerance (including metallic taste, anorexia, diarrhea) Hypothyroidism, especially when combined with ethionamide	Hepatitis Thyroid enlargement Allergic reactions Fever Increased prothrombin time Malabsorption syndrome (eg. Steatorrhea and low serum folate level)	

Contd...

Contd...

Drug	*Frequent*	*Occassional*	*Rare*
Linezolid	Gastrointestinal intolerance Rash Headache	Myelosuppression Peripheral neuropathy Optic neuropathy	
Clarithromycin	Gastrointestinal Intolerance (abdominal pain, nausea, vomiting, diarrhea) Hepatitis Ventricular arrhythmias		Hypersensitivity reaction Pseudomembranous colitis Fever Rash
Imipenem/ cilastatin	Gastrointestinal intolerance Hypersensitivity reaction Palpitation Tachycardia	Seizure Hypotension Anemia Thrombophlebitis	Renal failure Hemorrhagic colitis Pseudomembranous colitis
Thiacetazone	Gastrointestinal intolerance Rash Anemia	Hepatitis Exfoliative dermatitis Stevens-Johnson syndrome	Bone marrow depression Ototoxicity
Amoxicillin/ clavulanate	Diarrhea Rash Hypersensitivity reaction	*Candida stomatitis* Vaginitis	Hepatic injury

Occasional

- Vestibular and auditory damage (usually irreversible)
- Nephrotoxicity (dose related to cumulative and peak concentrations)
- Increased risk with renal insufficiency (often irreversible)
- Peripheral neuropathy
- Rash.

Ototoxicity potentiated by certain diuretics (especially loop diuretics), advanced age and prolonged use. The effect of nondepolarizing muscle relaxants may be increased.

Drug Interactions

- **Loop diuretics** (bumetanide, furosemide, ethacrynic acid, torsemide). Co-administration of aminoglycosides with loop diuretics may have an additive or synergistic auditory ototoxicity. Ototoxicity appears to be dose-dependent and may be increased with renal dysfunction. Irreversible ototoxicity has been reported.
  Avoid concomitant administration; if used together, careful dose adjustments in patients with renal failure and close monitoring for ototoxicity are required.
- **Nondepolarizing muscle relaxants** (atracurium, pancuronium, tubocurarine, gallamine triethiodide): Possible enhanced action of nondepolarizing muscle relaxant resulting in possible respiratory depression. Avoid co-administration; if concurrent administration is needed, titrate the non-depolarizing muscle relaxant slowly and monitor neuromuscular function closely.
- **Nephrotoxic agents** (amphotericin B, foscarnet, cidofovir): Additive nephrotoxicity. Avoid coadministration; if used together, monitor renal function closely and discontinue if warranted.

- **Penicillins:** In vitro inactivation (possible). Do not mix together before administration.

Contraindications

- Pregnancy (congenital deafness seen with streptomycin and kanamycin use in pregnancy)
- Hypersensitivity to aminoglycosides
- Use with caution in renal, hepatic, vestibular or auditory impairment.

Monitoring

Monthly creatinine and serum potassium in low-risk patients (young with no co-morbidities), more frequently in high-risk patients (elderly, diabetic, or HIV-positive patients, or patients with renal insufficiency). If potassium is low, check magnesium and calcium. Baseline audiometry and monthly monitoring in high-risk patients. For problems with balance, consider increasing dosing interval.

Alerting Symptoms

- Problems with hearing; dizziness
- Rash
- Trouble breathing
- Decreased urination
- Swelling, pain or redness at injection site
- Muscle twitching or weakness.

Management of Adverse Effects (Table 2.2)

Hearing loss can be prevented by:

1. Changing injectable to capreomycin if patient has documented susceptibility to capreomycin

TABLE 2.2: Common adverse effects, suspected agent(s) and management strategies of antituberculous drugs used in retreatment patients of TB

Adverse effect	*Suspected agent*	*Suggested management strategies*
Seizures	**Cs** H Fq	• Suspend suspected agent pending resolution of seizures • Initiate anticonvulsant therapy (e.g. phenytoin, valproic acid) • Increase pyridoxine to maximum daily dose (200 mg per day) • Restart suspected agent or reinitiate suspected agent at lower dose, if essential to the regimen • Discontinue suspected agent if this can be done without compromising regimen • Anticonvulsant is generally continued until MDR-TB treatment is completed or suspected agent discontinued • History of previous seizure disorder is not a contraindication to the use of agents listed here if a patient's seizures are well controlled and/or the patient is receiving anticonvulsant • Patients with history of previous seizures may be at increased risk for development of seizures during MDR-TB.

Contd...

Contd...

Adverse effect	*Suspected agent*	*Suggested management strategies*
Peripheral neuropathy	**Cs** **Lzd** **H** S Km Am Cm Eto/Pto Fq	• Increase pyridoxine to maximum daily dose (200 mg per day) • Change injectable to capreomycin if patient has documented susceptibility to capreomycin • Initiate therapy with tricyclic antidepressants such as amitriptyline. Nonsteroidal anti-inflammatory drugs or acetaminophen may help alleviate symptoms • Lower dose of suspected agent, if this can be done without compromising regimen • Discontinue suspected agent if this can be done without compromising regimen • Patients with comorbid disease (e.g. diabetes, HIV, alcohol (dependence) may be more likely to develop peripheral neuropathy, but these conditions are not contraindications to the use of the agents listed here • Neuropathy may be irreversible; however, some patients may experience improvement when offending agents are suspended
Hearing loss	**S** **Km** **Am** **Cm** Clr	• Document hearing loss and compare with baseline audiometry if available • Change parenteral treatment to capreomycin if patient has documented susceptibility to capreomycin • Decrease frequency and/or lower dose of suspected agent if this can be done without compromising the regimen (consider administration three times per week) • Discontinue suspected agent if this can be done without compromising the regimen • Patients with previous exposure to aminoglycosides may have baseline hearing loss. In such patients, audiometry may be helpful at the start of MDR-TB therapy • Hearing loss is generally not reversible • The risk of further hearing loss must be weighed against the risks of stopping the injectable in the treatment regimen • While the benefit of hearing aids is minimal to moderate in auditory toxicity, consider a trial use to determine if a patient with hearing loss can benefit from their use
Psychotic symptoms	**Cs** **H** Fq Eto/Pto	• Stop suspected agent for a short period of time (1–4 weeks) while psychotic symptoms are brought under control • Initiate antipsychotic therapy • Lower dose of suspected agent, if this can be done without compromising regimen • Discontinue suspected agent, if this can be done without compromising regimen • Some patients will need to continue antipsychotic treatment throughout MDR-TB therapy • Previous history of psychiatric disease is not a contraindication to the use of agents listed here but may increase the likelihood of psychotic symptoms developing during treatment • Psychotic symptoms are generally reversible upon completion of MDR-TB treatment or cessation of the offending agent

Contd...

Contd...

Adverse effect	*Suspected agent*	*Suggested management strategies*
Depression	**Cs** Fq Eto/Pto H	• Offer group or individual counseling • Initiate antidepressant therapy • Lower dose of suspected agent, if this can be done without compromising regimen • Discontinue suspected agent, if this can be done without compromising regimen • Socioeconomic conditions and chronic illness should not be underestimated as contributing factors to depression • Depressive symptoms may fluctuate during therapy and may improve as illness is successfully treated • History of previous depression is not a contraindication to the use of the agents listed but may increase the likelihood of depression developing during treatment
Hypothyroidism	**PAS** **Eto/Pto**	• Initiate thyroxine therapy • Completely reversible upon discontinuation of PAS or ethionamide/protionamide • The combination of ethionamide/protionamide with PAS is more frequently associated with hypothyroidism than the individual use of each drug
Nausea and vomiting	**Eto/Pto** **PAS** H E Z	• Assess for dehydration; initiate rehydration if indicated • Initiate antiemetic therapy • Lower dose of suspected agent, if this can be done without compromising regimen • Discontinue suspected agent, if this can be done without compromising regimen rarely necessary • Nausea and vomiting universal in early weeks of therapy and usually abate with time on treatment and adjunctive therapy • Electrolytes should be monitored, if vomiting is severe • Reversible upon discontinuation of suspected agent • Severe abdominal distress and acute abdomen have been reported with the use of clofazimine. Although these reports are rare, if this effect occurs, clofazimine should be suspended
Gastritis	**PAS** **Eto/Pto**	• H2-blockers, proton-pump inhibitors, or antacids • Stop suspected agent(s) for short periods of time (e.g, 1–7 days) • Lower dose of suspected agent, if this can be done without compromising regimen • Discontinue suspected agent, if this can be done without compromising regimen • Severe gastritis, as manifested by hematemesis, melena or hematechezia, is rare • Dosing of antacids should be carefully timed so as not to interfere with the absorption of antituberculosis drugs (take 2 hours before or 3 hours after antituberculosis medications) • Reversible upon discontinuation of suspected agent(s)

Contd...

Contd...

Adverse effect	*Suspected agent*	*Suggested management strategies*
Hepatitis	**Z** **H** **R** Eto/Pto PAS E Fq	• Stop all therapy pending resolution of hepatitis • Eliminate other potential causes of hepatitis • Consider suspending most likely agent permanently • Reintroduce remaining drugs, one at a time while monitoring liver function • History of previous hepatitis should be carefully analyzed to determine most likely causative agent(s); these should be avoided in future regimens • Generally reversible upon discontinuation of suspected agent
Renal toxicity	**S** **Km** **Am** **Cm**	• Discontinue suspected agent • Consider using capreomycin if an aminoglycoside had been the prior injectable in regimen • Consider dosing 2 to 3 times a week if drug is essential to the regimen and patient can tolerate (close monitoring of creatinine) • Adjust all antituberculosis medications according to the creatinine clearance • History of diabetes or renal disease is not a contraindication to the use of the agents listed here, although patients with these comorbidities may be at increased risk for developing renal failure • Renal impairment may be permanent
Electrolyte disturbances (hypokalaemia and hypomagnesaemia)	**Cm** **Km** **Am** S	• Check potassium • If potassium is low, also check magnesium (and calcium, if hypocalcemia is suspected) • Replace electrolytes as needed • If severe hypokalemia is present, consider hospitalization • Amiloride 5 to 10 mg QD or spironolactone 25 mg QD may decrease potassium and magnesium wasting and is useful in refractory cases • Oral potassium replacements can cause significant nausea and vomiting. Oral magnesium may cause diarrhea
Optic neuritis	**E** Eto/Pto	• Stop E • Refer patient to an ophthalmologist • Usually reverses with cessation of E • Rare case reports of optic neuritis have been attributed to streptomycin
Arthralgias	**Z** Fq	• Initiate therapy with nonsteroidal anti-inflammatory drugs • Lower dose of suspected agent, if this can be done without compromising regimen • Discontinue suspected agent, if this can be done without compromising regimen • Symptoms of arthralgia generally diminish over time, even without intervention • Uric acid levels may be elevated in patients on pyrazinamide. Allopurinol appears not to correct the uric acid levels in such cases

Isoniazid (H), Rifampicin (R), Ethambutol (E), Pyrazinamide (Z), Streptomycin (S), Kanamycin (Km), Amikacin (Am), Capreomycin (Cm), Fluoroquinolones (Fq), Ethionamide (Eto), Prothionamide (Pto), Para-aminosalicylic acid (PAS), Cycloserine (Cs), Clofazimine (Cfz), Linezolid (Lzd), Clarithromycin (Clr).
Drugs that the strongly associated with adverse effects shown in bold.

2. Discontinue suspected agents without compromising the regimen
3. Lower the dose of suspected agents without compromising the regimen.

In renal failure, dose reduction is needed and follow-up with serum creatinine and blood urea is required every one to two months regularly. If renal profile is uncontrolled despite of decreased dosage, then discontinue suspected agent and consider using capreomycin.

Amikacin

Drug class: Aminoglycoside

Activity against TB, mechanism of action and metabolism: Bactericidal, inhibit protein synthesis through disruption of ribosomal function; less effective in acidic pH, aminoglycosides are not metabolized in the liver, they are excreted unchanged in the urine.

Preparation and dose: Amikacin sulfate, colorless solution. 250 mg/mL (2 or 4 mL vials) and 50 mg/mL (2 mL vial). The optimal dose is 15–20 mg/kg body weight, usually 750 mg to 1 g given daily or 5–6 days per week by deep intramuscular injection. Rotation of injection sites avoids local discomfort. When necessary, it is possible to give the drug at the same total dose 2 or 3 times weekly during the continuation phase under close monitoring for adverse effects.

Storage: Solution is stable at room temperature (15°–25°C); diluted solution is stable at room temperature for at least 3 days or in the refrigerator for at least 60 days.

Oral absorption: There is no significant oral absorption. Intramuscular absorption may be delayed if the same site is used consistently.

CSF penetration: Penetrates inflamed meninges only.

Special Circumstances

- **Pregnancy/breastfeeding:** Safety class D. No reports linking the use of amikacin to congenital defects have been reported.
  Ototoxicity has not been reported as an effect of *in utero* exposure to amikacin; however, eighth cranial nerve toxicity in the fetus is well known following exposure to other aminoglycosides (kanamycin and streptomycin) and could potentially occur with amikacin. Only a trace amount of amikacin was found in some nursing infants. Given the poor absorption of aminoglycosides, systemic toxicity should not occur, but alteration in normal bowel flora may occur in nursing infants.
- **Renal disease:** Use with caution. Levels should be monitored for patients with impaired renal function. Interval adjustment (12–15 mg/kg—2 or 3 times per week) is recommended for creatinine clearance < 30 mL/min or hemodialysis.
- **Hepatic disease:** Drug levels not affected by hepatic disease (except a larger volume of distribution for alcoholic cirrhotic patients with ascites). Presumed to be safe in severe liver disease; however, some patients with severe liver disease may progress rapidly to hepatorenal syndrome.

Adverse Effects

Frequent

- Pain at injection site
- Proteinuria
- Serum electrolyte disturbances including hypokalemia and hypomagnesemia.

Occasional

- Cochlear ototoxicity (may be irreversible)
- Nephrotoxicity (often irreversible)
- Peripheral neuropathy
- Rash
- Vestibular toxicity (nausea, vomiting, vertigo, ataxia, nystagmus)
- Eosinophilia.

Ototoxicity potentiated by certain diuretics (especially loop diuretics), advanced age, and prolonged use. The effect of nondepolarizing muscle relaxants may be increased.

Drug Interactions

- **Loop diuretics** (bumetanide, furosemide, ethacrynic acid, torsemide).
  Coadministration of aminoglycosides with loop diuretics may have an additive or synergistic auditory ototoxicity.
  Ototoxicity appears to be dose-dependent and may be increased with renal dysfunction. Irreversible ototoxicity has been reported.
  Avoid concomitant administration; if used together, careful dose adjustments in patients with renal failure and close monitoring for ototoxicity are required.
- **Nondepolarizing muscle relaxants** (atracurium, pancuronium, tubocurarine, gallamine triethiodide): possible enhanced action of non-depolarizing muscle relaxants resulting in possible respiratory depression. Nephrotoxic agents (amphotericin B, foscarnet, cidofovir): additive nephrotoxicity.
- **Penicillins:** In vitro inactivation (possible). Do not mix together before administration.

Contraindications: Pregnancy (congenital deafness seen with streptomycin and kanamycin use in pregnancy). Hypersensitivity to aminoglycosides.
Use with caution in renal, hepatic, vestibular, or auditory impairment.
Monitoring: Monthly creatinine and serum potassium in low-risk patients (young with no comorbidities), more frequently in high-risk patients (elderly, diabetic, or HIV-positive patients, or patients with renal insufficiency). If potassium is low, check magnesium and calcium. Baseline audiometry and monthly monitoring in high-risk patients. For problems with balance, consider increasing dosing interval.

Alerting Symptoms

- Problems with hearing, dizziness or balance
- Rash or swelling of the face

- Trouble breathing
- Decreased urination
- Swelling, pain or redness at IM site
- Muscle twitching or weakness.

Management of Adverse Effects

Hearing loss can be prevented by:

1. Changing injectable to Capreomycin if patient has documented susceptibility to capreomycin
2. Discontinue suspected agents without compromising the regimen
3. Lower dose of suspected agents without compromising the regimen.

In renal failure, dose reduction is needed and follow-up with serum creatinine and blood urea nitrogen is required every one to two months regularly. If renal profile is uncontrolled despite a decreased dosage, then discontinue suspected agent and consider using capreomycin.

Capreomycin

Drug class: Cyclic polypeptide

Activity against TB, mechanism of action and metabolism: Bactericidal, polypeptides appear to inhibit translocation of the peptidyl-tRNA and the initiation of protein synthesis. No cross-resistance with the aminoglycosides. 50–60% excreted via glomerulofiltration. Small amount by biliary excretion. It is obtained from *Streptomyces capreolus*.[5]

Preparation and dose: Capreomycin sulfate is supplied as a sterile white powder for intramuscular injection in sealed vials each containing 1000 units, approximately equivalent to 1 g capreomycin base. This should be dissolved in 2 mL of 0.9% sodium chloride in water; 2–3 minutes should be allowed for complete solution.

Dose: 15–20 mg/kg daily. The usual dose is 1 g in a single dose daily. When necessary, it is possible to give the drug at the same dose 2 or 3 times weekly during the continuation phase, under close monitoring for adverse effects.

Storage: Reconstituted capreomycin can be stored in the refrigerator for upto 24 hours before use.

Oral absorption: There is no significant oral absorption. Intramuscular absorption may be delayed if the same site is used consistently.

CSF penetration: Penetrates inflamed meninges only.

Special Circumstances

- **Pregnancy/breastfeeding:** Less ototoxicity reported in adults with capreomycin than with aminoglycosides. Category C animal studies show teratogenic effect ('wavy ribs' when given 3.5 times the human dose). Avoid in pregnancy. Concentrations in breast milk unknown.
- **Renal disease:** Use with caution. Levels should be monitored for patients with impaired renal function. Interval adjustment (12–15 mg/kg—2 or 3

times per week) is recommended for creatinine clearance < 30 mL/min or hemodialysis.

Adverse Effects

Frequent

- Nephrotoxicity (20–25%)
- Tubular dysfunction
- Azotemia
- Proteinuria
- Urticaria
- Maculopapular rash.

Occasional

- Ototoxicity (vestibular > auditory)
- Electrolyte abnormalities (decreased blood levels of calcium, magnesium and potassium)
- Pain
- Induration
- Sterile abscesses at injection sites.

Drug Interactions

Avoid coadministration of nondepolarizing muscle relaxants. If concurrent administration is needed, titrate the nondepolarizing muscle relaxant slowly and monitor neuromuscular function closely. Though not reported with capreomycin, neuromuscular blockade has been reported with other polypeptide antibiotics when administered with nondepolarizing muscle relaxants. Avoid use with other nephro- or ototoxic agents because of the additive effect.

Contraindications: Patients with hypersensitivity to capreomycin and patients having myasthenia gravis. Great caution must be exercised in patients with renal insufficiency or pre-existing auditory impairment.

Monitoring: Monthly creatinine and serum potassium in low-risk patients (young with no comorbidities), more frequently in high-risk patients (elderly, diabetic, or HIV-positive patients, or patients with renal insufficiency). If potassium is low, check magnesium and calcium. Electrolyte disturbances are more common with capreomycin than other injectable agents. Baseline audiometry and monthly monitoring in high-risk patients. For problems with balance, consider increasing dosing interval.

Alerting Symptoms

- Rash
- Decreased urination
- Fever or chills
- Trouble breathing
- Bleeding or bruising
- Muscle weakness
- Problems with hearing, dizziness or balance
- Bleeding or lump at IM injection site.

Management of Adverse Effects

Hearing loss can be prevented by lowering the dose of drug, if this can be done without compromising the regimen and discontinuing the drug.

In renal failure, dose reduction is needed and follow-up with serum creatinine and blood urea is required every one to two months regularly. If renal profile is uncontrolled despite decreased dosage, then discontinue suspected agent.

Ethionamide and Prothionamide

Drug class: Carbothionamides group, derivatives of isonicotinic acid
Activity against TB, mechanism of action and metabolism: *Bactericidal,* ethionamide and prothionamide are bactericidal agents from the thioamide class.[6] The mechanism of action of thionamides has not been fully elucidated, but they appear to inhibit mycolic acid synthesis. Resistance develops rapidly if used alone and there is complete cross-resistance between ethionamide and prothionamide (partial cross-resistance with thioacetazone). Ethionamide is extensively metabolized, probably in the liver, to the active sulfoxide and other inactive metabolites and less than 1% of a dose appears in the urine as unchanged drug.

Most strains of *M. tuberculosis* are inhibited *in vitro* by concentration of 0.6 to 2.4 mcg/mL. A concentration of 10 mcg/mL or less will inhibit approximately 75% of photochromogenic mycobacteria, scotochromogen are more resistant.
Preparation and dose: Ethionamide and protionamide are normally administered in the form of tablets containing 125 mg or 250 mg of active drug. The maximum optimum daily dose is 15–20 mg/kg/day (maximum 1 g/day), usually 500–750 mg. For patients who are unable to tolerate a single dose, it may be divided into two doses.
Storage: Room temperature (15–25°C) in airtight containers.
Oral absorption: 100% absorbed but sometimes erratic absorption caused by gastrointestinal disturbances associated with the medication.
Distribution: Rapidly and widely distributed into body tissues and fluids, with concentrations in plasma and various organs being approximately equal. Significant concentrations also are present in CSF.

Special Circumstances

Pregnancy/breastfeeding: Safety class C. Animal studies have shown ethionamide to be teratogenic. Hence, it should not be given in pregnancy. Newborns, who are breastfed by mothers who are taking ethionamide, should be monitored for adverse effects.
Renal disease: Doses of the thionamides are only slightly modified for patients with severe renal impairment. When the creatinine clearance is less than 30 mL/minute, the recommended dosing is 250–500 mg daily.
Hepatic disease: Thionamides should not be used in severe hepatic impairment.
Porphyria: Ethionamide is considered to be unsafe in patients with porphyria because it has been shown to be porphyrinogenic in animals and *in vitro* systems.

Adverse Effects

Frequent

- Severe gastrointestinal intolerance (nausea, vomiting, diarrhea, abdominal pain, excessive salivation, metallic taste, stomatitis, anorexia and weight loss). Adverse gastrointestinal effects appear to be dose-related, with approximately 50% of patients unable to tolerate 1 g as a single dose. Gastrointestinal effects may be minimized by decreasing dosage, by changing the time of drug administration, or by the concurrent administration of an antiemetic agent. Gastric tolerance is better with protionamide as compared to ethionamide.

Occasional

- Allergic reactions
- Psychotic disturbances (including depression), drowsiness, dizziness, restlessness, headache and postural hypotension
- Neurotoxicity (administration of pyridoxine has been recommended to prevent or relieve neurotoxic effects)
- Increases in serum bilirubin; reversible hepatitis (2%) with jaundice (1–3%)
- Gynecomastia; menstrual irregularity
- Arthralgias
- Leukopenia
- Hypothyroidism especially when combined with PAS.

Rare

- Peripheral neuritis
- Optic neuritis, diplopia, blurred vision
- Pellagra-like syndrome, reactions including rash, photosensitivity
- Thrombocytopenia and purpura.

Drug Interactions

- **Cycloserine:** Potential increases incidence of neurotoxicity.
- **Ethionamide:** has been found to temporarily raise serum concentrations of isoniazid. Thionamides may potentiate the adverse effects of other antituberculosis drugs administered concomitantly. In particular, convulsions have been reported when ethionamide is administered with cycloserine. Excessive ethanol ingestion should be avoided because of possible psychotic reaction.
- **PAS:** Possible increase in liver toxicity, monitor liver enzymes; hypothyroidism in case of combined administration.

Contraindications

Thionamides are contraindicated in patients with severe hepatic impairment and in patients who are hypersensitive to these drugs.

Monitoring

Ophthalmological examinations should be performed before and periodically during the therapy. Periodic monitoring of blood glucose and thyroid function is desirable. Diabetic patients should be particularly alert for episodes of hypoglycemia. Liver function tests should be carried out before and during treatment with ethionamide.

Alerting Symptoms

- Any problems with eyes: eye pain, blurred vision, color blindness, or trouble seeing
- Numbness, tingling, or pain in hands and feet
- Unusual bruising or bleeding
- Personality changes such as depression, confusion or aggression
- Yellowing of skin
- Dark-colored urine
- Nausea and vomiting
- Dizziness.

Management of Adverse Effects

Gastrointestinal symptoms should be prevented by altering the timing of the drug administration and by prescribing antacids, antiemetics, withholding drugs for short periods, lowering dose of drug and discontinuing drug. An important factor that can influence tolerance of ethionamide is patient's determination not to give up treatment. Drug-induced neurotoxicity can be prevented by pyridoxine, 10 mg daily. Sometimes protionamide is better tolerated than ethionamide.

Cycloserine

Drug class: Analog of D-alanine

Activity against TB, mechanism of action and metabolism: Bacteriostatic, competitively blocks the enzyme that incorporates alanine into an alanyl-alanine dipeptide, an essential component of the mycobacterial cell wall. No cross-resistance with other antituberculosis drugs. 60–70% excreted unchanged in the urine via glomerular filtration; small amount excreted in feces; small amount metabolized. Cycloserine was valuable in preventing resistance to ethionamide in the retreatment cases. Most strains are inhibited *in vitro* by concentrations of 20 mcg/mL. Terizidone is a combination of two molecules of cycloserine.[7]

Preparation and dose: Cycloserine is supplied in the form of tablets of 250 mg. The dose for daily therapy being15–20 mg/kg,[8] i.e. 0.5 to 1.0 g daily and divided into two or three doses (some producers of terizidone make 300 mg capsule preparations, while others make 250 mg).

Storage: Room temperature (15–25°C) in airtight containers.

Oral absorption: Modestly decreased by food (best to take on an empty stomach); 70–90% absorbed.

Distribution: Widely distributed into body tissue and fluids such as lung, bile, ascitic fluid, pleural fluid, synovial fluid, lymph and sputum. Very good CSF penetration (80–100% of serum concentration attained in the CSF, higher level with inflamed meninges).

Special Circumstances

Pregnancy/breastfeeding: Safety class C. Cycloserine crosses the placental barrier. There are limited data on safety of drug in pregnancy. Breastfeeding with B6 supplement to the infant.
Renal disease: Doses of cycloserine should be reduced in patients with severe renal impairment. When the creatinine clearance is less than 30 mL/minute, the recommended dosing is 250 mg/day, or 500 mg/dose, three times per week. The appropriateness of 250 mg/day doses has not been established. There should be careful monitoring for evidence of neurotoxicity; if possible, measure serum concentrations and adjust regimen accordingly.

Adverse Effects

Frequent

- Neurological and psychiatric disturbances (headaches, irritability, sleep disturbances, aggression and tremors)
- Gum inflammation
- Pale skin
- Depression, confusion, dizziness, restlessness, anxiety, nightmares, severe headache, drowsiness.

Occasional

- Visual changes
- Skin rash
- Numbness, tingling or burning in hands and feet
- Jaundice
- Eye pain.

Rare

- Seizures
- Suicidal thoughts.

Drug Interactions

- **Ethionamide:** Additive nervous system side effects.
- **Isoniazid:** Additive nervous system side effects.
- **Phenytoin:** May increase phenytoin levels. Toxic effect if combined with alcohol, increases risk of seizures. Vitamin B6 decreases CNS effect.

Contraindications

- Hypersensitivity to cycloserine
- Epilepsy

- Depression, severe anxiety or psychosis
- Severe renal insufficiency
- Excessive concurrent use of alcohol.

Monitoring

When available, serum drug monitoring to establish optimal dosing (not higher than 30 μg/mL).

Alerting Symptoms

- Seizures
- Shakiness or trouble talking
- Depression or thoughts of intentional self-harm
- Anxiety, confusion or loss of memory
- Personality changes, such as aggressive behavior
- Rash or hives
- Headache.

Management of Adverse Effects

- For headache, rule out other causes of headache, like meningitis, migraine and cluster headache. Treatment includes analgesics—acetaminophen, ibuprofen, aspirin and increasing pyridoxine to 300 mg/day.
- Psychosocial support to relieve emotional components.
- Amitryptiline 100–150 mg at night. In psychosis, patient needs consultation by a psychiatrist.
- In case of seizure, it is necessary to rule out other causes (previous history of seizure or epilepsy, meningitis, encephalitis, alcohol abuse, metabolic disorder, like diabetes mellitus, hyper-/hypo-calcemia, cerebrovascular accident, malignancy with space-occupying lesions). Pyridoxine may be given in a dose of 100–200 mg/day to prevent and treat neurotoxic side effects.

Para-Aminosalicylic Acid (PAS)

Drug class: Salicylic acid; anti-folate. It was first used in 1944.[9]
Activity against TB, mechanism of action and metabolism: Bacteriostatic, disrupts folic acid metabolism. Acetylated in the liver to N-acetyl-p-aminosalicylic acid and p-aminosalicylic acid, which are excreted via glomerular filtration and tubular secretion. Over 80% of drug is excreted in urine. Most strains of *M. tuberculosis* are sensitive to a concentration of 1 mcg/mL. PAS prevents the emergence of isoniazid resistance when used in combination.
Preparation and dose: Tablets, sugar-coated, containing sodium salt: sodium p-aminosalicylate, 0.5 g of PAS.

Granules of PAS with an acid-resistant outer coating rapidly dissolved in neutral media, 4 g per packet.

150 mg/kg or 10–12 g daily in two divided doses.

Children: 200–300 mg/kg daily in 2–4 divided doses.

Storage: Packets should be kept in the refrigerator or freezer. Other formulations may not require refrigeration (consult manufacturer's recommendations).
Oral absorption: Incomplete absorption (usually 60–65%): sometimes requires increased doses to achieve therapeutic levels.
Distribution: Distributed in peritoneal fluid, pleural fluid and synovial fluid. Not well distributed in CSF (10–15%) and bile.
Special circumstances:

- **Pregnancy/breastfeeding:** Safety class C. Congenital defects in babies have been reported with exposure to PAS in the first trimester. PAS is secreted into human breast milk (1/70th of maternal plasma concentration).
- **Renal disease:** No dose adjustment is recommended. However, PAS can exacerbate acidosis associated with renal insufficiency and, if possible, should be avoided in patients with severe renal impairment due to crystalluria. Sodium PAS should also be avoided in patients with severe renal impairment.

Adverse Effects

Frequent

- Gastrointestinal intolerance (anorexia and diarrhea)
- Hypothyroidism (increased risk with concomitant use of ethionamide).

Occasional

- Hepatitis (0.3–0.5%)
- Allergic reactions
- Thyroid enlargement
- Malabsorption syndrome
- Increased prothrombin time
- Fever.

Careful use in patients with glucose-6-phosphate dehydrogenase (G6PD) deficiency.

Drug Interactions

Digoxin: Possible decrease in digoxin absorption; monitor digoxin level—may need to be increased.
Ethionamide: Possible increase in liver toxicity, monitor liver enzymes; hypothyroidism in case of combined administration.
Isoniazid: Decreased acetylation of isoniazid resulting in increased isoniazid level. Dose may need to be decreased.

Contraindications

Allergy to aspirin; severe renal disease; hypersensitivity to the drug.

Monitoring

Monitor TSH, electrolytes, blood counts and liver function tests.

Alerting Symptoms

- Skin rash, severe itching, or hives
- Severe abdominal pain, nausea or vomiting
- Unusual tiredness or loss of appetite
- Black stools as a result of intestinal bleeding.

Management of Adverse Effects

Gastrointestinal symptoms should be prevented by altering the timing of drug administration and by prescribing antacids, antiemetics, withholding drug for short periods, lowering dose of drug and discontinuing drug. Hypothyroidism can be prevented by initiating thyroxine therapy.

Levofloxacin

Drug class: Fluoroquinolone

Activity against TB, mechanism of action and metabolism: Bactericidal. The bactericidal action of fluroquinolone involves their interaction with DNA gyrase (Topoisomerase II), and its inhibition prevents replication and transcription process. Levofloxacin is generally considered to be about twice as active as its isomer, ofloxacin.[10–12] Minimal hepatic metabolism; 87% of dose excreted unchanged in the urine within 48 hours via glomerular filtration and tubular secretion.

Preparation and Dose: Tablets (250, 500, 750 mg). Aqueous solution or solution in 5% dextrose for IV administration vials (20, 30 mL) 500 or 750 mg and flexible containers (50,100, 150 mL) 250, 500 or 750 mg.

Usual dose: 750 mg/day.

Storage: Tablets: Room temperature (15°–25°C), airtight containers protected from light.

Oral absorption: Levofloxacin is rapidly and essentially completely absorbed after oral administration. Orally, should not be administered within 4 hours of other medications containing divalent cations (iron, magnesium, zinc, vitamins, didanosine, sucralfate). No interaction with milk or calcium.

Distribution: Distributes well in blister fluid and lung tissues, also widely distributed (kidneys, gallbladder, gynecological tissues, liver, lung, prostatic tissue, phagocytic cells, urine, sputum and bile). 30–50% of serum concentration is attained in CSF with inflamed meninges.

Special Circumstances:

- **Pregnancy/breastfeeding:** Safety class C. There are no adequate and well-controlled studies in pregnant women. Levofloxacin should be used during pregnancy only if the potential benefit justifies the potential risk to the fetus. Animal data demonstrated arthropathy in immature animals, with erosions in joint cartilage.

  Because of the potential for serious adverse effects from levofloxacin in nursing infants, a decision should be made whether to discontinue nursing or to discontinue the drug, taking into account the importance of the drug to the mother.

- **Renal disease:** Doses of levofloxacin should be reduced in patients with severe renal impairment. When the creatinine clearance is less than 30 mL/minute, the recommended dosing is 750–1000 mg three times per week.
- **Hepatic disease:** Given the limited extent of levofloxacin metabolism, the pharmacokinetics of levofloxacin are not expected to be affected by hepatic impairment.

Adverse Effects

Generally well tolerated.

Occasional

- Gastrointestinal intolerance
- CNS-headache, malaise, insomnia, restlessness, dizziness
- Allergic reactions
- Diarrhea
- Photosensitivity.

Rare

- QT prolongation
- Tendon rupture
- Peripheral neuropathy.

Drug Interactions

Should not be given to patients receiving Class Ia antiarrhythmic drugs (such as quinidine and procainamide) or Class III antiarrhythmics (such as amiodarone and sotalol).
Sucralfate: Decreased absorption of fluoroquinolones caused by the chelation by aluminum ions contained in the sucralfate.
Antacids (magnesium, aluminum, calcium, Al-Mg buffer found in didanosine): Antacid binding to fluoroquinolone antibiotics resulting in decreased absorption and loss of therapeutic efficacy.
Probenecid: Probenecid interferes with renal tubular secretion of fluoroquinolones, which may result in 50% increase in serum level of levofloxacin.
Vitamins and minerals containing divalent and trivalent cations such as zinc and iron: Formation of fluoroquinolone-ion complex results in decreased absorption of fluoroquinolones.
Mexiletine: Fluoroquinolones may inhibit cytochrome P450, resulting in increased mexiletine concentration.

Contraindications

- Pregnancy
- Hypersensitivity to fluoroquinolones
- Prolonged QT.

Monitoring

No specific laboratory monitoring requirements.

Alerting Symptoms

- Pain, swelling or tearing of a tendon or muscle or joint pain
- Rashes, hives, bruising or blistering, trouble breathing
- Diarrhea
- Yellow skin or eyes
- Anxiety, confusion or dizziness.

Management of Adverse Effects

Gastrointestinal symptom should be prevented by altering timing of drug administration and by prescribing antacids, antiemetics, withholding drug for short periods, lowering dose of drug and discontinuing drug. In case of headache, it is important to rule out other causes of headache including meningitis, migraine and cluster headache. Treatment includes supportive treatment only.

Moxifloxacin

Drug class: Fluoroquinolone

Activity against TB, mechanism of action and metabolism: Bactericidal. The bactericidal action of fluoroquinolone involves their interaction with DNA gyrase (Topoisomerase II),[10-12] and its inhibition prevents replication and transcription process. The cytochrome P450 system is not involved in moxifloxacin metabolism, and is not affected by moxifloxacin. Approximately 45% of an oral or intravenous dose of moxifloxacin is excreted as unchanged drug (~20% in urine and ~25% in feces).

Preparation and dose: Tablets 400 mg and intravenous solution 250mL containing 400 mg in 0.8% saline.

Usual dose: 400 mg/day.

Storage: Tablets: room temperature (15–25°C), airtight containers protected from light.

Oral absorption: Moxifloxacin, given as an oral tablet, is well absorbed from the gastrointestinal tract. The absolute bioavailability of moxifloxacin is approximately 90%. Coadministration with a high fat meal (e.g. 500 calories from fat) does not affect the absorption of moxifloxacin.

Distribution: Moxifloxacin has been detected in the saliva, nasal and bronchial secretions, mucosa of the sinuses, skin blister fluid, and subcutaneous tissue, and skeletal muscle following oral or intravenous administration of 400 mg.

Special Circumstances

- **Pregnancy/breastfeeding:** Safety class C. Since there are no adequate or well-controlled studies in pregnant women, moxifloxacin should be used during pregnancy only if the potential benefit justifies the potential risk to the fetus. Because of the potential for serious adverse effects in infants nursing from mothers taking moxifloxacin, a decision should be made whether to discontinue nursing or to discontinue the drug, taking into account the importance of the drug to the mother.

- **Renal disease:** No dosage adjustment is required in renally impaired patients, including those on either hemodialysis or continuous ambulatory peritoneal dialysis.
- **Hepatic disease:** No dosage adjustment is required in patients with mild or moderate hepatic insufficiency.

Adverse Effects

Generally well tolerated.

Occasional

- Gastrointestinal intolerance
- CNS-headache, malaise, insomnia, restlessness, dizziness
- Allergic reactions
- Diarrhea
- Photosensitivity.

Moxifloxacin has been found in isolated cases to prolong the QT interval.

Drug Interactions

Should not be given to patients receiving class Ia antiarrhythmic drugs (such as quinidine and procainamide) or Class III antiarrhythmics (such as amiodarone and sotalol).

Sucralfate: Decreased absorption of fluoroquinolones caused by the chelation by aluminum ions contained in the sucralfate.

Antacids (magnesium, aluminum, calcium, Al-Mg buffer found in didanosine): Antacid binding to fluoroquinolone antibiotics resulting in decreased absorption and loss of therapeutic efficacy.

Vitamins and minerals containing divalent and trivalent cations such as zinc and iron: Formation of fluoroquinolone-ion complex results in decreased absorption of fluoroquinolones.

Contraindications

- Pregnancy
- Hypersensitivity to fluoroquinolones
- Prolonged QT.

Monitoring

No specific laboratory monitoring requirements.

Alerting Symptoms

- Pain, swelling or tearing of a tendon or muscle or joint pain
- Rashes, hives, bruising or blistering, trouble breathing

- Diarrhea
- Yellow skin or eyes
- Anxiety, confusion or dizziness.

Management of Adverse Effects

Gastrointestinal symptom should be prevented by altering timing of drug administration and by prescribing antacids, antiemetics, withholding drug for short periods, lowering dose of drug and discontinuing drug. In case of headache, it is important to rule out other causes of headache including meningitis, migraine and cluster headache. Treatment includes supportive treatment only.

Ofloxacin

Drug class: Fluoroquinolones

Activity against TB, mechanism of action and metabolism: Bactericidal. The bactericidal action of fluoroquinolone involves their interaction with DNA gyrase (Topoisomerase II),[10-12] and its inhibition prevents replication and transcription process. There is no cross-resistance with other antituberculosis agents, but complete cross-resistance between ofloxacin and ciprofloxacin. There is limited metabolism to desmethyl and N-oxide metabolites; desmethylofloxacin has moderate antibacterial activity.

Ofloxacin is eliminated mainly by the kidneys. Excretion is by tubular secretion and glomerular filtration and 65–80% of a dose is excreted unchanged in the urine over 24–48 hours, resulting in high urinary concentrations.

Preparation and dose: Tablets (200, 300 or 400 mg). Vials (10 mL) or flexible containers (50 and 100 mL) with aqueous or 5% dextrose IV solutions equivalent to 200 and 400 mg.

Usual dose: 400 mg twice daily.

Storage: Room temperature (15–25°C), airtight containers protected from light.

Oral absorption: 90–98% oral absorption.

Distribution: About 25% is bound to plasma proteins. Ofloxacin is widely distributed in body fluids, including the CSF, and tissue penetration is good. It crosses the placenta and is distributed into breast milk. It also appears in the bile.

Special Circumstances

- **Pregnancy/breastfeeding:** Usually compatible with breastfeeding.
- **Renal disease:** Doses of ofloxacin should be reduced in patients with severe renal impairment. When the creatinine clearance is less than 30 mL/minute, the recommended dosing is 600–800 mg three times per week.

Adverse Effects

Generally well tolerated.

Occasional

- Gastrointestinal intolerance
- CNS-headache, malaise, insomnia, restlessness and dizziness.

Rare

- Allergic reactions
- Diarrhea
- Photosensitivity
- Increased LFTs
- Tendon rupture
- Peripheral neuropathy.

Drug Interactions

Fluoroquinolones are known to inhibit hepatic drug metabolism and may interfere with the clearance of drugs such as theophylline and caffeine that are metabolized by the liver. Cations such as aluminum, magnesium or iron reduce the absorption of ofloxacin and related drugs when given concomitantly. Changes in the pharmacokinetics of fluoroquinolones have been reported when given with histamine H2 antagonists, possibly due to changes in gastric pH, but do not seem to be of much clinical significance. The urinary excretion of ofloxacin and some other fluoroquinolones is reduced by probenecid; plasma concentrations are not necessarily increased.

Contraindications

Pregnancy, intolerance of fluoroquinolones.

Monitoring

No specific laboratory monitoring requirements.

Alerting Symptoms

- Pain, swelling or tearing of a tendon or muscle or joint pain
- Rashes, hives, bruising or blistering, trouble breathing
- Diarrhea
- Yellow skin or eyes
- Anxiety, confusion or dizziness.

Management of Adverse Effects

Gastrointestinal symptom should be prevented by altering timing of drug administration and by prescribing antacids, antiemetics, withholding drug for short periods, lowering dose of drug and discontinuing drug. In case of headache, it is important to rule out other causes of headache including meningitis, migraine and cluster headache. Treatment includes supportive treatment only.

Clofazimine

Drug class: Phenazine derivative
Clofazimine is a phenazinine dye.[13]
Activity against TB, mechanism of action and metabolism: Bacteriostatic against *M. leprae*, active *in vitro* against *M. tuberculosis*. Clinical effectiveness

against *M. tuberculosis* is not well established. It is bacteriostatic drug and acts by binding with GC-rich mycobacterium DNA and causing inhibition of transcription.[14] Excreted in feces as unabsorbed drug and via biliary elimination. Little urinary excretion.

Preparation and dose: Capsules (50 and 100 mg).

Storage: Store below 30°C, in airtight containers.

Oral absorption: 20–70% absorbed from gastrointestinal tract.

Distribution: Widely distributed principally to fatty tissue, reticuloendothelial system and macrophages. High concentrations found in mesenteric lymph nodes, adipose tissue, adrenals, liver, lungs, gallbladder, bile and spleen.

Special Circumstances

- **Pregnancy/breastfeeding:** Safety class C. Animal studies demonstrated teratogenicity (retardation of fetal skull ossification). Crosses placenta and is excreted in milk. Not recommended during breastfeeding.
- **Renal disease:** Usual dose.
- **Hepatic disease:** Dose adjustments should be considered in patients with severe hepatic insufficiency.

Adverse Effects

Frequent

- Ichthyosis and dry skin
- Pink to brownish-black discoloration of skin, cornea, retina and urine
- Anorexia
- Abdominal pain.

Drug interactions: May decrease absorption rate of rifampicin. Isoniazid increases clofazimine serum and urine concentrations and decreases skin concentrations. Ingestion of clofazimine with orange juice resulted in a modest reduction in clofazimine bioavailability.

Contraindications: Pregnancy, severe hepatic insufficiency, hypersensitivity to clofazimine.

Monitoring

No specific laboratory monitoring requirements.

Alerting Symptoms

- Nausea and vomiting
- Abdominal pain/distress (caused by crystal depositions and can present as an acute abdomen).

Management of Adverse Effects

Gastrointestinal symptom should be prevented by altering timing of drug administration and by prescribing antacids, antiemetics, withholding drug for short periods, lowering dose of drug and discontinuing drug. For skin discoloration, reassure the patients about reversal of effect after discontinuation of drug.

Thiacetazone

Drug class: Phenazine derivative. It is a thiosemicarbazone.
Activity against TB, mechanism of action and metabolism: It is a bacteriostatic drug of low efficacy. It delays resistance to other antitubercular drugs like streptomycin, isoniazid and ethambutol. It is orally active and primarily excreted unchanged in urine.
Preparation and dose: The daily dosage recommended is 2.5 mg/kg body weight daily; it is not effective when given intermittently.
Contraindications: In HIV-positive patients, the risk of major potentially fatal cutaneous reaction caused by thioacetazone is very high. It should never be used in patients who may be HIV-positive or in areas where HIV infection is common.

Adverse Effects

Frequent

- Cutaneous reactions
- Gastrointestinal intolerance
- Nausea, vomiting, abdominal discomfort
- Anemia.

Occassional

- Hepatitis
- Exfoliative dermatitis
- Stevens-Johnson syndrome.

Rare

- Bone marrow depression
- Ototoxicity
- Acute hepatic failure
- Cerebral edema
- Conjunctivitis
- Blurred vision.

Special Circumstances

- **Renal disease:** It should be avoided when renal impairment is present.
- **Pregnancy/breastfeeding:** Studies on the effects of thiacetazone in pregnancy and breastfeeding have not been done in humans or animals.

Monitoring

No specific laboratory monitoring requirements.

Management of Adverse Effect

If rash or other sign of hypersensitivity develops, all the treatment should be stopped and thioacetazone should not be used again. If there is itching with mild rash, then symptomatic treatment with antihistaminic may be tried. If there is severe rash or there is mucosal involvement with hypotension, then oral prednisolone 40–60 mg/day should be given until there is response; dose should be reduced gradually according to patient's response. Thioacetazone should not be administered in areas where HIV prevalence is high.

Clarithromycin

Drug class: It is a macrolide antibiotic.

Activity against TB, mechanism of action and metabolism: Clarithromycin is a semisynthetic derivative of erythromycin and is bacteriostatic in nature.[15] It is usually active against nontubercular mycobacterium particularly MAC.[12] It inhibits protein synthesis by binding reversibly to 50S ribosomal subunits. It is widely distributed and achieves high intracellular concentrations. It is metabolized in liver and excreted via urine.

Adverse Effects

Frequent

- Abdominal pain
- Nausea, vomiting and occasionally diarrhea.

Rare

- Hypersensitivity reaction
- Pseudomembranous colitis.

Drug Interactions

Several cases of QT prolongation, serious ventricular arrhythmias and death have been reported due to inhibition of CYP 3A4, resulting in high blood levels of concurrently administered terfinadine/astemizole/cisapride.

Special Circumstances

Renal and hepatic disease: Although the pharmacokinetics of clarithromycin are altered in patients with either hepatic or renal dysfunction, dose adjustment is not necessary until the creatinine clearance is < 30 mL/minute.

Pregnancy/breastfeeding: It is not recommended for routine use in patients with pregnancy. It should be used during pregnancy only when benefit outweighs risk. It should be used with caution in nursing mothers.

Monitoring

No specific laboratory monitoring requirements.

Management of Adverse Effects

Symptomatic management of adverse effects. Concurrent administration of drugs, namely, terfinadine, astemizole and cisapride, which are more prone to ventricular arrhythmias, should be avoided.

LINEZOLID

Drug class: Linezolid is a synthetic antimicrobial agent of oxazolidinone class.[16,17]

Mechanism of action, distribution, excretion: It inhibits protein synthesis by binding to the P-site of the 50S ribosomal subunit and preventing formation of the larger ribosomal-fMet-tRNA complex that initiates protein synthesis. It is 30% protein-bound and distributed widely. Approximately, 80% of the dose of Linezolid appears in the urine.

Adverse Effects

Frequent

- Gastrointestinal upset
- Rash.

Rare

- Myelosuppression
- Peripheral neuropathy
- Optic neuropathy.

Preparation and dose: Linezolid is supplied as 600 mg tablets. The dosage for daily therapy is 600 mg 12 hourly.

Special Circumstances

Renal disease: No modification in dosage required in patients with renal insufficiency.

Hepatic disease: No modification in dosage required in patients with mild to moderate hepatic disease.

Pregnancy/breastfeeding: It is not recommended for routine use in patients with pregnancy. It should be used during pregnancy only when benefit outweighs risk. It should be used with caution in nursing mothers.

Monitoring

No specific laboratory monitoring requirements.

Management of Adverse Effects

Gastrointestinal symptom should be prevented by altering timing of drug administration and by prescribing antacids, antiemetics, withholding drug for short periods, lowering dose of drug and discontinuing drug. In case of headache, it is important to rule out other causes of headache including meningitis, migraine and cluster headache. Treatment includes supportive treatment only.

IMIPENEM/CILASTATIN

Drug class: Imipenem belongs to the Carbapenem group of drugs. Carbapenems are beta-lactam antibiotics that have a broader spectrum of activity. Imipenem is derived from *Streptomyces cattleya*.

Mechanism of action: Beta-lactam antibiotics interfere with the synthesis of bacterial cell wall. The beta-lactam antibiotics inhibit the transpeptidases so that cross-linking of the adjacent peptide chains does not take place. Imipenem is very resistant to hydrolysis by most beta lactamases. Activity of Imipenem is excellent *in vitro* for a wide variety of aerobic and anaerobic microorganisms.

Pharmacokinetics: Imipenem is not absorbed orally. Imipenem is rapidly hydrolyzed by the enzyme dehydropeptidase I located on the brush border of renal tubular cells. Hence, Imipenem is combined with Cilastatin which is a reversible inhibitor of dehydropeptidase and, thus, imipenem is protected from hydrolysis.

Adverse Effects

Frequent

- Gastrointestinal upset
- Hypersensitivity reactions
- Palpitation and tachycardia.

Occassional

- Hypotension
- Thrombophlebitis
- Seizures
- Anemia.

Special Circumstances

Renal disease: Dosage should be modified for patients with renal insufficiency.

Hepatic disease: No modification in dosage required in patients with hepatic disease.

Pregnancy/breastfeeding: It should be used with caution in patients with pregnancy and breastfeeding.

Monitoring

No specific laboratory monitoring requirements.

AMOXICILLIN CLAVULANATE

Drug class: Amoxicillin is an extended spectrum semisynthetic penicillin which is penicillinase susceptible. It is an Aminopenicillin.

Mechanism of action: Beta-lactam antibiotics interfere with the synthesis of bacterial cell wall. The beta-lactam antibiotics inhibit the transpeptidases so that cross-linking of the adjacent peptide chains does not take place.

Pharmacokinetics: It is not degraded by gastric acid. Primary channel of excretion is kidney.

Adverse Effects

- Diarrhea
- Rash
- Hypersensitivity reaction.

Drug class: Clavulanate is a beta lactamase inhibitor. It is obtained from *Streptomyces clavuligerus*. It has a beta-lactam ring but no antibacterial activity of its own.

Pharmacokinetics: It is eliminated mainly by glomerular filtration. Its elimination and tissue distribution matches amoxicillin with which it is used.

Adverse Effects

Frequent

- Diarrhea
- Rash
- Hypersensitivity reaction.

Occasional

- *Candida stomatitis* and vaginitis.

Special Circumstances

Renal disease: Dosage should be modified for patients with renal insufficiency.

Hepatic disease: No modification in dosage required in patients with hepatic disease.

Pregnancy/breastfeeding: It should be used with caution in patients with pregnancy and breastfeeding.

Monitoring

No specific laboratory monitoring requirements.

References

1. Grosset J.18 National congres de la Tuberculose et des Maladaise Respiratoires, Clermont-Ferrand. Pris, Masson,1974.
2. Kucer A, Bennet NM, et al. The use of antibiotics: a comprehensive review with clinical emphasis. Philadelphia:Lippincott;1988;pp.585-1436.
3. United States Pharmacopeil Dispencing Information for healthcare professional. Vol. I. Englewood, CO; Micro-medex; 1999;pp.69-1419.
4. Meyer RD. Amikacin. Ann Intern Med 1981;95:328-32.
5. Sutton WB, Gordee RS, et al. In vitro and in vivo laboratory study on the antitubercular activity of capreomycin. Ann N Y Sci. 1966;135:947-59.
6. Davidson PJ, Le HQ. Drug treatment of tuberculosis-1992. Drugs.1992;43:651-73.
7. Chopra I, Brennam P. Molecular action of antimycobacterial agents. Tubercle Lung Dis. 1998;78:89-98.

8. Freidman TR, Sherman LF, Maw KL, Fujiwara, Craford JT. A multi-institutional outbreak of highly drug-resistant tuberculosis: epidemiology and clinical outcome. JAMA. 1996;276: 1229-35.
9. Lehman J. Para-aminosalicyclic acid in treatment of tuberculosis. Lancet. 1946;1:15-6.
10. Pan X-S, Amber J, et al. Involvement of topoisomerase and DNA gyrase as ciprofloxacin targets. Antimicrob Agent Chemother. 1996;40:2321-6.
11. Tsukamura M, Nakamura E, et al. Therapeutic effect of new antibacterial substance ofloxacin. Am Rev Respir Dis. 1987;136:1339-42.
12. Hong Kong Chest Service/BMRC. A controlled dose of ofloxacin in the treatment of pulmonary tuberculosis resistant to streptomycin, rifampicin, isoniazid. Tubercle Lung Dis. 1998;78: 89-98.
13. Jagannath C, Venkta Reddy M, et al. Chemotherapeutic activity of clofazimine and its analog against *M. tuberculosis* in vitro and in vivo. Am J Respir Crit Care Med. 1995;151:1083-6?
14. Hong Kong Chest Service/BMRC. Five year follow-up of a controlled trial of five 6-month regimen for chemotherapy for pulmonary tuberculosis. Am Rev Respir Dis. 1987;136: 1339-42.
15. Casal M, Gutierrez J, Gonzalez J, et al. In vitro susceptibility of *Mycobacterium tuberculosis* to a new macrolide. Am J Respir Crit Care Med. 1995;151:1083-6.
16. Cynamon MH, Klemens SP. et al. Activity of several novel oxazolidinones against *Mycobacterium tuberculosis* in a murine model. Antimicrob. Agents Chemother. 1999;43:1189-91.
17. Jones RN, Jhonson DM, et al. In vitro antimicrobial activity and spectra of U-100592 and U-100766, the two novel fluorinated oxazolidine group. Antimicrob Agents Chemother. 1996;40:720-6.

Chapter 3

Management of Retreatment Cases in Tuberculosis

Introduction

Tuberculosis retreatment refers to treatment in a patient of tuberculosis, who has been previously treated for more than four weeks with antituberculosis drugs and who are now smear or culture positive for *Mycobacterium tuberculosis.*[1] The management of retreatment cases in tuberculosis (TB) involves management of entities like relapse, failure and treatment after default and poor adherence to previous treatment. All of these entities may imply different approaches and physician handling these problems requires adequate knowledge of appropriate retreatment regimens. Retreatment patients correspond to the greater part of the problem and the major source of complications. In the two largest high-tuberculosis burden countries (China and India), re treatment cases accounted for up to 20% of sputum smear-positive cases.[2] Retreatment forms the most complex part of the problem because these patients have already had the opportunity to receive a curative treatment; therefore, excluding relapse cases, most retreatment cases arise due to errors during the implementation or administration of the previous treatment regimen.[3] This chapter aims at management of retreatment cases in tuberculosis.

The retreatment of TB involves entities such as relapse, failure, treatment after default, and poor patient adherence to the previous treatment.

Relapse

Relapse is defined as a patient previously treated for TB who has been declared cured or treatment completed, and is diagnosed with bacteriologically positive (smear or culture) tuberculosis.[1,4] However, there can be certainty that a patient has completed all their medication only when treatment administration is directly observed. If the treatment was not supervized, the authenticity of a relapse can be questioned. The rapidly dividing population of bacilli is eliminated early in effective therapy as shown by early clinical responses and clearing of live bacilli from sputum within 2 months in 80% of patients. The remaining subpopulations i.e. mainly the persisters of *M. tuberculosis* account for relapse cases. For this reason, it is theoretically accepted that relapses exhibit the same pattern of resistance as that of the patient's initial TB; hence, the same initial treatment could be administered. If the relapse occurs several years after the initial treatment, re-infection is more likely than relapse.[5,6] Though this is not simple to demonstrate, but the indication for the same initial treatment scheme still applies. Although relapses are usually due to susceptible bacilli, it is still advisable to carry out Drug Susceptibility Test (DST) to first-line anti-TB drugs before the commencement of treatment for relapse cases. However, when DST is conducted in the field, the incidence of resistance among relapse patients increases significantly compared to that seen in initial cases. This might be explained by irregularities in drug intake but also by selection of initial single or multiple resistances. This situation has led to the recommendation that, in low- and middle-income countries like India and under Revised National Tuberculosis Control Program (RNTCP) conditions, relapses be treated with a reinforced first-line drug regimen,[3] administered for a longer period of time, which is in the form of Category II regimen of WHO (2SRHEZ/RHEZ/5RHE either daily or thrice weekly).

Defaulters or Treatment after Default

A person who returns to treatment, positive bacteriologically, following interruption of treatment for 2 months or more of anti-TB treatment.[1] There are two different kinds of defaulters: one who abandons all of his/her drugs, and others who omit one of them. Those who abandon all of their drugs usually do not incur an elevated risk of selection of resistance, since the drugs were effective when the patient took the treatment, and there were no favorable conditions for selection of the naturally resistance mutants. When the effect of the treatment was interrupted due to default, the entire bacillary population resumes growth, as before the initial treatment. Thus, in these cases, it is adequate to reintroduce the initial treatment regimen or better with a reinforced first-line drug regimen or a Category II regimen. The situation is entirely different when the patient abandons one of the drugs while undergoing treatment. It generates the conditions for the selection of microorganisms spontaneously resistant to the drugs the patient continues taking.[4] This is the reason why fixed dose combinations (multiple drugs incorporated into one) are superior to individual drugs, and are strongly recommended in international recommendations of WHO and IUALTD when DOTS (Directly Observed Treatment Short-Course) is not possible since drug resistance may be less likely to develop and further, because when treatment is interrupted,[7] simultaneously all drugs will be stopped together and this would prevent resistant organisms being selected.

Failure

Failure is defined on the basis of two aspects bacteriologically, i.e. on sputum smear and culture status. In low- and middle-income countries like India, where cultures are less frequently used, sputum smears are used to define failures. Failure for initially smear-positive patients (Category I and Category II) is defined as sputum smear-positive at the end of the fifth month of treatment or later.[1] Failure for initially smear-negative patients (Category III) regimen is defined as who became smear-positive during treatment.[1]

Based on culture, failure is defined as the reappearance, while the patient is receiving treatment and after the negative conversion of cultures, of bacteriological activity.[1,4] It is also considered treatment failure when cultures do not become negative during the course of treatment. For the initial 6-month treatment scheme with Rifampicin (R) in both phases, i.e. Category I, failure is considered when sputum cultures are still positive at the end of the fourth month. For the 8-month treatment scheme, without R in the continuation phase, i.e. 2RHEZ/6HE, failure is not diagnosed before the end of the fifth month.[1,8] The failure is due to a population of bacilli that is metabolically active and proliferates during the treatment, which creates favorable conditions for selection of naturally resistant mutant bacilli present in the original population. Therefore, the failure situation should imply resistance to all the drugs being administered at the time when failure was diagnosed; hence the importance of carrying out DST to first-line drugs. However, some studies show that up to 50% of failures exhibit drug susceptibility in drug susceptibility testing,[9,10] and can be cured with an initial or reinforced first-line-drug-based scheme, i.e. Category II regimen.[11] The contributing factors for this could be the imperfect correlation between DST results and the behavior of bacilli in vivo, and the extremely small fraction of patients in whom negative conversion of cultures take > 4 months despite well-documented susceptibility to drugs.

Poor Adherence to Treatment

This may be much more common than thought especially in the latter months of treatment, when most of the patients are already relieved of symptoms. When this situation is continued over a period of time, it results in creating a favorable environment for naturally resistant mutant bacilli to develop.[3]

Drug Resistant Tuberculosis

Drug Resistance in New Cases

The management of new patients suspected of having contracted drug-resistant strains of *M. Tuberculosis* i.e. primary resistance or now known as 'resistance in new cases' should be essentially similar to the lines of treatment of other new patients. They should be given the same initial standardized treatment recommended by the National Tuberculosis Programme (NTP), i.e. Category I regimen; however, as resistance is highly suspected, drug susceptibility testing (DST) to first-line drugs should be carried out. If these tests confirm MDR, but if the patient shows a favorable clinical progression, the initial regimen should perhaps remain unchanged, since some reports have demonstrated that 20 to 50% of these new patients with MDR-TB are cured by standard regimens.[11] If the clinical response is not favorable, the initial treatment must be interrupted in favor of a new regimen following the basic principles of drug resistance treatment detailed later. Nonetheless, some authors advocate the administration of empirical treatments with up to seven drugs until DST results are available, with further adaptation of the regimen subsequent to these results.

Drug Resistance in Retreatment Cases

First and foremost requirement before starting a retreatment regimen is to assess the possibility whether the person carries resistance strain or not. The two basic approaches for this is by establishment of prior TB treatments and DST reports.[3] In the case of failure, partial default on medication, sustained poor compliance of the patient, or chronicity with multiple previous treatments, the presence of resistance to one or more drugs is very likely, whereas, in the case of relapse or total treatment default, it can be assumed that there is no resistance. A comprehensive history of previous TB treatments requires complete chronology of the previous introduction and cessation of drugs, including administered doses and pharmacological associations of prior regimens. This allows the evaluation of real or masked monotherapies previously received by the patient. The main predictor of resistance to a particular drug is the demonstration of its prior use in monotherapy for more than one month.[3,12] Sometimes resistance develops if the patient was on the functional equivalent of two drugs, depending on the drugs concerned. For example, pyrazinamide is not considered a good companion drug to prevent resistance. If a patient was receiving functionally only rifampicin and pyrazinamide in the initial phase (because of resistance to isoniazid and ethambutol), resistance to rifampicin may develop. Thus, it is crucial to consider which functional drugs the patient received between the time of DST specimen collection and the time of the new regimen design (i.e. consider whether resistance has developed to any of the functional drugs).

In practice, the quality of information collected through this medical history is better than that from DST, which can take >3 months (when carried out by conventional methods on solid media) and may also fail due to insufficient growth of cultures. Susceptibility testing for isoniazid, rifampicin, the fluoroquinolones, and the injectable agents is fairly reliable. For other agents, it is less reliable, and basing individualized treatments on DST for these agents should be avoided. The clinical effectiveness or ineffectiveness of a drug cannot be predicted by DST with 100% certainty.[16,17] DST to pyrazinamide (Z) requires BACTEC, a radiometric method not available in most low-income countries.[13-17] It should be pointed out that drug resistance, as detected in the DST, reflects the inefficacy of this drug in culture media, but drug susceptibility does not necessarily correspond to the efficacy of the drug within a new regimen; the latter can be estimated in view of the history of previous treatments. Labs too vary in reliability and errors may occur in lab also and it is often seen that different sensitivity pattern reports are obtained from different labs at different times. Therefore, the DST results should not be relied uncritically especially without the background of previous drug history. At present, it appears that DST results concerning second-line drugs such as kanamycin and ofloxacin/ciprofloxacin could be of great help, but not DST to other drugs.[16]

Category II Regimen for Retreatment of TB Patients

In the case of failure, partial default on medication, or chronicity with multiple previous treatments, the presence of resistance to one or more drugs is very likely. The reinforced first-line drug 8- to 9-month regimen (Category II regimen employed in India) can cure most relapses and treatment defaults (the most common sources of patients for retreatment) and a variable proportion of initial failures. The difficulty with the 8- to 9-month regimen is the group representing failure of the initial treatment and patients carrying multidrug-resistant strains of *Mycobacterium tuberculosis*. Short-course chemotherapy (SCC) for patients infected with drug-resistant strains may create even more resistance to the drugs in use. This has been termed the "amplifier effect" of SCC[18] which implies that resistant strains in bacterial population are selected repeatedly when a regimen is used continuously over a long period in a given community and these become dominant strains. The argument against Category II regimen for retreatment cases by many physicians is the fear of adding a single drug to a failing regimen, causing emergence of further drug resistance, particularly MDR. Therefore, in the case of failure of an initial 6-month regimen, i.e. Category I regimen, there is a high risk of resistance to H and R and so, if an 8-month regimen or Category II regimen is prescribed, it would amount to masked monotherapy with Ethambutol during the last five months of treatment.[3] This entails a high risk of amplifying resistance to ethambutol and will not cure the patient. Likewise, if the patient has been initially infected with an MDR strain of *M. tuberculosis* (primary MDR) and fails to respond to the initial 6-month regimen, selection of resistance to Ethambutol and Pyrazinamide during the initial two months of treatment is very likely, because the combination of these two drugs is weak, in the context of inefficiency of H and R. In this case, administration of the 8-month treatment regimen would be equivalent to masked monotherapy with Streptomycin in the initial phase, with a high risk of amplifying resistance to Streptomycin.[3] No sufficient data are available on the response of patients with TB who have multidrug resistance to SCC with first-line drugs under routine countrywide control program conditions. Currently, the only few available data are from patients treated in limited or special settings[19,20] or in few clinical trials.[21-23] A retrospective study to assess the results of treatment with first-line drugs for patients enrolled in the WHO and the International Union Against Tuberculosis and Lung Disease's global project on drug-resistance surveillance was carried out in six countries. These data suggest that standard short-course chemotherapy, based on first-line drugs, was an inadequate treatment for some patients with drug-resistant TB.[10] A study from Vietnam[22] had reported 80% of Category I failure cases to have MDR-TB. A recent study done from a rural area of Tamil Nadu showed that out of Category I regimen using DOTS treatment; only 17% (10 of 60) had organisms resistant to isoniazid and rifampicin (MDR-TB) from sputum collected of 60 patients out of 74 cases declared as failures (smear positive at five/six months of treatment) to Category I regimen.[23]

These findings suggest that the current WHO policy of administration of the five first-line drugs as standard retreatment regimens needs to be revisited according to the availability of resources and DST, the prevalence of multidrug-resistant TB, and the prevailing quality of TB control. Although the proportion of failures is small, in a high-burden country such as India, the absolute number of failures is high. A change in the present policy to use 'stronger regimens' for these patients will have other implications. Providing culture and drug susceptibility testing for such a large number of patients across the country is logistically and economically nonfeasible in low-income countries like India. Under the new guidelines of RNTCP (Revised National Tuberculosis Control Programme in India), any patient, who fails a Category I or III treatment regimen or any Category II patient, who remains smear positive at the end of the fourth month of treatment or later, will be identified as "MDR-TB suspect" and will be subjected to sputum culture and DST.[24] Timely identification of DR-TB and adequate second-line treatment regimens (Category IV regimens—see below) administered early in the course of the disease are essential to stop primary transmission. Experience has shown that implementing a DR-TB control program substantially strengthens overall TB control for both drug-susceptible and drug-resistant cases.[25]

Non-MDR-TB

These include patients with mono-resistant TB and patients with poly-resistant TB other than MDR-TB. Mono-resistance refers to resistance to a single first-line drug, and poly-resistance refers to resistance to two or more first-line drugs but not to both isoniazid and rifampicin. Cases with mono- or poly-resistance will be identified during the course of case-finding for MDR-TB. Treatment of patients infected with mono- or poly-resistant strains using standardized SCC has been associated with increased risk of treatment failure and further acquired resistance, including the development of MDR-TB.[22,26]

Treatment of such patients includes using regimens which are considered "modifications" of Category I or Category II treatment and the adjusted treatment continued for the indicated length of time.[18] When a decision has been made to modify standardized SCC, the most effective regimen should be chosen from the start to maximize the likelihood of cure; effective drugs should not be withheld for later use. They are not classified as Category IV treatments, which are regimens designed to treat MDR-TB. Definitive randomized or controlled studies have not been performed to determine the best treatment for various patterns of drug resistance, except for streptomycin resistance.[18]

Chronic TB Case

A Chronic case of TB is defined as a TB patient who remains smear-positive after completing a retreatment regimen.[1] Chronic cases form the most complex part of problems encompassing patients undergoing retreatment because they, having received multiple treatments, are thought to carry higher degree of resistance strains to primary-line drugs and second-line drugs (SLDs) depending on their usage. The management of this high-risk group entails DST for atleast the primary-line drugs and DST for SLD if there is previous history of treatment with SLD and commencement of standardized or individualized regimen based on resource setting as detailed below.

MDR-TB

Among the few drugs available for the treatment of tuberculosis (TB), only isoniazid (H) and rifampicin (R) are highly effective. Curing TB patients with resistance to at least both of these drugs, multidrug-resistant tuberculosis (MDR-TB), is, therefore, very difficult and presents huge challenges worldwide. As per RNTCP report, the number of patients who were registered under Category II during the year 2006 was 185,718 (RNTCP Central TB Division, India: Personal Communication). Out of these, the total number of patients declared cured was 113,845, i.e. 61.3% and the number of patients who were classified as failure, treatment default and died during Category II treatment were 10,400 (5.6%), 30,643 (16.5%), and 3157 (1.7%) respectively. Based on the studies done, assuming that approximate 50% of Category II failures have MDR pattern of resistance, then according to this report, the probable number of MDR patients would then be approximately 5200 (i.e. 50% of 10,400). Also taking into account the possibility that MDR strains would have been present in patients who died and defaulted during the course of treatment, so then assuming that 50% of these two categories were also MDR, the total number of MDR patients in the year 2006 in India under RNTCP would be around 27,671 (50% of total of Category II Failure + Died + Default). According to the WHO/IUATLD 4th global survey, the estimated prevalence of primary and acquired MDR-TB in India is 2.8% (95% CI, 2.3–3.4%) and 17.2% (95% CI, 15.0–19.7) respectively[27] and the number of estimated cases of MDR-TB in India during 2006 was 1,10,132 (95% CI, 79,975–1,42,386).[27] This huge deficit between the two figures speaks volumes of huge number of patients being treated outside the tuberculosis control program of our country and also throws light on the grim situation our country faces when it comes to discrepancies in the management of DR-TB between the private and government sector.

The diagnosis of MDR-TB should be based on the patient's treatment history (failure of standard regimens, exposure to patients with MDR-TB, etc.) and on the results of DST[28] against H and R, for which reliability approaches 100%.[29] Even then, it takes three months or more to confirm the diagnosis. During this period, they can spread the multidrug-resistant disease to others. WHO with the Stop TB Partnership, UNITAID and the Foundation for Innovative New Diagnostics (FIND) together unveiled a new policy endorsing the use of Line Probe Assays[30] and GeneXpert MTB/RIF[31] in low-resource countries like India. The advantages include rapid screening of patients with MDR-TB risk within 2 hours to 2 days as compared to 2 to 3 months for conventional cultures.

The number of drugs needed to constitute a good retreatment regimen in the patients with MDR-TB is one of the most controversial topics debated and the conclusion is that clinical trials, comparing different number and type of drugs, are necessary to develop the evidence base for the most appropriate treatment of

MDR-TB. The statement from the American Thoracic Society/Centres for Disease Control and Prevention/Infectious Diseases Society of America (ATS/CDC/IDSA) states that regimens employing four to six medications appear to be associated with better results.[32] They concluded that acceptable results have been obtained using more than four drugs, with favorable responses varying between 65%[33] and 85.5%.[34] However, the problem with administration of four, six or more drugs is a high probability of intolerance by the patient who will default from treatment or will refuse to take it when faced with the appearance of severe side effects. It is not insignificant that the 30% to 54.4% of patients experienced side effects that compelled them to discontinue one or two drugs.[33,35] A study from India showed that 16 out of 39 patients, i.e. 41% developed side effects and out of which 8 patients (21.1%) developed significant side effects that required the stoppage/change of drugs.[36] Given the significant global increase in MDR-TB in recent years, more solid evidence validating the various recommendations will certainly come to light in the near future.

Now for the treatment of MDR-TB patients, whether to use individualized or standardized regimen, the main principles of individualized regimen being the selection of treatment based on the individual DST results and elaboration of aggressive therapeutic regimens in settings that allow close follow-up of patients by skilled professionals. Several published studies have reported the efficacy of this strategy.[37-43] This is, however, a highly expensive approach that is difficult to implement in the majority of middle- and low-income countries like India which bear the high burden of MDR-TB. As many countries have employed very few second-line drugs in recent years, the micro-organisms would be expected to be more susceptible to these than would be assumed from the often unreliable DST results.[3] For this reason, the WHO recommendations for the treatment of MDR-TB favored the use of standardized treatment regimens in such circumstances.[44,45] Standard treatment regimens for these MDR-TB patients facilitate their management, reduce the number of specialist physicians needed and reduce the overall cost of treatment by five to ten times. The efficacy of this strategy has been confirmed by reports in the literature.[46]

DOTS-Plus is an integral component of RNTCP to manage MDR-TB to be implemented through program infrastructure.[24] The strategy is designed to manage MDR-TB using second-line anti-TB drugs within the DOTS strategy in low- and middle-income countries like India. Therefore, in every DOTS-implementing unit of the country, DOTS would be prioritized above DOTS-Plus with the view that DOTS reduces the emergence of MDR-TB, and, therefore, the need for DOTS-Plus over time. The RNTCP under DOTS-Plus will be using a standardized treatment regimen (STR), Category IV regimen, comprising of 6 drugs (kanamycin, ofloxacin, ethionamide, cycloserine, pyrazinamide and ethambutol) during 6–9 months of the Intensive Phase and four drugs (ofloxacin, ethionamide, cycloserine and ethambutol) during the 18 months of the Continuation Phase. *p*-aminosalicylic acid (PAS) is included in the regimen as a substitute drug if any bactericidal drug (kanamycin, ofloxacin, ethionamide and pyrazinamide) or any two bacteriostatic (ethambutol and cycloserine) drugs are not tolerated.

This Category IV regimen is highly suitable for high TB prevalence as well in low- to middle-income countries like India. Injectable agent should be given atleast six months and the whole treatment duration is minimum of 18 months beyond sputum conversion. Fully standardized second-line treatment have shown to be feasible and cost-effective in MDR-TB treatment.[47]

Prevention of Retreatment Cases

TB is still a curable disease and the main crux is the initial treatment, which is said to be the most important and the safest bet in curing the disease without any relapse and preventing drug-resistant strains from developing. However, the irony of the fact is the irrational and improper use of ATT, be it in dosage, duration, quality of drugs or even in the number of drugs which is still rampant in our country. Even though by March 2006, nationwide DOTS coverage had been achieved, however, the ground reality is that private sector in India[48] still continues to play a big role in the management of TB patients. A recent study in India to analyze the prescription patterns of private doctors for TB patients found that 33 different regimens were prescribed by 449 doctors and 45% doctors did not practice current NTP/WHO-recommended regimens and 75% doctors made prescription errors.[49] This is probably an area which our country can be benefitted by proper education of both practioners and public alike. Sensing this need, WHO came up with the Stop TB Strategy (which aims to reduce dramatically the burden of TB by 2015) and one of the main components of this strategy is by scaling up public-private mix (PPM) to bridge down the gap between the private and government sector by engaging all care providers, including public, nongovernmental and private providers, and other approaches to ensure adherence to international standards of TB care.

Conclusion

Presently, in our country, which is still lacking in resources, all retreatment cases should be given Category II regimen under DOTS (2SRHEZ/RHEZ/5RHE either daily or thrice weekly) and ideally, if possible, their sputum cultures should be sent for DST even before the start of the retreatment regimen to identify the drug-resistant strains at the earliest. Efforts to ensure that good, reliable and adequate number of laboratory services for the timely diagnosis of drug- resistant strains be made available throughout the country. Now that DOTS has been implemented throughout our country and the foremost aim at present is the fast implementation of DOTS-Plus program throughout the country at the earliest. Along with this, proper education on the management aspects of retreatment cases including drug-resistant and multi-drug-resistant TB should be imparted to all the practioners of the country. The proper use of second-line drugs must be ensured to cure the existing multi-drug-resistant tuberculosis, to reduce transmission of MDR-TB and to prevent the emergence of XDR-TB.

References

1. World Health Organization. Treatment of TB Guidelines; 4th edn. WHO/HTM/TB/2009.420.
2. Global tuberculosis control: surveillance, planning, financing. WHO report 2008. Geneva, World Health Organization, 2008 (WHO/HTM/TB/2008.393).
3. Caminero JA. Management of multidrug-resistant tuberculosis and patients in retreatment Eur Respir J. 2005;25:928-36.
4. Caminero JA. Guía de la Tuberculosis para Médicos Especialistas. [Tuberculosis Guide for Specialist Physicians]. Paris, International Union Against Tuberculosis and Lung Disease, 2003.
5. Caminero JA, Pena MJ, Campos-Herrero MI, et al. Exogenous reinfection with tuberculosis on an European island with a moderate incidence of disease. Am J Respir Crit Care Med. 2001;163:717-20.
6. Van Rie A, Warren R, Richardson M, et al. Exogenous reinfection as a cause of recurrent tuberculosis after curative treatment. N Engl J Med. 1999;341:1174-9.
7. Moulding T, Putt A, Reichman L. Fixed dose combinations of tuberculosis medications to prevent drug resistance. Annals of internal medicine.1995;122:951-4.
8. Enarson DA, Rieder HL, Arnadottir T, Trébucq A. Management of tuberculosis: a guide for low-income countries; 5th edn. Paris, International Union Against Tuberculosis and Lung Disease, 2000.
9. Tuberculosis Research Centre, Indian Council of Medical Research. Low rate of emergence of drug resistance in sputum-positive patients treated with short course chemotherapy. Int J Tuberc Lung Dis. 2001;5:40-5.
10. Prasad R, Verma SK, Garg R, Jain A, Anand SC, Hosmane GB, et al. Drug susceptibility pattern of Mycobacterium tuberculosis isolates from patients of Category-II failure of pulmonary tuberculosis under directly observed treatment short-course from north India, Biosci Trends. 2012;6:110-4.
11. Espinal MA, Kim SJ, Suarez PG, et al. Standard short-course chemotherapy for drug-resistant tuberculosis: treatment outcomes in six countries. JAMA. 2000;283:2537-45.
12. Mitchison DA. The segregation of streptomycin-resistant variants of *Mycobacterium tuberculosis* into groups with characteristic levels of resistance. J gen microbiol. 1951;5:596-604.
13. Caminero JA. Guía de la tuberculosis para médicos especialistas. [Tuberculosis guide for specialist physicians]. Paris, International Union Against Tuberculosis and Lung Disease. 2003.
14. Iseman MD. Treatment of multi-drug-resistant tuberculosis. N Engl J Med. 1993;329:784-91.
15. Ortega A. Retratamientos en tuberculosis. [Retreatment in tuberculosis]. Rev Clin Esp. 1987;180:269-74.
16. Kim SJ. Drug-susceptibility testing in tuberculosis: methods and reliability of the results. Eur Respir J. 2005;25:564-9.
17. Canetti G. Present aspects of bacterial resistance in tuberculosis. Am Rev Respir Dis. 1965;92:687-703.
18. Guidelines for the programmatic management of drug-resistant tuberculosis. WHO, 2008.
19. Garcia-Garcia M, Ponce-de-Leon A, Jiménez-Corona M, et al. Clinical consequences and transmissibility of drug-resistant tuberculosis in Southern Mexico. Arch Intern Med. 2000;160:630-6.

20. Coninx R, Mathieu C, Debacker M, et al. First-line tuberculosis therapy and drug-resistant *Mycobacterium tuberculosis* in prisons. Lancet. 1999;353:969-73.
21. Mitchinson D, Nunn AJ. Influence of initial drug resistance on the response to short-course chemotherapy of pulmonary tuberculosis. Am Rev Respir Dis. 1986;133:423-30.
22. Quy HWT, Lan NTN, Borgdoff MW, et al. Drug susceptibility among failures and relapse cases of tuberculosis: Is standard retreatment regimen adequate? Int J Tub Lung Dis. 2003;7:631-6.
23. Santha T, Gopi PG, Rajeswari R, Selvakumar N, Subramani R, Chandrasekaran V, et al. Is it worth treating Category I failure patients with Category II regimen? Indian J Tuberc. 2005;52:203-6.
24. DOTS-Plus guidelines, Revised National Tuberculosis Control Programme, Central TB Division Directorate General Health Services, Ministry of Health & Family Welfare, Nirman Bhawan, New Delhi. Sep. 2008.
25. Kim JY, et al. From multi-drug-resistant tuberculosis to DOTS expansion and beyond: making the most of a paradigm shift. Tuberculosis (Edinb). 2003;83:59-65.
26. Tuberculosis Research Centre, Chennai, India. Low rate of emergence of drug resistance in sputum-positive patients treated with short-course chemotherapy. Int J of Tub and Lung Dis. 2001;5:40-5.
27. WHO-IUALTD Global Project on Anti-Tuberculosis Drug Resistance Surveillance (2002–2007), Fourth Global Report (2008).
28. American Thoracic Society. Treatment of drug-resistant tuberculosis. Am Rev Respir Dis. 1966;94:125-7.
29. Kim SJ. Drug-susceptibility testing in tuberculosis: methods and reliability of results. Eur Respir J. 2005;25:564-9.
30. WHO Press Release New Rapid Test for DR-TB for Developing Countries. Geneva, June 30, 2008.
31. Towards universal access to diagnosis and treatment of multi-drug-resistant and extensively drug-resistant tuberculosis by 2015. WHO Progress Report, 2011. WHO/HTM/TB/2011.3.
32. American Thoracic Society Documents. American Thoracic Society/Centers for Disease Control and Prevention/Infectious Diseases Society of America: treatment of tuberculosis. Am J Respir Crit Care Med. 2003;167:603-62.
33. Goble M, Iseman MD, Madsen LA, Waite D, Ackerson L, Horsburgh R. Treatment of 171 patients with pulmonary tuberculosis resistant to isoniazid and rifampicin. N Engl J Med. 1993;328:527-32.
34. Park SK, Kim CT, Song SD. Outcome of chemotherapy in 107 patients with pulmonary tuberculosis resistant to isoniazid and rifampicin. Int J Tuberc Lung Dis. 1998;2:877-84.
35. Geerligs WA, Altena R, de Lange WCM, Van Soolingen D, Van der Werf TS. Multi-drug-resistant tuberculosis: long-term treatment outcome in the Netherlands. Int J Tuberc Lung Dis. 2000;4:758-64.
36. Prasad R, Verma SK, Sahai S, Kumar S, Jain A. Efficacy and safety of kanamycin, Ethionamide, PAS, and Cycloserine in Multi-drug-resistant Pulmonary Tuberculosis Patients. Ind J Chest Dis Allied Sci. 2006;48:183-6.
37. Mukherjee J, Socci A, Acha J, et al. The PIH guide to management of multi-drug-resistant tuberculosis. International edition. Boston, MA, USA: Partners in Health, 2003.
38. Mukherjee JS, Rich ML, Socci AR, et al. Programs and principles in treatment for multi-drug-resistant tuberculosis. Lancet. 2004;363:474-81.
39. Tahaoglu K, Törün T, Sevim T, et al. The treatment of multi-drug-resistant tuberculosis in Turkey. N Engl J Med. 2001;345:170-4.

40. Narita M, Alonso P, Lauzardo M, Hollender ES, Pitchenik AE, Ashkin D. Treatment experience of multi-drug-resistant tuberculosis in Florida, 1994–1997. Chest 2001;120:343-8.
41. Chan ED, Laurel V, Strand MJ, et al. Treatment and outcome analysis of 205 patients with multi-drug-resistant tuberculosis. Am J Respir Crit Care Med. 2004;169:1103-9.
42. Park SK, Lee CM, Heu JP, Song SD. A retrospective study for the outcome of pulmonary resection in 49 patients with multi-drug-resistant tuberculosis. Int J Tuberc Lung Dis. 2002;6:143-9.
43. Evan W, Orenstein BS, Sanjay Basu, N Sarita Shah, et al. Treatment outcomes among patients with multi-drug-resistant tuberculosis: systematic review and meta-analysis. Lancet Infect Dis. 2009;9:153-61.
44. Crofton J, Chaulet P, Maher D, et al. Guidelines for the management of drug-resistant tuberculosis. WHO/TB/96.210. Geneva, Switzerland: WHO, 1997.
45. Prasad R. Management of Multi-drug-Resistant Tuberculosis: Practitioner's viewpoint. Indian J Tub. 2007;54:3-11.
46. Van Deun A, Hamid Salim MA, Kumar Das AP, Bastian I, Portaels F. Results of a standardized regimen for multi-drug-resistant tuberculosis in Bangladesh. Int J Tuberc Lung Dis. 2004;8:560-7.
47. Suarez PG, et al. Feasibility and cost effectiveness of standardized secondline drug treatment for chronic tuberculosis patients; a national cohort study in Peru. Lancet. 2002;359:1980-9.
48. Uplekar MW, Shepard DS. Treatment of tuberculosis by private general practitioners in India. Tubercle. 1991;72:284-90.
49. Prasad R, Nautiyal RG, Mukherji PK, Jain A, et al. Treatment of new pulmonary tuberculosis patients : What Do Allopathic Doctors Do in India? Int J Tuberc Lung Dis. 2002;6:895-902.

Chapter 4

Mono- and Poly-drug-resistant Tuberculosis: Current Status

Introduction

Drug-resistant tuberculosis has been reported since the early days of introduction of antitubercular chemotherapy. Cases with mono- or poly-resistance will be identified during the course of case-finding for MDR-TB. Treatment of patients infected with mono- or poly-resistant strains using standardized Short Course Chemotherapy has been associated with increased risk of treatment failure and further acquired resistance, including the development of MDR-TB. Therefore, this current chapter aims to review the present scenario of mono- and poly-drug-resistant TB.

Definition

Drug-resistant tuberculosis is defined as a case of tuberculosis excreting bacilli resistant to one or more antitubercular drugs. Drug-resistant tuberculosis is defined as a case of tuberculosis excreting bacilli resistant to one or more antitubercular drugs. Mono-resistance is defined as resistance to one anti-tuberculosis drug, whereas poly-resistance is defined as resistance to more than one antituberculosis drug, other than both isoniazid and rifampicin.

Types of Drug Resistance

Drug resistance may be of two types—primary and acquired. Primary drug resistance may be defined as drug resistance in a patient who has not received any antitubercular treatment in the past. The resistance that develops in a patient who has received prior chemotherapy is defined as acquired drug resistance. Recently the terms "resistance in new cases" and "resistance in previously treated cases" have been proposed for use because of the difficulty to confirm the validity of the patient's past history of treatment. When one is not sure whether the resistance is primary or acquired due to concealed history of previous treatment or unawareness of treatment taken before, it is known as "initial drug resistance". Combined resistance is defined as the sum of primary and acquired resistance.

Prevalence of Mono- and Poly-drug Resistance: Global Scenario

A review by WHO of a series of 63 surveys of drug-resistant TB carried out between 1985 and 1994 led to the conclusion that the problem of drug resistance was global.[2] The overall percentages of resistance to different antituberculosis drugs obtained from different surveys done throughout the world are shown in Tables 4.1 and 4.2. The available information shows that the levels of primary resistance to Isoniazid (H) as single agent ranged from 0 to 16.9%. High rates of primary resistance to Isoniazid have been reported from Kenya, India, Haiti while it is reported to be low in South-eastern England, Melbourne and Argentina. The rates of primary resistance to streptomycin range from 0.1 to 23.5%. High rates of resistance to streptomycin (S) were reported in Zaire, Pakistan and Brazil and low levels of resistance were reported from China, Ethiopia and Bosnia-Herzegovina. Primary resistance to Rifampicin (R) as a single agent was unusual with a rate ranging from 0 to 3% and the rates of resistance to ethambutol were similarly low, ranging from 0 to 4.2%.[2] There are fewer surveys of acquired drug resistance and the rates of acquired resistance are usually higher than those of primary resistance. The rates of acquired resistance to H ranged from 4 to 53.7%, to S from 0 to 19.4%, to R from 0 to 14.5% and to ethambutol (E) from 0 to 13.7%.[2] Resistance to multiple drugs also varied by geographical region

TABLE 4.1: Global primary/initial drug resistance

Study	*Any Drug*	*Any H %*	*Any S %*	*Any R %*	*Any E %*
Cohn et al. review of 63 surveys (1985-1994)[2]	-	0–16.9	0.1–23.5	0–3.0	0–4.2
WHO-IUATLD 1994 –1997 surveillance[3]	9.9 (2.0–40.6)	7.3 (1.5–31.7)	6.5 (0.3–8.0)	1.8 (0–16.8)	1.0 (0–9.9)
WHO-IUATLD 1996–1999 surveillance[5]	10.7 (1.7–36.9)	6.2 (0–28.1)	5.2 (0.3–32.4)	1.2 (0–15.8)	0.6 (0–11.1)
WHO-IUATLD 1999–2002 surveillance[10]	10.2 (0–57.1)	5.7 (0–42.6)	6.3 (0–51.5)	1.4 (0–15.6)	0.8 (0–24.8)
WHO-IUATLD 2002–2007 surveillance[11]	17 (0–56.3)	10.3 (0–42.4)	10.9 (0–51.5)	3.7 (0–22.7)	2.5 (0–24.8)

TABLE 4.2: Global acquired drug resistance

Study	*Any Drug*	*Any H %*	*Any S %*	*Any R %*	*Any E %*
Cohn et al. review of 63 surveys (1985-1994)[2]	-	4–53.7	0–19.4	0–14.5	0–13.7
WHO-IUATLD 1994–1997 surveillance[3]	36.0 (5.3–100.0)	-	-	-	-
WHO-IUATLD 1996–1999 surveillance[5]	23.3 (0.0–93.8)	19.6 (0.0–50.0)	12.4 (0.0–53.4)	12.0 (0.0–50.0)	5.9 (0.0–32.1)
WHO-IUATLD 1999–2002 surveillance[10]	18.4 (0–82.1)	14.4 (0–71.0)	11.4 (0–77.1)	8.7 (0–61.4)	3.5 (0–54.2)
WHO-IUATLD 2002–2007 surveillance[11]	35 (0–85.9)	27.7 (0–81.2)	20.1 (0–83.5)	17.5 (0–62.5)	10.3 (0–54.3)

and was more common in patients with acquired resistance. It is evident that prevalence of drug-resistant tuberculosis varied considerably throughout the world. The reasons for this variation in different surveys were the degree of selection of patients studied, the degree of misuse of drugs, the quality of enquiry regarding previous treatment and the inadequate culture and drug susceptibility facilities in many parts of the world. Considering the limitation of the previous studies, a WHO/IUATLD global project of drug resistance surveillance spread over 35 countries in five continents was carried out between 1994 and 1997[3] and observed that the median prevalence of primary and acquired resistance to any of the four first-line antitubercular drugs was 9.9% (95% CI, 2–40.6%) and 36% (95% CI, 5.3–100%) respectively. The report concluded that resistance to anti-TB drugs was found in all 35 countries and regions surveyed, suggesting again that the problem was global.

A second WHO/IUATLD global project on drug resistance surveillance in 58 countries/geographical sites was carried out from 1996 to 1999.[4] Trends of drug resistance were also observed from 28 sites. The overall percentages of resistance to different antituberculosis drugs obtained from different surveys done throughout the world are shown in Tables 4.1and 4.2. Median prevalence of primary and acquired resistance to at least one drug was 10.7% (95% CI, 2–36%) and 23% (95% CI, 0–94%) respectively. Of the 58 sites surveyed, drug resistance among new and previously treated cases were reported in 54 and 48 sites respectively. This global survey tested a total of 61,415 patients with tuberculosis (Median per site 661; range 41–12,675). These sites accounted for 610,000 (18%) of 3.3 million cases of tuberculosis reported to WHO in 1997and 1.5 billion (26%) of the world's 5.8 billion inhabitants. Several countries including 11 of the 22 world tuberculosis high-burdened countries had not yet been surveyed. Trend analysis showed an increasing prevalence of resistance to at least one drug and MDR-TB among new cases in countries like Estonia and Denmark.[4-6] Statistically significant decrease in prevalence of resistance to at least one drug had been found in Cuba, Peru, Wales, Korea and England as in developed countries with long history of TB control, such as Australia, Canada, Denmark, France, the Netherlands, the United States and the United Kingdom.[4,5,7-9]

A Third WHO/IUATLD global project on drug resistance surveillance in 77 countries/geographical sites was carried out in 1999–2002,[10] representing 20% of the global total of new smear-positive TB cases. It included 39 settings not previously included in Global Project and report trends for 46 settings. Median prevalence of primary and acquired resistance to at least one drug was 10.2% (95% CI, 0–57.1%) and 18.4% (95% CI, 0–82.1%) respectively. Trends in drug resistance in new cases were determined in 46 settings. There was significant increase in prevalence of any resistance in Botswana, New Zealand, Poland, and Tomsk Oblast (Russian Federation), whereas Thailand reported decrease prevalence. Drug resistance trends in previously treated cases were determined in 43 settings. A significant increase in prevalence of any resistance was observed in Botswana. Cuba, Switzerland and the USA showed a significant decrease. Despite the expansion in coverage of drug-resistance surveillance for both new and previously treated cases in recent years, data on drug resistance are still not available for >100 countries.

A Fourth WHO/IUATLD global project on drug resistance surveillance includes drug susceptibility test results (DST) from 91,577 patients from 93 settings in 81 countries and two special administrative regions (SARs) of China collected between 2002 and 2007, and representing 35% of the global total of notified new smear-positive TB cases.[11] It included data from 33 countries that have never been previously reported. New data were included from the high TB-burden countries like India, China, Russian Federation, Indonesia, Ethiopia, Philippines, Vietnam, Thailand and Myanmar. Between 1994 and 2007, a total of 138 settings in 114 countries and 2 SARs of China had reported data to the global project. The reported Median prevalence of primary and acquired resistance to at least one drug was 17% (95% CI 13.6–20.4%) and 35% (95% CI 24.1–45.8%) respectively. Median prevalence of primary and acquired resistance to Isoniazid was 10.3% (95% CI 8.4–12.1%) and 27.7% (95% CI 18.7–36.7%) respectively. Trends in drug resistance were determined in 47 countries with three or more data points. Trend data show a range of scenarios. The majority of low TB-burden countries reporting surveillance data showed stable proportions of resistance as well as an absolute number of cases.

The Global Project has collected data from 114 countries and 2 SARs of China and trend analysis includes data from all global reports between 1994 and 2007, as well as data provided between the publication of Reports. Analyses were limited to countries reporting three data points or more. In countries conducting surveillance on all TB cases, trends were reported on both new and combined cases. In conducting surveys, trends were reported on new cases only. Proportions of Isoniazid resistance, and any resistance were examined. Trends were declining, stable or having an increasing direction. Declining trends in DR-TB resistance were noted in the USA, Hong Kong, SAR, China among all TB cases. Hong Kong, SAR, China also showed significant decrease in any resistance among all cases and Isoniazid resistance among new cases. Both the countries reported declining TB notifications. Denmark showed significant declines in any drug resistance in both new and combined TB cases. Puerto Rico showed declining trends in any resistance and MDR-TB among combined cases.

Prevalence of Mono- and Poly-Drug Resistance: India

Though the development of drug resistance in India was noted since the beginning of the chemotherapeutic era, it was based on clinical perception and several isolated reports, which failed to give an idea of the national situation as a whole. The first definite step was taken in this direction in 1965 to 67, when the ICMR conducted two surveys to estimate the prevalence of drug resistance.[12,13] Since then, several studies have been conducted by various authors in different parts of the country. The total prevalence of primary/initial drug resistance (Table 4.3) was observed to be about 18.8% (7.9%–27.1%).[5,10-26] The overall impression as seen in Table 4.3 is that the primary and initial drug resistance has remained more or less constant over the years. According to the third Global Report of WHO, total prevalence of drug resistance among new cases in India (Wardha) is 19.8%.

TABLE 4.3: Primary/initial drug resistance (India)

Study		*Total Prevalence*	*H %*	*S %*	*R %*
ICMR (1968)[12]		20.4	14.7	12.5	-
ICMR (1969)[13]		22	15.5	13.8	-
Krishnan Swamy KV, et al. (1976)[15]		-	10.6	9.5	-
Trivedi, et al. (1988)[14]		20	13.9	7.4	0
Chandrasekharan, et al. (1990)[16]		21.2	17.4	5.7	3
Chandrasekharan, et al. (1992)[17]	Rural	34.9	32.8	5.1	4.4
	Urban				
Parmasivan, et al. (1993)[18]	North Arcet of (1985–89)	20.5	17.3	4.1	2.9
	Pondicherry (1985–91)	13.9	6.0	4.0	0.9
Gupta, et al. (1993)[19]		19.5	10.1	7.6	3
Jain, et al. (1993)[20]		-	18.5	-	0.6
Jena, et al. (1996)[21]		7.9	2.9	4.9	1
Parmasivan, et al. (2000)[22] (Tamil Nadu)		18.8	15.4	6.8	4.4
R Prasad, et al. (2001)[23]		27.4	15.6	11.7	3.9
WHO-IUATLD (1996–1999)[5]		18.8	15.4	6.8	4.4
Paramasivan et al. (2002)[24]	North Arcot (South) 1999	27.7	23.4	12.4	2.8
	Raichur (South) 1999–2000	21.9	18.7	7.2	2.5
WHO-IUATLD (1999–2002)[10]	Wardha	19.8	15.2	7.6	0.5
Sofia, et al. (2004)[25] Bangalore City		27.7	13.7	22.5	2.6
Mahadeo, et al. (2005)[26]	Mayurbhanj 2000–2002	5.3	2.5	3.9	0.7
	Hoogli 2000–2001	16.7	10.3	13.7	3.0
WHO/IUATLD (2002–2007)[11]		-	11.7	9.9	2.2

The prevalence of acquired drug resistance (Table 4.4) ranged from 25 to 100%[3,5,10-11,13,14,20,24,27-31] in several studies. In a study conducted in Gujarat, it was found that 95% of the R-resistant strains were also resistant to H or S or both. The WHO-IUATLD surveillance[3] in India noted the combined prevalence of drug resistance to be 13.3% (95% CI, 10.9–14.9%) in 1998; however, this was done on a small sample of 2240 people around Delhi city and, therefore, was not representative of the country.[3] Study conducted in two districts of South India showed that acquired drug resistance ranged from 69 to 100%.[18] Although variable rates of acquired drug resistance have been obtained, the message is very clear that the prevalence of acquired drug resistance is high and that it is not in isolated pockets but in the country as a whole. These studies were conducted in different states mostly in institutions and tertiary care centers and they do not reflect the overall status of drug resistance problem in India. It is, therefore, necessary to conduct a countrywide multi-center drug resistance surveillance comprising both rural and urban areas in order to have a picture of the total situation in the country.

TABLE 4.4: Acquired drug resistance (India)

Study	*Total Prevalence %*	*H %*	*S %*	*R %*
ICMR (1969)[13]	32 (22–74)	15–69	12–63	-
Trivedi, et al. (1988)[14]				
1980	50.1	34.5	26	2.8
1986	65.3	55.8	-	37.3
Dutta M, et al. 1993[27]	-	67.0	26.0	12.0
Jain, et al. (1992)[20] Delhi	50.7	50.7	-	33.3
Outside Delhi	78.8	78.8	-	61.5
Chowgule, et al. (1998)[28]	25.6	15	53.6	66.8
WHO-IUATLD Surveillance (1994–1997)[3]	32.4	28.8	18.1	14
WHO-IUATLD Surveillance (1999–2002)[5]	50.0	50.0	12.5	25.0
Shah AR, et al. (2002)[29]	58.67	57.18	35.58	37.47
Deivanayagam (2002)[30]	71.0	66.3	35.6	55.5
Paramasivan, et al. (2002)[24]	81.0	81.0	56.2	69.0
North Arcot (South) Raichur (South)	100.0	100.0	36.4	100.0
R. Prasad, et al. (2003)[31]	79.2	48.6	36.6	34.4
WHO-IUATLD (2002–2007) surveillance[11]	-	36.8	26.2	18.1

Mechanism of Drug Resistance

Drug resistance in tuberculosis occurs by random single-step spontaneous mutation at a low but predictable frequency in large bacterial populations. There is no convincing evidence for the role of plasmids or transposons as in other bacterial pathogens. The probability of drug-resistant mutants in the case of Rifampicin is 10^{-8}, for INH, Streptomycin and Ethambutol is 10^{-6} and for Ethionamide, Cycloserine, Capreomycin and Thiacetazone 10^{-3}. The probability of resistance developing in a 2.5 cm cavity which harbors 10^8 to 10^9 bacilli is 10^6 for INH and 10^8 for Rifampicin and 10^{14} for INH and Rifampicin together. In reality, therefore, only one of the bacilli in 10^{14} organisms will be resistant to both Isoniazid and Rifampicin. This illustrates a very fundamental principle that drug-resistant and multi-drug-resistant tuberculosis is a man made problem.

HIV Infection and Drug-resistant Tuberculosis

There is a well-documented association between TB and human immunodeficiency virus (HIV), and although outbreaks of drug-resistant forms of tuberculosis among HIV-infected patients have been widely documented in nosocomial and other congregate settings, little information is available about the association of HIV and drug-resistant TB on a population level. The primary reason for the lack of information is that HIV and anti-TB drug susceptibility testing have not been sufficiently accessible for joint surveys under routine conditions. The accelerating and amplifying influence of HIV infection and the delay in recognition and diagnosis of tuberculosis were found to contribute to outbreaks of DR-TB among HIV-infected patients in the USA.[32-36] An association between HIV/AIDS and drug-resistant tuberculosis may be due to the following reasons:[32-34] (i) Increase in the number of cases of tuberculosis due to HIV/AIDS will give rise to an increase in the number of cases with primary drug resistance; (ii) Overloading of the tuberculosis treatment services because of the expected increase in the number of cases will give rise to more cases with acquired drug resistance; (iii) Immunocompromised status of HIV patients may lead to decreased efficacy of antituberculosis treatment regimens, and, thereby, increasing the chance of acquired drug resistance; (iv) The malabsorption of antituberculosis drugs has been shown to occur with high frequency among persons with AIDS, presumably because of various HIV-caused, parasitic or other enteropathies. Potentially, this could lead to grossly disparate drug levels, resulting in acquired resistance despite adherence to the prescribed regimen. Acquired rifamycin resistance has been associated with HIV infection among TB patients under treatment and anti-TB drug malabsorption has been documented in patient cohorts in settings of high HIV prevalence. In addition, HIV-infected patients and drug-resistant TB patients may have similar risk factors such as history of hospitalization. Lately, however, several studies in India and other South-East Asian countries, having high prevalence of HIV seropositivity, have reported very low prevalence of drug-resistant TB including MDR-TB in HIV-seropositive patients contrary to western literature. HIV-infected TB cases are more likely to be smear-negative, and delayed diagnosis of drug resistance as well as unavailability of treatment have led to high death rates in people living with HIV. Both these factors may suggest a lower rate of transmission.

In the fourth WHO/IUATLD global drug surveillance report, eight settings in seven countries reported data on drug resistance stratified by HIV status: Cuba, Honduras, Latvia, the Russian Federation (Tomsk Oblast), Spain (Barcelona and Galicia), Ukraine (Donetsk Oblast) and Uruguay. Four countries were not able to discriminate between negative and unknown HIV status. The data reported from the majority of countries were not strong enough to examine an association between HIV and drug resistance. Currently, most TB control programs in high-burden countries do not have the diagnostic infrastructure to either detect an outbreak nor the programmatic capacity to manage an outbreak. The development of infection control measures in congregate settings as well as diagnostic screening tools to rapidly identify drug-resistant TB are a priority, for all countries. From a global perspective, routine diagnosis of both HIV and drug-resistant TB should be scaled up for patient's benefit. Better surveillance data may help in developing an understanding of the relationship between these epidemics; however, additional studies should be undertaken in several settings in order to answer the questions which surveys cannot.

Risk Factors of Mono- and Poly-drug Resistance

Several risk factors have been identified in the causation of drug-resistant tuberculosis of which the three most important are—previous treatment with antitubercular drugs which may be inappropriate, incomplete or erratic, high prevalence of drug-resistant tuberculosis in the community and contact with a patient known to have drug-resistant tuberculosis. In patients with previous treatment or disease, the odds of resistant tuberculosis were 4 to 7 times higher than for persons with no history of past treatment. However, standardized short- course chemotherapy carries only a minimal risk of emergence of DR-TB.[31] Other factors that may be responsible for increased risk of resistant tuberculosis are: coinfection with HIV, socioeconomically deprived groups in slums, prisons, correctional facilities, daycare centers, intravenous drug abusers and other immunocompromised states as in transplant recipients, anticancer therapy patients, and patients with diabetes mellitus. Radiologically, far advanced pulmonary tuberculosis with cavitary lesions were four times as likely to harbor drug-resistant organisms.

Sources and Causes of Mono- and Poly-drug Resistance

Though unfortunate, yet a reality is that drug-resistant tuberculosis including multi-drug resistance is a manmade problem. The sources are many and the causes multifactorial. To blame for this are the government, the pharmaceutical industry, doctors, patients and their families, each of whom contribute in their own way to add up to the problem. The government plays its share by providing poor infrastructure in the National Tuberculosis Control Program, unnecessary administrative control on purchase and distribution of drugs with no proper mechanism on quality control and bioavailability tests. The pharmaceutical industry in its turn contributes by manufacturing drugs of uncertain bioavailability in fixed dose or inappropriate drug combinations, poor storage condition of drugs and substitution by inferior quality drugs by pharmacies. The doctor, by his lack of knowledge regarding doses, duration of treatment, side effects and standard regimens, frequent change of brand names and poor patient motivation, contributes the lion's share to the problem. In one of the studies, where prescriptions of 449 doctors were analyzed, 75% of the doctors were found to have made some prescription error.[37] Added to this are the poor teaching and training facilities for them. Noncompliant patients due to monetary lack, lack of information, side effects of drugs and social myths and misconceptions often do not adhere to treatment. Comorbid conditions like diabetes, HIV, psychiatric conditions, the habits of smoking and alcoholism make the patient more vulnerable.

References

1. Multidrug-resistant tuberculosis. ICMR. 1999;29(10 and 11):105-14.
2. Cohn DL, Bustreo F, Raviglione MC. Drug-resistant tuberculosis. Review of the world-wide situation and the WHO/IUATLD Global Surveillance Project. International Union Against Tuberculosis and Lung Disease. Clin Infect Dis. 1997;24 (Suppl 1):S121-30.
3. Pablos-Mendez A, Biokin N, Rieder HL, Bustreo F, Cohn DL, Lambregts van Weezenbeek CS, et al. Global surveillance for antituberculosis drug resistance, 1994–97. World Health Organization—International Union Against Tuberculosis and

Lung Disease Working Group on Antituberculosis Drug Resistance Surveillance. N Engl J Med. 1998;338:1641-9.
4. Espinal MA, Laszlo A, Simonsen L, et al. Global trends in resistance to antituberculosis drugs. N Engl J Med. 2001;344:1294-303.
5. World Health Organization. Antituberculosis drug resistance in the world: prevalence and trends. Report No. 2. WHO/CDS/TB/2000. 278. Geneva: WHO, 2000.
6. Dye C, William BG, Espinal MA, Raviglione MC. Erasing the world's slow strain: strategies to beat multi-drug-resistant tuberculosis. Science. 2002;295:2042-6.
7. Robert J, Trystram D, Pernot-Truffot C, Jarlier V. Surveillance de la tuberculose a bacilles multiresistants en France en 1998. Bull Epidemiol Hebdo. 2002;16-17:71-2.
8. Robert J,Trystram D, Truffot-Pernot C, Carbonelle B. Surveillance of *Mycobacterium tuberculosis* drug resistance in France, 1995-97. Int J Tuberc Lung Dis. 2000;4:665-72.
9. Centers for Disease Control. Reported tuberculosis in the United States 2000. Atlanta, GA: US Department of Health and Human Services, CDC, August 2001.
10. WHO/IUALTD Global Project on Antituberculosis Drug Resistance Surveillance (1999–2002), Third Global Report (2003).
11. WHO/IUALTD Global Project on Antituberculosis Drug Resistance Surveillance (2002–2007), Fourth Global Report (2008).
12. ICMR, Prevalence of drug resistance in patients with pulmonary tuberculosis presenting for the first time with symptoms at chest clinics in India. I. Findings in urban clinics among patients giving no history of previous chemotherapy. Indian J. Med Res. 1968;56:1617-30.
13. ICMR, Prevalence of drug resistance in patients with pulmonary tuberculosis presenting for the first time with symptoms at chest clinics in India II. Findings in urban clinics among all patients, with or without history of previous chemotherapy. Indian J Med Res. 1969;57:823-35.
14. Trivedi SS, Desai SC. Primary antituberculosis drug resistance and acquired rifampicin resistance in Gujarat, India. Tubercle. 1988;69:37-42.
15. Krishnaswamy KV, Rahim MA. Primary drug resistance in pulmonary tuberculosis. Indian J Chest Dis. 1976;28:233-337.
16. Chandrasekaran S, Chauhan MM, Rajalakshmi R, Chaudhuri K, Mahadev B. Initial drug resistance to anti-tuberculosis drugs in patients attending an urban district tuberculosis centre. Ind J Tub. 1990;37:215-6.
17. Chandrasekaran S, Jagota P, Chaudhuri K. Initial drug resistance to antituberculosis drugs in urban and rural district tuberculosis program. Ind J Tub. 1992;39:171-5.
18. Paramasivan CN, Chandrasekaran V, Santha T, Sudarsanam NM, Prabhakar R. Bacteriological investigations for short course chemotherapy under the tuberculosis program in two districts in India. Tuber Lung Dis. 1993;74:23-7.
19. Gupta PR, Singhal B, Sharma TN, Gupta RB. Prevalence of initial drug resistance in tuberculosis patients attending a chest hospital. Ind J Med Res. 1993;97:102-3.
20. Jain NK, Chopra KK, Prasad G. Initial and acquired isoniazid and rifampicin resistance to M. tuberculosis and its implications for treatment. Ind J Tub. 1992;39:121-4.
21. Jena J, Panda BN, Nema SK, Ohri VC, Pahwa RS. Drug resistance pattern of Mycobacterium tuberculosis in a chest disease hospital of armed forces. Lung India. 1995;13:56-9.
22. Parmasivan CN, Bhaskaran K, Venkataraman P, Chandrasekhran V, Narayanan PR. Survilence of drug resistance in tuberculosis in the state of Tamil Nadu. Ind. J. Tub. 2000;47:27-33.
23. Prasad R, Suryakant, Mukerji PK, Gupta AK, Garg R, Rizvi DM, et al. Initial drug resistance in patients of pulmonary tuberculosis attending a tertiary care center. Ind J Tub. 2001;48:159.

24. Paramasivan CN, Venkataraman P, Chandrashekhran V, Bhatt S, Narayanan PR. Surveillance of drug resistance in tuberculosis in two districts of south India. Int J Tuberc Lung Dis. 2002;6:479-84.
25. Sofia V, Balasangameshwara VH, Jagannatha PS, Kumar P. Initial drug resistance among tuberculosis patients under DOTS program in Bengaluru city. Ind J Tuberc. 2004;52:17-21.
26. Mahadeo B, Kumar P, Agrawal SP, Chauhan LS, Sriknataramu N, Surveillance of drug resistance to antituberculosis drugs in districts of Hoogli in West Bengal and Mayurbhanj in Orissa. Ind J Tuberc. 2005:52;5-10.
27. Datta M, Radhamani MP, Selvaraj R, Paramasivan CN, Gopalan BN, Sudeendra CR, et al. Critical assessment of smear-positive pulmonary tuberculosis patients after chemotherapy under the district tuberculosis program. Tub Lung Dis. 1993;74:180-6.
28. Chowgule RV, Deodhar L. Pattern of secondary acquired drug resistance to antituberculosis drug in Mumbai, India—1991–1995. Ind J Chest Dis Allied and Sci. 1998;40:23-31.
29. Shah AR, Agarawal SK, Shah KV. Study of drug resistance in previously treated tuberculosis patients in Gujarat, India. Int J Tuberc Lung Dis. 2002;6:1098-101.
30. Deivanayagam CN, Rajasekaran S, Venkatesan R, et al. Prevalence of acquired MDR-TB and HIV Coinfection. Ind J Chest Dis Allied Sci. 2002;44:237-42.
31. Prasad R, Suryakant, Mukerji PK, Gupta AK, Garg R, Rizvi DM, et al. Acquire drug resistance in patients of pulmonary tuberculosis attending a tertiary care center. Int J Tuberc Lung Dis. 2003;11(Suppl):S3O3.
32. Edlin BR, Tokars, JI, Grieco MH, et al. An outbreak of multi-drug-resistant tuberculosis among hospitalized patients with the acquired immunodeficiency syndrome. N Engl J Med. 1992;326:1514-21.
33. Frieden TR, Sterling T, Pablos-Mendez A, Kilburn JO, Cauthen GM, Dooley SW. The mergence of drug-resistant tuberculosis in New York City. N Engl J med. 1993;328:521-6.
34. Coronado VG, Beck-Sague CM, Hutton MD, et al. Transmission of multi-drug-resistant *Mycobacterium tuberculosis* among persons with human immunodeficiency virus infection in an urban hospital: epidemiologic and restriction fragment length polymorphism analysis. J Infect Dis. 1993;168:1052-5.
35. Busillo C, Lessnau K-D, Sanjana V, et al. Multi-drug-resistant *Mycobacterium tuberculosis* in patients with human immunodeficiency virus infection. Chest. 1992;102:797-801.
36. Shafer RW, Small PM, Larkin C, et al. Temporal trends and transmission patterns during the emergence of multi-drug-resistant tuberculosis in New York City: a molecular epidemiologic assessment. J Infect Dis. 1995;152:171-6.
37. R. Prasad, Nautiyal RG, Ahuja RC, et al. Treatment of new pulmonary tuberculosis patients: what do allopathic doctors do in India? Int J Tuberc Lung Dis. 2002; 6: 895-902.

Chapter 5

Mono- and Poly-drug-resistant Tuberculosis: Treatment

Introduction

Drug-resistant tuberculosis (DR-TB) has been reported since the early days of introduction of antitubercular chemotherapy. These include patients with mono-resistant TB and patients with poly-resistant TB other than MDR-TB. Mono-resistance refers to resistance to a single first-line drug, and poly-resistance refers to resistance to two or more first-line drugs but not to both isoniazid and rifampicin. Cases with mono- or poly-resistance will be identified during the course of case-finding for MDR-TB. The current chapter deals with the treatment of patients with mono- and poly-drug-resistant tuberculosis other than MDR-TB.

Impact of Mono- and Poly-drug Resistance on the Outcome of Chemotherapy

In early treatment era, it was recognized that the resistance with isoniazid (H) and streptomycin (S) was associated with increased risk of treatment failure,[1] but in the current situation, the loss of single drug to resistance is potentially less significant because of the availability and use of potent agents such as Rifampicin, Pyrazinamide, and Ethambutol (E). The most reliable data on treatment outcome were derived from British Medical Research Council (BMRC) short course chemotherapy trials performed in East Africa, Hong Kong, Singapore.[2] Failure rate of Isoniazid (H), Rifampicin (R), Pyrazinamide (Z) and Streptomycin (S) containing regimen among such cases was less than 5% in contrast to approximately 20% failure rate among cases assigned to less potent regimens. Thus, it is possible to obtain good result with use of six months short course chemotherapy with isoniazid, rifampin, pyrazinamide and streptomycin or ethambutol when initial susceptibility test indicates resistance to isoniazid and/or streptomycin. It was also confirmed in Indian study that strains resistant to isoniazid, streptomycin, or both neither pose a major problem nor affect the result of treatment in a big way, provided proper regimens are used. On the contrary, patients infected with organisms resistant to rifampicin, isoniazid and both have a high rate of treatment failure[3-5] and this forms a major threat to tuberculosis control programs particularly for countries like India with poor resources.[6] Resistance to Rifampicin is a relatively rare event and leads to selection of mutants that are already resistant to other components of short-course treatment. It is, therefore, regarded as excellent surrogate marker of Multi-drug-resistant TB.

General Principles for Designing Treatment Regimen for Mono- and Poly-drug-resistant TB

Treatment of patients infected with mono- or poly-drug-resistant strains using standardized short-course chemotherapy has been associated with increased risk of treatment failure and further acquired resistance, including the development of MDR-TB.[7,8] While the likelihood of poor outcomes is relatively low with many types of mono- and poly-resistance and majority of patients with mono- or poly-resistant strains will be cured with short course chemotherapy. The design of regimens for mono- and poly-resistant cases of TB requires experience. Individually designing treatment for mono- and poly-resistance are often determined based on previous treatment history, DST patterns and the possibility of strains of *M. tuberculosis* having acquired new resistance. Modification of regimens for mono- and poly-drug resistance requires careful clinical evaluation and is prone to error if the DST result is not reliable or the possibility of changing drug resistance patterns due to further drug exposure is not taken into consideration. This is particularly important for flouroquinolones, as they play a crucial role in the treatment of MDR-TB, and bacilli may become resistant after a short period of exposure. The prevalence of flouroquinolone (FQ) resistance among isolates without resistance to first-line antituberculosis drugs as well as among isolates with resistance to any first-line drug, but not MDR-TB, is also increasing.[9] The frequently asked clinical question in the management of mono- and poly-drug resistance is whether to modify regimens by adding second-line drugs, including the fluoroquinolones. These drugs may have the potential to shorten the duration of TB treatment. Protection of these second-line drugs requires restrictions in the indiscriminate use of these drugs in the management of mono- and poly-drug-resistant tuberculosis. Unfortunately, there are till date no clear international recommendations on protecting the fluoroquinolones.

Definitive randomized or control studies have not been performed to determine the best treatment for various patterns of drug resistance except for streptomycin resistance. WHO has suggested regimen (Table 5.1) for mono- and poly-drug resistance when Drug Susceptibility Testing (DST) results are highly reliable and further acquired resistance while awaiting DST results is not a factor.[10]

These recommendations are based on evidences from the prerifampicin era, observational studies, general principles of microbiology and therapeutics in TB, extrapolations from established evidence and expert opinion. The objectives in the management of mono-drug and poly-drug resistance are to successfully cure these patients and to avoid amplifying resistance, especially Rifampicin resistance. When a decision has been made to modify standard short-course

TABLE 5.1: Suggested regimen for mono- and poly-drug-resistance

Pattern of drug resistance	*Suggested Regimen*	*Minimum Duration of Treatment (months)*	*Comments*
H (± S)	R, Z and E	6–9	A fluoroquinolone may strengthen the regimen for patients with extensive disease.
H and Z	R, E and fluoroquinolones	9–12	A longer duration of treatment should be used for patients with extensive disease.
H and E	R, Z and fluoroquinolones	9–12	A longer duration of treatment should be used for patients with extensive disease.
R	H, E, fluoroquinolones, plus at least 2 months of Z	12–18	An injectable agent may strengthen the regimen for patients with extensive disease.
R and E (± S)	H, Z, fluoroquinolones, plus an injectable agent for at least the first 2 to 3 months	18	A longer course (6 months) of the injectable agent may strengthen the regimen for patients with extensive disease.
R and Z (± S)	H, E, fluoroquinolones, plus an injectable agent for at least the first 2 to 3 months	18	A longer course (6 months) of the injectable agent may strengthen the regimen for patients with extensive disease.
H, E, Z (± S)	R, fluoroquinolones, plus an oral second-line agent, plus an injectable agent for the first 2 to 3 months	18	A longer course (6 months) of the injectable agent may strengthen the regimen for patients with extensive disease.

H = isoniazid; R = rifampicin; E = ethambutol; Z = pyrazinamide; S = streptomycin

chemotherapy, the most effective regimen should be chosen from the start to maximize the likelihood of cure. Effective drugs should not be withheld for later use. The regimen should be based on previous treatment history, DST pattern and the possibility of strain of *M. tuberculosis*, having acquired new resistance while awaiting DST result. When using such type of regimens, it is essential to consider whether resistance has been acquired to any of the drugs that will be used in the recommended regimen.

In our Indian set-up, most of the time either DST results are not available or, if available, they are usually not reliable. The author has treated such mono- and poly-drug-resistant cases with either five drug regimens (2–3 RHEZ and/or S followed by 6–7 RHE and/or Z or 2–3 SRHEZ followed by 6–7 RHE and/or Z) and has observed good outcome (personal experience).

Development of Further Resistance

Further resistance should be suspected if the patient was on the functional equivalent of only one drug for one month or more, but even periods of less than one month on inadequate therapy can lead to resistance. Sometimes resistance develops if the patient was on the functional equivalent of two drugs, depending on the drugs concerned. For example, pyrazinamide is not considered a good companion drug to prevent resistance. If a patient was receiving functionally only rifampicin and pyrazinamide in the initial phase because of resistance to isoniazid and ethambutol, resistance to rifampicin may develop.

References

1. Stewart SM, Crofton JW. The clinical significance of low degrees of drug resistance in pulmonary tuberculosis. Am Rev Respir Dis. 1964;89:811-29.
2. Mitchison DA, Nunn AJ. Influence of initial drug-resistance on the response to short-course chemotherapy of pulmonary tuberculosis. Am Rev Respir Dis. 1986;133:423-30.
3. Chandrasekaran S, Jagota P, Chaudhuri K. Initial drug resistance to antituberculosis drugs in urban and rural district tuberculosis programme. Ind J Tub. 1992; 39:171-5.
4. Paramasivan CN, Chandrasekaran V, Santha T, Sudarsanam NM, Prabhakar R. Bacteriological investigations for short-course chemotherapy under the tuberculosis programme in two districts in India. Tuber Lung Dis. 1993;74:23-7.
5. Jain NK, Chopra KK, Prasad G. Initial and acquired isoniazid and rifampicin resistance to M. tuberculosis and its implications for treatment. Ind J Tub. 1992;39:121-4.
6. Mathew R, Santha T, Parthasarathy R, Rajaram K, Paramasivan CN, Janardhanam B, et al. Response of patients with initially drug-resistant organisms to treatment with short-course chemotherapy. Indian J Tuberc. 1993;40:119-23.
7. Quy HT, et al. Drug resistance among failure and relapse cases of tuberculosis: is the standard re-treatment regimen adequate? Int J Tuberc Lung Dis. 2003;7(7):631-6.
8. Tuberculosis Research Centre, Chennai, India. Low rate of emergence of drug resistance in sputum-positive patients treated with short-course chemotherapy. International Journal of Tuberculosis and Lung Disease. 2001;5(1):40-5.
9. Jeon CY, Hwang SH, Min JH, et al. Extensively drug-resistant tuberculosis in South Korea: risk factors and treatment outcomes among patients at a tertiary referral hospital. Clin Infect Dis. 2008;46:42-9.
10. Drug-resistant tuberculosis: a survival guide for clinicians. San Francisco, Francis J. Curry National Tuberculosis Center and California Department of Health Services, 2004.

Chapter 6

Multi-drug-resistant Tuberculosis: Current Status

Introduction

Drug-resistant tuberculosis has been reported since the early days of introduction of antitubercular chemotherapy, but multi-drug-resistant tuberculosis (MDR-TB) has been an area of growing concern, and is posing threat to global efforts of tuberculosis control. The exact magnitude of the problem of MDR-TB worldwide was not known till the 1994 to 1997 global project on antituberculosis drug resistance surveillance initiated by WHO and IUAT-LD. Prevalence of MDR-TB mirrors the functional state and efficacy of tuberculosis control programs and realistic attitude of the community towards implementation of such programs.[1] With potent antitubercular drugs and effective treatment strategies like DOTS presently available worldwide, we hope to prevent the further development of MDR-TB. More than 400,000 cases of MDR-TB emerge every year as a result of poor management of drug-sensitive as well as drug-resistant TB. This chapter aims to review the present scenario of Multi-drug-resistant tuberculosis.

Definition

Drug-resistant tuberculosis is defined as a case of tuberculosis excreting bacilli resistant to one or more antitubercular drugs. Multi-drug-resistant tuberculosis (MDR-TB) is defined as disease due to *M. tuberculosis* that is resistant to isoniazid and rifampicin with or without resistance to other drugs (the culture and drug susceptibility test result being from an RNTCP-accredited laboratory). Mono-resistance is defined as resistance to one antituberculosis drug whereas poly-resistance is defined as resistance to more than one antituberculosis drug, other than both isoniazid and rifampicin.

Types of Drug Resistance

Drug resistance may be of two types—primary and acquired. Primary drug resistance may be defined as drug resistance in a patient who has not received any antitubercular treatment in the past. The resistance that develops in a patient who has received prior chemotherapy is defined as acquired drug resistance. Recently, the terms "resistance in new cases" and "resistance in previously treated cases" have been proposed for use because of the difficulty to confirm the validity of the patient's past history of treatment. When one is not sure whether the resistance is primary or acquired due to concealed history of previous treatment or unawareness of treatment taken before, it is known as initial drug resistance. Thus, initial resistance is primary resistance plus some undisclosed acquired resistance. Combined resistance is defined as the sum of primary and acquired resistance.

Prevalence of MDR-TB: Global Scenario

A review by WHO of a series of 63 surveys of drug-resistant TB carried out between 1985 and 1994 led to the conclusion that the problem of drug resistance was global.[2] The overall percentages of resistance to different antituberculosis drugs obtained from different surveys done throughout the world are shown in Tables 6.1 and 6.2. The rate of MDR-TB was very low in most of the surveys ranging from 0 to 10.8% in the case of primary resistance and from 0 to 48% for acquired resistance. Multi-drug resistance was reported to range from 0.5 to 14.3% in surveys where there was no distinction between primary and acquired resistance. In most regions of the world, the rates of MDR-TB were very low,[2] except in New York and Nepal, where high rates of acquired type MDR-TB were reported. It is evident that prevalence of drug-resistant tuberculosis varied considerably throughout the world. The reasons for this variation in different surveys were the degree of selection of patient studied, the degree of misuse of drugs, the quality of enquiry regarding previous treatment and the inadequate culture and drug susceptibility facilities in many parts of the world.

Considering the limitation of the previous studies, a WHO/IUATLD global project of drug resistance surveillance spread over 35 countries in five continents was carried out between 1994 and 1997.[3] Median prevalence of primary and acquired multi-drug resistance was reported to be 1.4% (0–14.4%) and 13% (0–54.4%) respectively (Tables 6.1 and 6.2). Particularly high prevalence of multi-drug resistance was found in the former Soviet Union, Asia, Argentina and the Dominican Republic. The WHO for the first time introduced the term 'MDR hotspot', where high prevalence of MDR has been observed. The 'hotspots' referred to the countries or regions where the combined prevalence of MDR-TB exceeded 5%. The report concluded that resistance to anti-TB drugs was found in all 35 countries and regions surveyed, suggesting again that the problem was global.

A second WHO/IUATLD global project on drug resistance surveillance in 58 countries/geographical sites was carried out in 1996 to 1999.[4] Trends of drug resistance were also observed from 28 sites. Median prevalence of primary and acquired multi-drug resistance was reported in 1% (0–14%) and 9% (0–48%) respectively. Of the 58 sites surveyed, drug resistance among new and previously treated cases were reported in 54 and 48 sites respectively. Most of the previous 'hotspots' of MDR-TB were confirmed again; however, new areas in Russia and China were added. This global survey tested a total of 61,415 patients with

TABLE 6.1: Global primary/initial drug resistance

Study	*Any Drug*	*Any H %*	*Any S %*	*Any R %*	*Any E %*	*H+R %*
Cohn, et al. review of 63 surveys (1985–1994)[2]	–	0–16.9	0.1–23.5	0–3.0	0–4.2	0–10.8
WHO-IUATLD 1994–1997 surveillance[3]	9.9 (2.0–40.6)	7.3 (1.5–31.7)	6.5 (0.3–8.0)	1.8 (0–16.8)	1.0 (0–9.9)	1.4 (0–14.4)
WHO-IUATLD 1996–1999 surveillance[6]	10.7 (1.7–36.9)	6.2 (0–28.1)	5.2 (0.3–32.4)	1.2 (0–15.8)	0.6 (0–11.1)	1.0 (0–14.1)
WHO-IUATLD 1999–2002 surveillance[12]	10.2 (0–57.1)	5.7 (0–42.6)	6.3 (0.5–1.5)	1.4 (0–15.6)	0.8 (0–24.8)	1.1 (0–4.2)
WHO-IUATLD 2002–2007 surveillance[14]	17 (0–56.3)	10.3 (0–42.4)	10.9 (0–51.5)	3.7 (0–22.7)	2.5 (0–24.8)	2.9 (0–22.3)
M/XDR-TB Global report on surveillance and response 2010[14]						1.5 (0–28.3)
Global TB report 2012[15]						3.7 (0–32.3)

TABLE 6.2: Global acquired drug resistance

Study	*Any Drug*	*Any H %*	*Any S %*	*Any R %*	*Any E %*	*H+R %*
Cohn, et al. review of 63 surveys (1985–1994)[2]	-	4–53.7	0–19.4	0–14.5	0–13.7	0–48.0
WHO-IUATLD 1994–1997 surveillance[3]	36.0 (5.3–100.0)	-	-	-	-	13.0 (0–54.4)
WHO-IUATLD 1996–1999 surveillance[6]	23.3 (0.0–93.8)	19.6 (0.0–0.0)	12.4 (0.0–53.4)	12.0 (0.0–50.0)	5.9 (0.0–32.1)	9.3 (0.0–48.2)
WHO-IUATLD 1999–2002 surveillance[12]	18.4 (0–82.1)	14.4 (0–71.0)	11.4 (0–77.1)	8.7 (0–61.4)	3.5 (0–54.2)	7.0 (0–58.3)
WHO-IUATLD 2002–2007 surveillance[14]	35 (0–85.9)	27.7 (0–81.2)	20.1 (0–83.5)	17.5 (0–62.5)	10.3 (0–54.3)	15.3 (0–62.5)
M/XDR-TB Global report on surveillance and response 2010[14]						7.9 (0–61.6)
Global TB report 2012–2015						20 (0–65)

tuberculosis (Median per site 661; range 41-12,675). These sites accounted for 610,000 (18%) of 3.3 million cases of tuberculosis reported to WHO in 1997 and 1.5 billion (26%) of the world's 5.8 billion inhabitants. Several countries including 11 of the 22 world tuberculosis high-burdened countries had not yet been surveyed. A mathematical model had estimated the magnitude of MDR-TB worldwide and suggested that in the year 2000, 3% (273,000; 95% CI, 185,000–414,000) of all new and previously treated TB cases were MDR-TB.[5] The trend analysis confirmed that MDR-TB was not a major problem in countries implementing TB control according to international guidelines for several years. Botswana, Chile, Cuba, and Czech Republic and Uruguay have all showed very low prevalence of MDR-TB confirming that efficient TB control prevents the outset and spread of MDR-TB.[4,6-11]

A third WHO/IUATLD global project on drug resistance surveillance in 77 countries/geographical sites was carried out in 1999 to 2002[12] representing 20% of the global total of new smear-positive TB cases. It included 39 settings not previously included in Global Project and reported trends for 46 settings. Median prevalence of primary and acquired multi-drug resistance was reported in 1.1% (0–14.2%) and 7% (0–58.3%) respectively (Tables 6.1 and 6.2). This report analyzed the distribution of MDR Prevalence (among new cases) from 74 settings. After analysis the cut off value for hot spots was reset to MDR prevalence of more than 6.5% among new cases. There were 10 countries regarded as hot spots with MDR-TB prevalence viz. Ecuador (6.6%), Henan (7.8%), Latvia (9.3%), Lithuania (9.4%), Liaoning (10.4%), Estonia (12.2%), Uzbekistan (13.2%), Tomsk Oblast (13.7%), Israel (14.2%) and Kazakhastan (14.2%). Despite the expansion in coverage of drug-resistance surveillance for both new and previously treated cases in recent years, data on drug resistance are still not available for more than 100 countries. To estimate the levels of drug resistance in places where direct data are not available, Matteo Zignol et al,[13] had developed statistical models for settings where data were available and applied them to places where they are not. After their analysis, they have revealed the total number of MDR-TB cases estimated to have occurred worldwide in 2004 is 424,203 (95% CI, 376,019–620, 061), or 4.3% (95% CI, 3.8%–6.1%) of all new and previously treated TB cases. Three countries—China, India and the Russian Federation—accounted for 261,362 (95% CI, 180,779–414,749) MDR-TB cases, or 62% of the estimated global burden. In the same year, the total number of MDR-TB cases was 2.7% (95% CI, 2.4% –3.8%) of 8,987,743 new cases (242,794, 95% CI, 209,363–350,291) and 18.4% (95% CI, 14.2%–31.7%) of previously treated cases (181,408, 95% CI, 135,276–319,017). This study provides a new comprehensive set of estimates of the incidence of MDR-TB in 184 countries and globally. They have found lower rates of MDR-TB in countries of Central Europe such as Hungary, Macedonia and Turkey in comparison to previous studies. Their study showed a positive correlation between proportion of patients, who had previously received treatment and proportion of MDR-TB cases among the new cases.

A fourth WHO/IUATLD global project on drug resistance surveillance included drug susceptibility test results (DST) from 91,577 patients from 93 settings in 81 countries and two special administrative regions (SARs) of China collected between 2002 and 2007, and representing 35% of the global total of notified new smear-positive TB cases.[14] It included data from 33 countries that have never been previously reported. New data were included from the high-TB burden countries like India, China, Russian Federation, Indonesia, Ethiopia, Philippines, Vietnam, Thailand and Myanmar. Between 1994 and 2007, a total of 138 settings in 114 countries and 2 SARs of China had reported data to the global project. The median prevalence of primary and acquired MDR-TB globally was 2.9% (95% CI, 2.2–3.6%) and 15.3% (95% CI, 9.6–21.1%) respectively. The global population weighted proportion of multi-drug resistance among all TB cases was 5.3% (95% CI, 3.9–6.6%). It is estimated that 489,139 MDR-TB cases emerged in 2006 globally and the global proportion of multi-drug resistance among all new and previously treated cases is 4.8%. According to the new data, China and India carry approximately 50% of the global burden and Russia a further 7% in 2008. Multi-drug and extensively drug-resistant TB (M/XDR-TB) 2010 Global Report on Surveillance and Response, estimated that 440,000 (95% CI, 390,000–510,000) cases of MDR-TB emerged globally in 2008. Among all the incident TB cases globally, 3.6% (95% CI, 3.0%–4.4%) are estimated to have MDR-TB. These estimates, which lie in the same range as the previous ones, are based on more data and a revised methodology. Almost 50% of MDR-TB cases worldwide are estimated to occur in China and India. In 2008, MDR-TB caused an estimated 150,000 deaths.[14]

The Global Tuberculosis Report, 2012 summarizes the latest status of progress in global surveillance of anti-TB drug resistance, using the most recent data on multi-drug resistance TB (MDR-TB), extensively drug-resistant TB (XDR-TB). Data on drug resistance has been systematically collected and analyzed from 135 countries worldwide (70% of WHO's 194 Member States). This includes 63 countries that have continuous surveillance systems based on routine diagnostic drug susceptibility testing (DST) of all TB patients and 72 countries that rely on special surveys of representative samples of patients. During the past 4 years, most of the 27 high MDR-TB and 22 high TB-burden countries have expanded coverage of surveillance of drug resistance to obtain more accurate estimates of the burden of MDR-TB. Globally, 3.7% (95% CI, 2.1–5.2%) of new cases and 20% (95% CI, 13–26%) of previously treated cases estimated to have MDR-TB. Proportions of MDR-TB in new TB cases ranged from 0% to 32.3% and were highest in Belarus (32.3%), Estonia (22.9%), Kazakhstan (30.3%), Kyrgyzstan (26.4%), the Republic of Moldova (19.4%) and Uzbekistan (23.2%). The proportion of MDR-TB in previously treated TB cases at country level ranged from 0% to 65.1%. Countries or subnational areas with the highest reported proportions were Azerbaijan (Baku City, 55.8% in 2007), Belarus (75.6% in 2011), Estonia (57.7% in 2011), Kazakhstan (51.3% in 2011), Kyrgyzstan (51.6% in 2011), the Republic of Moldova (63.5% in 2011), Tajikistan (53.6% in 2011) and Uzbekistan (62.0% in 2011). There is an estimated number of 310,000 cases of MDR-TB among the notified cases of TB across the globe in 2011. India, China and Russian Federation contribute to almost 60% of the estimated global burden of MDR-TB.[15]

Trends in MDR-TB: Global Scenario

The Global Project has collected data from 114 countries and two SARs of China and trend analysis includes data from all global reports between 1994 and 2007, as well as data provided between the publication of Reports. Analysis were limited to countries reporting three data points or more. Proportions of MDR-TB, isoniazid resistance, and any resistance were examined. Declining trends in MDR-TB were noted in USA, Hong Kong, SAR, China among all TB cases. Hong Kong, SAR, China also showed significant decreases in any resistance among all cases and isoniazid resistance and MDR-TB among new cases. Both countries reported declining TB notifications. Denmark showed significant declines in any drug resistance in both new and combined TB cases. Puerto Rico showed declining trends in any resistance and MDR-TB among combined cases. Singapore showed a significant decrease in prevalence of MDR-TB among all TB cases; however, numbers were very small. Countries of the Baltic region (Estonia, Latvia and Lithuania) showed relatively stable trends in MDR-TB among new cases, with a slow but significant increase in MDR-TB among new cases in Lithuania. The proportion of resistance remained high in these countries, ranging from 9.8% (95% CI, 8.2–11.7) in Lithuania to 13.2% (95% CI, 9.7–17.5) in Estonia. These trends in MDR-TB were coupled with declining TB notification rates in all three countries. Estonia has shown the most rapid decline at about 8% per year. Increasing trends in resistance were reported to the global project from Orel and Tomsk Oblasts of the Russian Federation. These countries showed a statistically significant increase in the proportion of MDR-TB among new TB cases as well as increases in absolute number of cases. Both regions showed increase in isoniazid resistance though neither were statistically significant. Both regions showed a slowly declining TB notification rate. During this same time period, TB notification rates for the whole of the Russian Federation have remained stable. The Republic of Korea and Peru have shown increasing trends in MDR-TB, any resistance and isoniazid resistance among new cases. In Peru and the Republic of Korea, increase in isoniazid and any resistance were found to be statistically significant. The increase in MDR-TB was statistically significant in the Republic of Korea. The Republic of Korea has shown a steadily declining TB notification rate from 1994 until 2003. From 2004, the TB notification rate has increased slowly; however, this is likely due to expansion of the national surveillance system into the private sector.

The Russian Federation, which was able to provide high-quality continuous surveillance data from 12 of its oblasts and republics, reported proportions of 23.8 to 28.3% MDR-TB among new TB cases in three of its oblasts in the north-west part of the country. Other Russian oblasts were found to have proportions of MDR-TB as low as 5.4% among new TB cases. Tajikistan, in its first ever survey, found proportions of 16.5% MDR-TB among new TB cases and 61.6% MDR-TB among previously treated TB patients in Dushanbe city and Rudaki district, the highest proportion ever reported among previously treated TB patients. To date, 12 countries have reported nationwide or subnational proportions of MDR-TB of 6% or more among new TB cases. Five of these countries also report MDR-TB proportions of 50% or more among previously treated cases. All these settings are located in the eastern part of Europe or in Central Asia. [14]

Prevalence of MDR-TB: India

Though the development of drug resistance in India was noted since the beginning of the chemotherapeutic era, it was based on clinical perception and several isolated reports, which failed to give an idea of the national situation as a whole. The first definite step was taken in this direction in 1965 to 1967, when the ICMR conducted two surveys to estimate the prevalence of drug resistance.[16,17] Since then, several studies have been conducted by various authors in different parts of the country. The total prevalence of primary/initial drug resistance (Table 6.3) was observed to be about 20.49% (5.3% to 34.9%)[6,12-14,16-30] and Multi-drug resistance

TABLE 6.3: Primary/initial drug resistance (India)

Study		*Total Prevalence*	*H %*	*S %*	*R %*	*H+R %*
ICMR (1968)[16]		20.4	14.7	12.5	-	-
ICMR (1969)[17]		22	15.5	13.8	-	-
Krishnan Swamy KV, et al. 1976[19]		-	10.6	9.5	-	-
Trivedi, et al. (1988)[18]		20	13.9	7.4	0	0
Chandrasekharan, et al. (1990)[20]		21.2	17.4	5.7	3	1.3
Chandrasekharan, et al. (1992)[21]	Rural	34.9	32.8	5.1	4.4	3.4
	Urban	20.5	17.3	4.1	2.9	1.4
Parmasivan, et al. (1993)[22]	North Arcot (1985–89)	25.0	13.0	4.0	2.0	1.6
	Pondicherry (1985–91)	13.9	6.0	4.0	0.9	0.7
Gupta, et al. (1993)[23]		19.5	10.1	7.6	3	0.7
Jain, et al. (1993)[24]		-	18.5	-	0.6	0.4
Jena, et al. (1996)[25]		7.9	2.9	4.9	1	0.4
Parmasivan, et al. (2000)[26] (Tamil Nadu)		18.8	15.4	6.8	4.4	3.4
R. Prasad, et al. (2001)[27]		27.4	15.6	11.7	3.9	5.0
WHO-IUAT (1996-1999)[6]		18.8	15.4	6.8	4.4	3.4
Paramasivan, et al. (2002)[28]	North Arcot (South) 1999	27.7	23.4	12.4	2.8	2.8
	Raichur (South) 1999–2000	21.9	18.7	7.2	2.5	2.5
WHO-IUATLD (1999-2002)[12]	Wardha	19.8	15.2	7.6	0.5	0.5
Sofia, et al. (2004)[29] Bengaluru city		27.7	13.7	22.5	2.6	2.2
Mahadeo, et al. (2005)[30]	Mayurbhanj (2000–2002)	5.3	2.5	3.9	0.7	0.7
	Hoogli (2000–2001)	16.7	10.3	13.7	3.0	3.0
Zignol M, et al. (2006)[13]	-	-	-	-	-	2.4
WHO/IUATLD (2002–2007)[14]		-	11.7	9.9	2.2	2.8
M/XDR-TB Global report on surveillance and response 2010[14]						2.3
WHO-TB report 2012[15]						2.1

among new cases varied between 0 and 5%.[20-30] A study conducted by Tuberculosis Research Centre, Chennai in collaboration with the National Tuberculosis Institute, Bengaluru using WHO/IUATLD guidelines between 1999-2002 including 6 districts in India showed that incidence of primary MDR-TB ranged from 0.7 to 2.8%.[28-30] The overall impression as seen in Table 6.3 is that the primary and initial drug resistance has remained more or less constant over the years, including initial multi-drug resistance. According to the third Global Report of WHO, total prevalence of drug resistance among new cases in India (Wardha) is 19.8% and MDR is 0.5 %.[12]

The prevalence of acquired drug resistance (Table 6.4) ranged from 25 to 100%[3,6,12-14,17,18,24,28,31-35] in several studies. The acquired multi-drug resistance rates

TABLE 6.4: Acquired drug resistance (India)

Study	*Total Prevalence %*	*H %*	*S %*	*R %*	*H+R %*
ICMR (1969)[16]	32 (22-74)	15-69	12-63	-	-
Trivedi, et al. (1988)[18]					
1980	50.1	34.5	26	2.8	95% of R-resistant were resistant to H or S or both
1986	65.3	55.8	-	37.3	-
Dutta M, et al. (1993)[31]	-	67.0	26.0	12.0	6.0
Jain, et al. (1992)[24] Delhi	50.7	50.7	-	33.3	33.3
Outside Delhi	78.8	78.8	-	61.5	61.5
Chowgule, et al. (1998)[32]	25.6	15	53.6	66.8	10.7
WHO-IUATLD Surveillance (1994–1997)[3]	32.4	28.8	18.1	14	13.3
WHO-IUATLD Surveillance (1999–2002)[6]	50.0	50.0	12.5	25.0	25.0
Shah AR, et al. (2002)[33]	58.67	57.18	35.58	37.47	35.1
Deivanayagam (2002)[34]	71.0	66.3	35.6	55.5	54. 8
Paramasivan, et al. (2002)[28] North Arcot (South) Raichur (South)	81.0	81.0	56.2	69.0	69.0
	100.0	100.0	36.4	100.0	100.0
R Prasad, et al. (2003)[35]	79.2	48.6	36.6	34.4	29.5
Zignol M, et al. (2006)[13]	-	-	-	-	14.7
WHO-IUATLD (2002–2007) surveillance[14]	-	36.8	26.2	18.1	17.2
M/XDR-TB Global report on surveillance and response 2010[14]					17.2
WHO-TB report 2012[15]					15.0

also varied from 6 to 100%[24,28,32-35] in the same time period. In a study conducted in Gujarat, it was found that 95% of the R-resistant strains were also resistant to H or S or both. The WHO-IUATLD surveillance[3] in India noted the combined prevalence of drug resistance to be 13.3% (95% CI, 10.9–14.9%) in 1998; however, this was done on a small sample of 2240 people around Delhi city and, therefore, was not representative of the country.[3] The WHO-IUATLD global drug resistance surveillance carried out between 1996 and 1999 reported that the median prevalence of primary and acquired MDR-TB to be 3.4% (95% CI, 1.8–5.7%) and 25% (95% CI, 7.3–52.3%) respectively.[4] Study conducted in two districts of South India showed that acquired drug resistance ranged from 69 to100%.[22] Zignol, et al estimated the incidence of primary and acquired MDR-TB cases to be 44,653 cases (95% CI,13, 547–85,068) among 1,824,395 new cases or 2.4% (95% CI,1–5%) and 42,760 cases (95% CI, 6068-171,774) among 290,019 previously treated cases or 14.7% (95% CI, 2.1–56.9%) respectively. The estimated incidence of MDR-TB among new and previously treated cases was 87,413 (4.1%) of all the TB cases in India.[13] The fourth global surveillance of WHO-IUATLD, carried out in 2002–2007 also reported new data from Gujarat giving the first reliable source of data with regard to MDR-TB among previously treated cases in India. Data from nine sites in India show that drug resistance among new cases is relatively low; however, new data from Gujarat indicate that 17.2% MDR among retreatment cases is higher than previously anticipated and it is estimated that 110,132 (95% CI, 79,975–142,386) MDR-TB cases emerged in India in 2006, representing over 20% of the global burden. The estimated prevalence of primary and acquired MDR- TB in India is 2.8% (95% CI, 2.3–3.4%) and 17.2% (95% CI, 15.0–19.7%) respectively. The estimated prevalence among all TB cases is 4.9% (95% CI, 3.9-6.2%).[14] In India, estimates based on subnational drug resistance data showed that percentage of MDR among new TB cases is 2.3 (1.8–2.8), and in previously treated patients is 17.2 (14.9–19.5). Estimated number of MDR-TB patients in India is 99,000 (95% CI, 79,000–120,000).[14] In India, estimates based on subnational drug resistance data showed that percentage of MDR among new TB cases is 2.3 (1.8–2.8), and in previously treated patients is 17.2 (14.9–19.5). Estimated number of MDR-TB patients in India is 99,000 (95% CI, 79,000–120,000).[14] The estimated prevalence of MDR-TB among notified pulmonary TB patients in India is 5.3% (95% CI, 3.6–6.2%). The estimated prevalence among notified new pulmonary TB patients in 2.1% (95% CI, 1.5–2.7%) and in retreatment pulmonary TB patients is 15% (95% CI, 13–17%). India accounted for an estimated 64,000 cases of MDR-TB among the notified TB cases in 2011.[15] These studies were conducted in different states, mostly in institutions and tertiary care centers and they do not reflect the overall status of drug resistance problem in India. It is, therefore, necessary to conduct a countrywide multi-center drug resistance surveillance comprising both rural and urban areas in order to have a picture of the total situation in the country.

HIV Infection and Multi-drug-Resistant Tuberculosis

There is a well-documented association between TB and human immunodeficiency virus (HIV). Outbreaks of drug-resistant forms of tuberculosis among

HIV-infected patients have been widely documented in nosocomial and other congregate settings[36,37] but little information is available about the association of HIV and drug-resistant TB on a population level.[38,39] The primary reason for the lack of information is that HIV and anti-TB drug susceptibility testing have not been sufficiently accessible for joint surveys under routine conditions. The accelerating and amplifying influence of HIV infection and the delay in recognition and diagnosis of tuberculosis were found to contribute to outbreaks of MDR-TB among HIV-infected patients in USA.[36,40-42] Shafer, et al.[43] studied temporal trends and transmission patterns in New York City using restriction fragment length polymorphism (RFLP) and found clustering of MDR-TB cases, particularly among HIV-infected persons who suffered disproportionately from drug-resistant disease, findings consistent with the above scenario. A subsequent survey of 167 consecutive cases of tuberculosis seen at five New York hospitals during 1992 and 1993 demonstrated that HIV-infected persons were significantly more likely to have been recently infected with MDR-TB; indeed, 79% of the drug-resistant cases were shown by RFLP to be clustered with the clear implication of recent transmission.[43] In the fourth WHO/IUATLD global drug surveillance report,[14] eight settings in seven countries reported data on drug resistance stratified by HIV status: Cuba, Honduras, Latvia, the Russian Federation (Tomsk Oblast), Spain (Barcelona and Galicia), Ukraine (Donetsk Oblast) and Uruguay. Four countries were not able to discriminate between negative and unknown HIV status. The data reported from the majority of countries were not strong enough to examine an association between HIV and drug resistance. However, the data available from Donetsk Oblast, Ukraine and Latvia indicated a significant association between HIV and MDR-TB. Additional information on risk factors including history of hospitalization or imprisonment were not available for this analysis. So, the specific reasons for the association are not known. Both the countries have a high underlying prevalence of MDR-TB, as well as an emerging HIV epidemic, that initially was concentrated among risk groups, but has now become more generalized. However, several studies in India and other South-East Asian countries, having high prevalence of HIV seropositivity, have reported very low prevalence of MDR-TB in HIV-seropositive patients contrary to western literature. Main reasons for an association between HIV/AIDS and multi-drug-resistant tuberculosis may be because of the acquired rifamycin resistance associated with HIV infection among TB patients under treatment and anti-TB drug malabsorption, which has been documented in patient cohorts in settings of high HIV prevalence. In addition, HIV-infected patients and drug-resistant TB patients may have similar risk factors such as history of hospitalization. It is also possible that HIV-infected TB cases may be more susceptible to infection once exposed. HIV-infected TB cases are more likely to be smear-negative, and delayed diagnosis of drug resistance as well as unavailability of treatment have led to high death rates in people living with HIV. Both these factors may suggest a lower rate of transmission. However, HIV-infected cases progress rapidly to disease, and in settings where MDR-TB is prevalent, this may lead to rapid development of a pool of drug-resistant TB patients or an outbreak. Despite some of the weakness in these data and subsequent analysis, the association between HIV and MDR-TB is concerning particularly given the implications for the clinical management of these patients. Rapid progression to death in HIV-infected MDR-TB patients in both outbreaks and treatment cohorts has been widely documented.[36,44] Antiretroviral treatment for HIV does appear to benefit coinfected MDR-TB patients; however, comanagement of treatment for both diseases is very complicated.

Currently, most TB control programs in high-burden countries do neither have the diagnostic infrastructure to either detect an outbreak nor the programmatic capacity to manage an outbreak. Given the impact on mortality, outbreaks should be avoided at all costs. The development of infection control measures in congregate settings as well as diagnostic screening tools to rapidly identify drug-resistant TB are a priority, for all countries, but particularly for those with high prevalence of HIV or MDR-TB. From a global perspective, routine diagnosis of both HIV and drug-resistant TB should be scaled up for patient benefit. Better surveillance data may help in developing an understanding of the relationship between HIV and MDR-TB.

Risk Factors of MDR-TB

Several risk factors have been identified in the causation of multi-drug-resistant tuberculosis, of which the three most important are—previous treatment with antitubercular drugs, which may be inappropriate, incomplete or erratic, high prevalence of drug-resistant tuberculosis in the community and contact with a patient known to have drug-resistant tuberculosis. In patients with previous treatment or disease, the odds of resistant tuberculosis were 4 to 7 times higher than for persons with no history of past treatment. Other factors that may be responsible for increased risk of MDR-TB are—coinfection with HIV, socioeconomically deprived groups in slums, prisons, correctional facilities, daycare centers, intravenous drug abusers and other immunocompromised states as in transplant recipients, anticancer therapy patients, and patients with diabetes mellitus. Radiologically far advanced pulmonary tuberculosis with cavitary lesions were four times as likely to harbor drug-resistant organisms.

Sources and Causes of MDR-TB

Though unfortunate, yet a reality is that multi-drug resistance is a manmade problem. Drug-resistant Tuberculosis results largely from poorly managed care of TB.[45] The sources are many and the causes multifactorial. To blame for this are the government, the pharmaceutical industry, doctors, patients and their families, each of whom contribute in their own way to add up to the problem. The government plays its share by providing poor infrastructure in the National Tuberculosis Control Program, unnecessary administrative control on purchase and distribution of drugs with no proper mechanism on quality control and bioavailability tests. The pharmaceutical industry, in its turn, contributes by manufacturing drugs of uncertain bioavailability in fixed dose or inappropriate drug combinations, poor storage condition of drugs and substitution by inferior quality drugs by pharmacies. The doctor, by his lack of knowledge regarding doses, duration of treatment, side effects and standard regimens, frequent change of brand names and poor patient motivation, contributes the lion's share to the problem. In one of the studies, where prescriptions of 449 doctors were analyzed, 75% of the doctors were found to have made some prescription error. [46] Added to this is the poor teaching and training facilities for them. Noncompliant patients due to monetary lack, lack of information, side effects of drugs and social myths and misconceptions often do not adhere to treatment. Comorbid conditions like diabetes, HIV, psychiatric conditions, the habits of smoking and alcoholism make the patient more vulnerable. To sum up, multi-drug-resistant tuberculosis usually result from inadequate drug therapy in multibacillary cases of tuberculosis, addition of single drug in cases of failure, difficulty in obtaining drugs by the poor due to lack of financial resources or social insurances, frequent shortage of second-line antituberculous drugs by poor management and/or financial constrains, use of drugs or combination of drugs (FDC) with unproven bioavailability, lack of motivation at the beginning of treatment and inadequate self-administration of drugs without direct observation in the intensive phase of therapy.

Control of MDR-TB

The primary aim in the control of multi-drug-resistant tuberculosis is to prevent its development in the first place. This can be done by Directly Observed Treatment Short Course (DOTS), which is the most cost-effective way of treatment and prevention of MDR tuberculosis. At the same time, since MDR-TB cases respond poorly to short-course chemotherapy, careful introduction of second-line drugs to treat MDR-TB to reduce further transmission of such strains will be required.[47] To control the emergence of drug-resistant and multi-drug-resistant tuberculosis, WHO in 1998 had proposed the work plan known as 'DOTS-Plus' for which WHO had established Green Light Committee.[48] The primary aims of committee were to approve, conduct and oversee pilot projects based on guidelines for establishing 'DOTS-Plus' pilot projects. 'Dots-Plus' is a comprehensive management strategy to control tuberculosis and multi-drug-resistant tuberculosis. Following the roll-out and successful implementation of "DOTS-Plus" pilot projects for the management of drug-resistant TB between 2000 and 2005, a new Stop TB Strategy was launched in 2006. The New Stop TB Strategy includes the diagnosis and management of drug-resistant TB.[49] The launch of the Stop TB Strategy was followed by the Global Plan to Stop TB, 2006 to 2015 that provided targets for scaling up and budgets required for the implementation of the strategy Stop TB partnership.[50] To combat the threat of XDR-TB, WHO convened a Global Task Force on XDR-TB in October 2006 and recommended to strengthen basic activities to control TB and HIV/AIDS, to avoid additional emergence of M/XDR-TB as well as acceleration of treatment of MDR and XDR -TB cases with universal access to sound management of M/XDR-TB by 2015 in all countries and near to universal access in the high-burden countries by 2010.[51] The revised plan recommended the treatment of 1.6 million M/XDR-TB cases by 2015 instead of 800,000 MDR-TB cases. It will require integration of M/XDR-TB activities into general TB control activities. It will include the strengthening of laboratory services for adequate and timely diagnosis of M/XDR-TB, surveillance of M/XDR-TB, development and implementation of sound TB infection control policies, Advocacy Communication and Social Mobilization to sustain political commitment and resource mobilization and the promotion of research and development into new diagnostics, drugs, vaccines and operational research on MDR-TB management. It is expected that full implementation of this response plan will save the lives of thousands of people infected by M/XDR-TB and will be able to prevent and control M/XDR-TB.

Conclusion

MDR-TB has been an area of growing concern and posing threat to control of TB. It is estimated that more than 400,000 cases of MDR-TB emerge every year globally as a result of poor management of sensitive as well as drug-resistant TB cases. MDR-TB is a manmade problem and its emergence can be prevented by prompt diagnosis and effective treatment of all TB cases. The DOTS-Plus proposed by WHO highlights the comprehensive management strategy to control MDR-TB. Laboratory services for adequate and timely diagnosis of MDR-TB must be strengthened and programmatic management of MDR-TB must be scaled up as per the target set by global plan. It must be emphasized that optimal treatment of MDR-TB alone will not curb the epidemic. Efforts must be focused on the effective use of first-line drugs in every new patient so as to prevent the ultimate emergence of multi-drug resistance. The proper use of second-line drugs must be ensured to cure existing multi-drug-resistant tuberculosis, to reduce transmission of MDR-TB and to prevent XDR-TB. Sound infection control measures to avoid further transmission of MDR-TB and research towards development of new diagnostics, drugs and vaccines should be promoted to control MDR-TB.

References

1. Multi-drug-resistant tuberculosis. ICMR. 1999;29:105-14.
2. Cohn DL, Bustreo F, Raviglione MC. Drug-resistant tuberculosis. Review of the world-wide situation and the WHO/IUATLD Global Surveillance Project. International Union Against Tuberculosis and Lung Disease. Clin Infect Dis. 1997;24:S121-30.
3. Pablos-Mendez A, Biokin N, Rieder HL, Bustreo F, Cohn DL, Lambregts van Weezenbeek CS, et al. Global surveillance for antituberculosis drug resistance, 1994-97. World Health Organization—International union against tuberculosis and lung disease; Working Group on Anti-Tuberculosis Drug Resistance Surveillance. N Engl J Med. 1998;338:1641-9.
4. Espinal MA, Laszlo A, Simonsen L, et al. Global trends in resistance to anti-tuberculosis drugs. N Engl J Med. 2001;344:1294-303.
5. Dye C, Espinal MA, Watt CJ, Mbiaga C, Williams BG. Worldwide incidence of multi-drug-resistant tuberculosis. J Infect Dis. 2002;185:1197-202.
6. World Health Organization. Antituberculosis drug resistance in the world: prevalence and trends. Report No. 2. WHO/CDS/TB/2000. 278. Geneva: WHO, 2000.

7. Dye C, William BG, Espinal MA, Raviglione MC. Erasing the world's slow strain: Strategies to beat multi-drug-resistant tuberculosis. Science. 2002;295:2042-6.
8. National Tuberculosis Programme. Tuberculosis in Latvia 1991-2000. Riga. 2001;21-3.
9. Robert J, Trystram D, Pernot-Truffot C, Jarlier V. Surveillance de la tuberculose a bacilles multiresistants en France en 1998. Bull Epidemiol Hebdo. 2002;16:71-2.
10. Robert J, Trystram D, Pernot-Truffot C, Carbonelle B. Surveillance of *Mycobacterium tuberculosis* drug resistance in France, 1995-1997. Int J Tuberc Lung Dis. 2000;4:665-72.
11. Centers for Disease Control. Reported tuberculosis in the United States 2000. Atlanta, GA: US Department of Health and Human Services, CDC, August 2001.
12. WHO/IUALTD Global Project on Anti-Tuberculosis Drug Resistance Surveillance (1999-2002), Third Global Report (2003).
13. Zignol M, Hosseini MS, Wright A, Weezenbeek CL, Nunn P, Watt CJ, et al. Global incidence of multi-drug-resistant tuberculosis. J Infect Dis. 2006;194:479-85.
14. WHO/IUALTD Global Project on Anti-Tuberculosis Drug Resistance Surveillance (2002-2007), Fourth Global Report (2008), updated 2010.
15. Global Tuberculosis Report 2012. WHO/HTM/TB/2012.6.
16. ICMR, Prevalence of drug resistance in patients with pulmonary tuberculosis presenting for the first time with symptoms at chest clinics in India—I. Findings in urban clinics among patients giving no history of previous chemotherapy. Indian J Med Res. 1968;56:1617-30.
17. ICMR, Prevalence of drug resistance in patients with pulmonary tuberculosis presenting for the first time with symptoms at chest clinics in India—II. Findings in urban clinics among all patients, with or without history of previous chemotherapy. Indian J Med Res. 1969;57:823-35.
18. Trivedi SS, Desai SC. Primary antituberculosis drug resistance and acquired rifampicin resistance in Gujarat, India Tubercle. 1988;69:37-42.
19. Krishnaswamy KV, Rahim MA. Primary drug resistance in pulmonary tuberculosis. Indian J Chest Dis. 1976;28:233-7.
20. Chandrasekaran S, Chauhan MM, Rajalaksmi R, Chaudhuri K, Mahadev B. Initial drug resistance to anti-tuberculosis drugs in patients attending an urban district tuberculosis centre. Ind J Tub. 1990;37:215-6.
21. Chandrasekaran S, Jagota P, Chaudhuri K. Initial drug resistance to antituberculosis drugs in urban and rural district tuberculosis programme. Ind J Tub. 1992;39:171-5.
22. Paramasivan CN, Chandrasekaran V, Santha T, Sudarsanam NM, Prabhakar R. Bacteriological investigations for short course chemotherapy under the tuberculosis programme in two districts in India Tuber Lung Dis. 1993;74:23-7.
23. Gupta PR, Singhal B, Sharma TN, Gupta RB. Prevalence of initial drug resistance in tuberculosis patients attending a chest hospital. Ind J Med Res. 1993;97:102-3.
24. Jain NK, Chopra KK, Prasad G. Initial and acquired isoniazid and rifampicin resistance to *M. tuberculosis* and its implications for treatment. Ind J Tub. 1992;39:121-4.
25. Jena J, Panda BN, Nema SK, Ohri VC, Pahwa RS. Drug resistance pattern of *Mycobacterium tuberculosis* in a chest disease hospital of armed forces. Lung India. 1995;13:56-9.
26. Parmasivan CN, Bhaskaran K, Venkataraman, Chandrasekhran V, Narayanan PR. Survilence of drug resistance in tuberculosis in the state of Tamil Nadu. Ind J Tub. 2000;47:27-33.
27. Prasad R, Suryakant, Mukerji PK, Gupta AK, Garg R, Rizvi DM, et al. Initial drug resistance in patients of pulmonary tuberculosis attending a tertiary care center. Ind J Tub. 2001;48:159.

28. Paramasivan CN, Venkata Raman P, Chandrashekhran V, Bhatt S, Narayanan PR. Surveillance of drug resistance in tuberculosis in two districts of south India. Int J Tuberc Lung Dis. 2002;6:479-84.
29. Sofia V, Balasangameshwara VH, Jagannatha PS, Kumar P. Initial drug resistance among tuberculosis patients under DOTS programme in Bengaluru city. Ind J Tuberc. 2004;52:17-21.
30. Mahadeo B, Kumar P, Agrawal SP, Chauhan LS, Sriknataramu N. Surveillance of drug resistance to antituberculosis drugs in districts of Hoogli in West Bengal and Mayurbhanj in Orissa.Indian J Tuberc. 2005:52;5-10.
31. Datta M, Radhamani MP, Selvaraj R, Paramasivan CN, Gopalan BN, Sudeendra CR, et al. Critical assessment of smear-positive pulmonary tuberculosis patients after chemotherapy under the district tuberculosis programme. Tub Lung Dis. 1993;74:180-6.
32. Chowgule RV, Deodhar L. Pattern of secondary acquired drug resistance to antituberculosis drug in Mumbai, India—1991–1995. Indian J Chest Dis Allied and Sci. 1998;40:23-31.
33. Shah AR, Agarawal SK, Shah KV. Study of drug resistance in previously treated tuberculosis patients in Gujarat, India. Int J Tuberc Lung Dis. 2002;6:1098-101.
34. Deivanayagam CN, Rajasekaran S, Venkatesan R, et al. Prevalence of acquired MDR-TB and HIV Co-Infection. Indian J Chest Dis Allied Sci. 2002;44:237-42.
35. Prasad R, Suryakant, Mukerji PK, Gupta AK, Garg R, Rizvi DM, et al. Acquired drug resistance in patients of pulmonary tuberculosis attending a tertiary care center. Int J Tuberc Lung Dis. 2003;11(Suppl):S3O3.
36. Edlin BR, Tokars JI, Grieco MH, et al. An outbreak of multidrug-resistant tuberculosis among hospitalized patients with the acquired immunodeficiency syndrome. N Engl J Med. 1992;326:1514-21.
37. Moro ML, et al. An outbreak of multidrug-resistant tuberculosis involving HIV-infected patients of two hospitals in Milan, Italy. AIDS. 1998;12:1095-102.
38. Kenyon TA, et al. Low levels of drug resistance amidst rapidly increasing tuberculosis and human immunodeficiency virus coepidemics in Botswana. Int.J Tuberc.Lung Dis. 1999;3:4-11.
39. Chum HJ, et al. An epidemiological study of tuberculosis and HIV infection in Tanzania, 1991-1993. AIDS. 1996;10:299-309.
40. Frieden TR, Sterling T, Pablos-Mendez A, Kilburn JO, Cauthen GM, Dooley SW. The emergence of drug-resistant tuberculosis in New York City. N Engl J med. 1993;328:521-6.
41. Coronado VG, Beck-Sague CM, Hutton MD, et al. Transmission of multi-drug-resistant mycobacterium tuberculosis among persons with human immunodeficiency virus infection in an urban hospital: epidemiologic and restriction fragment length polymorphism analysis. J Infect Dis. 1993;168:1052-5.
42. Busillo C, Lessnau KD, Sanjana V, et al. Multi-drug-resistant *Mycobacterium tuberculosis* in patients with human immunodeficiency virus infection. Chest. 1992;102:797-801.
43. Shafer RW, Small PM, Larkin C, et al. Temporal trends and transmission patterns during the emergence of multi-drug-resistant tuberculosis in New York City: a molecular epidemiologic assessment. J Infect Dis. 1995;152:171-6.
44. Mac-Arthur A Jr, et al. Characteristics of drug resistance and HIV among tuberculosis patients in Mozambique. Int.J Tuberc. Lung Dis. 2001;5:894-902.
45. Philip C Hopewell, Madhukar Pai, Dermot Maher, Mukund Uplekar, Mario C Raviglione: International standards for tuberculosis care. Lancet Infect Dis. 2006;6:710-25.
46. Prasad R, Nautiyal RG, Ahuja RC, et al. Treatment of new pulmonary tuberculosis patients: What do allopathic doctors do in India? Int J Tuberc Lung Dis. 2002;6;895-902.

47. Espinal MA, Kim SJ, Surarez PG, et al. Standard short-course chemotherapy for drug-resistant tuberculosis: treatment outcome in six countries JAMA. 2000;283:2537-45.
48. DOTS-Plus and Green Light Committee, www.who.int/gtb/policyrd/dotsplus.htm.
49. The Global MDR-TB and XDR-TB Response Plan 2007-2008. World Health Organization Document, 2007 WHO/HTM/TB/2007.387.
50. Stop TB Partnership and World Heath Organization. The global plan to Stop TB 2006–2015, Geneva, Switzerland: World Health Organization, 2006.
51. WHO Global XDR-TB task force meeting, Oct 2006: Available at:http://www.who.int/tb/xdr/taskforcereport_oct06.pdf.

Chapter 7

Multi-drug-resistant Tuberculosis: Case Finding Strategies

Introduction

Timely identification and prompt initiation of treatment of pulmonary tuberculosis cases prevent the patient from spreading the disease to others, acquiring further resistance and progressing to a state of permanent lung damage. It is strongly recommended that programs have representative Drug Resistance Surveillance (DRS) data for new patients and for the different categories of retreatment patients (failure of Category I, failure of retreatment, default and relapse) as well as other high-risk groups. This chapter aims to address strategies for case-finding and diagnosis of patients with either suspected or confirmed drug-resistant tuberculosis (DR-TB).

Targeting Risk Groups for Drug Susceptibility Test (DST)

Routine DST at the start of treatment may be indicated for all TB patients or only in specific groups of patients at increased risk for drug resistance. Specific elements of the history that suggest an increased risk for drug resistance are listed below in tabulated form. Stronger risk factors are placed higher in Table 7.1.

TABLE 7.1: Target groups for DST

Risk factors for drug-resistant TB	*Comments*
Failure of retreatment regimens and chronic TB cases	Chronic TB cases are defined as patients who are still sputum smear-positive at the end of a retreatment regimen. These patients have perhaps the highest Multi-drug-resistant tuberculosis (MDR-TB) rates of any group.[1,2]
Exposure to a known DR-TB case	Most studies have shown close contacts of MDR-TB patients to have very high rates of MDR-TB
Failures of Category I	Failures of Category I are patients who while on treatment are sputum smear-positive at month 5 or later during the course of treatment. Not all patients in whom a regimen fails have MDR-TB, and the percentage may depend on a number of factors, including whether rifampicin was used in the continuation phase and whether DOT was used throughout the treatment

Contd...

Contd...

Risk factors for drug-resistant TB	*Comments*
Failure of Antituberculosis regimens from the private sector	Antituberculosis regimens from the private sector can vary greatly A detailed history of drugs used is essential if both isoniazid and rifampicin were used, the chances of MDR-TB may be high. Sometimes second-line antituberculosis drugs may have been used, and this is an important information for designing the retreatment regimen.
Patients who remain sputum smear-positive at month 2 or 3 of short-course chemotherapy (SCC)	Many may choose to do culture and DST on patients who remain sputum smear-positive at months 2 and 3. This group of patients is at risk for DR-TB, but rates can vary considerably.
Relapse and return after default without recent treatment failure	Evidence suggests that most relapse and return after default cases do not have MDR-TB. However, certain histories may point more strongly to possible MDR-TB; for example, erratic drug use or early relapses.
Exposure in institutions that have MDR-TB outbreaks or a high MDR-TB prevalence	Patients who frequently stay in homeless shelters, prisoners in many countries and healthcare workers in clinics, laboratories and hospitals can have high rates of MDR-TB.
Residence in areas with high MDR-TB prevalence	MDR-TB rates in many areas of the world can be high enough to justify routine DST testing in all new cases.
History of using antituberculosis drugs of poor or unknown quality	The percentage of MDR-TB caused by use of poor-quality drugs is unknown but considered significant. It is known that poor-quality drugs are prevalent in all countries. All drugs should comply with quality-assured WHO standards.
Treatment in programs that operate poorly	These are usually non-DOTS or DOTS programs with poor drug management and distribution systems.
Comorbid conditions associated with malabsorption or rapid-transit diarrhea	Malabsorption may result in selective low-serum drug levels and may occur in either HIV non-infected or infected patients
HIV in some settings	Data from the 2002 to 2006 Global Surveillance projects[3] suggest an association between HIV and MDR-TB in some parts of the world, and numerous MDR-TB outbreaks have been documented in HIV patients. The data are still limited and specific factors involved in this association have not been determined.

The prevalence of resistance in specific risk groups can vary greatly across different settings. The routine use of DST and Category IV treatment for patients with any risk factor listed in tabulated form above is, therefore, not recommended. Programs should instead examine DRS data from risk groups, together with their technical capacity and resources, to determine which groups of patients should get routine DST and/or inclusion into Category IV regimens.

Strategies for Programs with Minimal Access to DST and Limited Resources

Access to DST is required in all programs. Under exceptional circumstances, and while building the laboratory capacity to perform DST, programs may use strategies to enrol patients with a very high risk of MDR-TB in Category IV regimens without individual DST. The three groups that are most likely to be considered for direct enrolment in Category IV regimens are discussed as follows:

- **Category II failures (chronic TB cases):**[4,5] Patients in whom Category II treatment has failed in sound National Tuberculosis Control Programs (NTPs) often have MDR-TB.[1,2] If the quality of DOTS is poor or unknown, patients may fail in Category II treatment for reasons other than MDR-TB.
- **Close contacts of MDR-TB cases who develop active TB disease:** Close contacts of MDR-TB patients who develop active TB disease can be enrolled for treatment with Category IV regimens.
- **Category I failures:** Since the prevalence of MDR-TB in this group of patients may vary greatly,[5-9] the rate in this group must be documented before deciding whether enrolment in DR-TB control programs can take place without DST. Programs should conduct DRS surveys in this group to determine whether the routine use of Category II regimens provides an adequate retreatment regimen for patients in whom Category I treatment failed.

The rate of MDR-TB in these three groups can vary. These guidelines strongly recommend confirming treatment failure by culture and testing for DR-TB through the use of DST to at least isoniazid and rifampicin for all patients who start a Category IV regimen following this strategy. All programs should, therefore, have capacity for DST of at least isoniazid and rifampicin.

DST Specimen Collection

If DST is chosen as part of the case-finding strategy, it is recommended that two sputum specimens be obtained for culture and that DST be performed with the specimen that produces the best culture. DST does not routinely need to be carried out in duplicate. Procedures for collecting and managing specimens for culture and DST are described in laboratory diagnosis, which also addresses different techniques, limitations, quality assurance requirements and other issues of culture and DST. Previously treated patients may have had DST in the past but it may no longer reflect the resistance pattern of the strain they had at the time of enrolment in the DR-TB control program. Programs that base treatment on DST should repeat DST in all patients who have received treatment since the collection of their previous DST specimen.

Case-finding in Pediatric Patients

Pediatric cases require adjustments in diagnostic criteria and indications for treatment. Younger children in particular may not be able to produce sputum specimens on demand. Smear- and culture-negative children with active TB, who are close contacts of patients with MDR-TB, can be started on Category IV regimens.

Case-finding in HIV-infected Patients

Cases of HIV infection also require adjustment in diagnostic criteria and indications for treatment. The diagnosis of TB in HIV-infected people is more difficult and may be confused with other pulmonary or systemic infections. People living with HIV are more likely to have smear-negative TB or extrapulmonary TB. WHO guideline[10] recommend the use of clinical algorithms that include the use of chest X-ray and culture to improve the ability to diagnose TB in smear-negative patients living with HIV. Because unrecognized MDR- and XDR-TB are associated with such high mortality in these patients, many programs perform culture and DST testing for all patients living with HIV and with active TB. Programs without facilities or resources to screen all patients living with HIV for MDR-TB should put significant efforts into obtaining them, especially if MDR-TB rates are moderate or high. Some programs may adopt a strategy of targeted DST for patients with increased risk of MDR-TB or low CD4 count. Rapid diagnostic techniques for people living with HIV with active TB can be very useful to promptly identify those with MDR-TB.

If XDR-TB is prevalent, people living with HIV, who have MDR-TB, should be screened for XDR-TB with the use of liquid media or another validated rapid technique for DST of second-line injectable agents and a fluoroquinolone.

Case Finding of Patients with Mono- and Poly-drug Resistance

Mono- and poly-drug-resistant strains are strains that are resistant to anti-tuberculosis drugs but not to both isoniazid and rifampicin. Most diagnostic strategies used by DR-TB control programs will also identify cases of mono- and poly-drug resistance, in addition to MDR-TB cases. Patients with Mono- or poly-drug resistance may require modifications to their SCC regimens or to be moved to Category IV regimens.

Use of Rapid Drug-resistance Testing

Case-finding strategies can be greatly enhanced with rapid drug resistance testing, which significantly improves the ability to identify cases of MDR-TB earlier that can be isolated and started on treatment. Rifampicin is the most potent antituberculosis drug of the first-line regimen, and rifampicin resistance most commonly occurs with concomitant isoniazid resistance. A positive rapid test for rifampicin resitance is a strong indicator that a patient may have MDR-TB,[11,12] while a negative test makes a final diagnosis of MDR-TB highly unlikely. Administrative infection control measures including isolation should start as soon as a patient is identified as a TB suspect. Rapid testing can identify MDR-TB quickly and allows patients to be taken off general TB wards where they may infect others with resistant strains.

Use of Second-line DST in Case-finding and Diagnosing XDR-TB

Not all DR-TB control programs have the capacity to perform DST of second-line drugs. These guidelines recommend that all programs develop the ability to do DST to isoniazid and rifampicin and, when proficient at those, to develop the ability to test the second-line injectable agents (kanamycin, amikacin and capreomycin) and a fluoroquinolone. This will enable programs to perform case-finding for XDR-TB and to assure proper treatment.The two strongest risk factors for XDR-TB are:

i. Failure of an anti-TB regimen that contains second-line drugs including an injectable agent and a fluoroquinolone.
ii. Close contact with an individual with documented XDR-TB or with an individual for whom treatment with a regimen including second-line drugs is failing or has failed.

All suspects of XDR-TB should have DST of isoniazid and rifampicin, the second-line injectable agents and a fluoroquinolone. For people living with HIV, who are at risk of XDR-TB, given the high and rapid risk of death with co-infection, liquid or other validated rapid techniques for DST of first- and second-line drugs is recommended.

References

1. Treatment of tuberculosis: guidelines for national programmes, 3rd ed. Geneva, World Health Organization, 2003 (WHO/CDS/TB/2003.313).
2. Ait-Khaled N, Enarson DA. Tuberculosis: a manual for medical students. Geneva, World Health Organization, 2003 (WHO/CDS/TB/99.272).
3. Anti-tuberculosis drug resistance in the world. Fourth global report. The WHO/IUATLD global project on anti-tuberculosis drug resistance surveillance, 2002–2007. Geneva, World Health Organization, 2008 (WHO/HTM/TB/2008.394).
4. Heldal E, Arnadottir T, Cruz JR, Tardencilla A, Chacon L. Low failure rate in standardised retreatment of tuberculosis in Nicaragua: patient category, drug resistance and survival of 'chronic' patients. In J Tuber Lung Dis. 2001;5:129-36.
5. Saravia JC, Appleton SC, Rich ML, Sarria M, Bayona J, Becerra MC. Retreatment management strategies when first-line tuberculosis therapy fails. International Journal of Tuberculosis and Lung Disease. 2005;9:421-9.
6. Harries AD, Nyierenda TE, Kemp JR, Squire BS, Godfrey-Faussett P and Salaniponi FML. Management and outcome of tuberculosis patients who fail treatment under routine program conditions in Malawi. International Journal of Tuberculosis and Lung Disease. 2003;7:1040-4.
7. Quy HTW, Lan NTN, Borgdorff MW, Grosset J, Linh PD, et al. Drug resistance among failure and relapse cases of tuberculosis: Is the standard retreatment regimen adequate? Interational Journal of Tuberculosis and Lung Disease. 2003;7:631-6.
8. Trebucq A, Anagonou S, Gninafon M, et al. Prevalence of primary and acquired resistance of *Mycobacterium tuberculosis* to antituberculosis drugs in Benin after 12 years of short-course chemotherapy. Int J Tuber Lung Dis. 1999;3:466-70.
9. Kritski AL, Rodrigues de Jesus LS, Andrade MK, Werneck-Barroso E, Vieira MA, Haffner A, et al. Retreatment tuberculosis cases. Factors associated with drug resistance and adverse outcomes. Chest. 1997;111:1162-7.
10. Improving the diagnosis and treatment of smear-negative pulmonary and extrapulmonary tuberculosis among adults and adolescents: recommendations for HIV-prevalent and resource-constrained settings. Geneva, World Health Organization, 2007 (WHO/HTM/TB/2007.379, WHO/HIV/2007.01).
11. Skenders G, Fry AM, Prokopovica I, Greckoseja S, Broka L, Metchock B, et al. Multi-drug-resistant tuberculosis detection, Latvia. Emerging Infectious Diseases. 2005;11:1461-3.
12. Abdel Aziz M, Laszlo A De Muynck, Portaels F, Van Deun A, Wells C, Nunn P, et al. Epidemiology of antituberculosis drug resistance (the Global Project on Antituberculosis Drug Resistance Surveillance): an updated analysis. Lancet. 2006;368:2142-54.

Chapter 8

Multi-drug-resistant Tuberculosis: Laboratory Issues

Introduction

A definitive diagnosis of drug-resistant tuberculosis (DR-TB) requires that *M. tuberculosis* be isolated on culture, identified and Drug Susceptibility Testing (DST) completed. Major challenges remain around the capacity of laboratories to meet the demand for scaling up. Laboratory constraints relate to infrastructure, equipment, quality assurance and biosafety. Compounded by an urgent need for reliable and reproducible methodologies, especially for second-line DST, rational use of culture and DST is, therefore, imperative. This chapter aims to describe standards for laboratory services needed to diagnose and treat DR-TB.

General Considerations

Procedures for microscopy, culture and DST of first-line antituberculosis drugs have been standardized internationally. On the other hand, surveys on practices for second-line DST in specialized laboratories and a few multi-center laboratory studies have revealed important methodological differences. No studies have systematically evaluated all available DST methods for all available second-line drugs, established critical concentrations for all available second-line drugs, or evaluated a large number of clinical isolates for microbiological and clinical end-points. Most importantly, the correlation of in vitro DST results with clinical outcome has not been established, and the prognostic value of in vitro resistance to second-line antituberculosis drugs is, therefore, not known. Given the urgent need for expansion of laboratory services in support of DR-TB control programs, WHO recently issued new policies on the expanded use of liquid culture and interim policy guidance on second-line DST, outlining the current evidence for reliability and reproducibility of DST methods, consensus agreement on critical drug concentrations to define resistance and providing recommendations for rational use of DST under programmatic conditions.[1–5]

Essential Laboratory Services and Infrastructure

Optimal management of DR-TB requires both mycobacterial and clinical laboratory services. At a minimum, the mycobacteriology laboratory service should provide culture, confirmation of *M. tuberculosis* and DST of isoniazid and rifampicin. Clinical laboratory services should provide basic hematology, biochemistry, serology and urine analysis, required for the adequate evaluation and monitoring of patients. In addition to diagnostic services, laboratories supporting DR-TB control programs have a critical role in surveillance of the prevailing drug resistance patterns and trends. Surveillance of antituberculosis drug resistance is essential for providing information on the magnitude of and trends in drug resistance, for developing appropriate treatment modalities and for evaluating the impact of control program interventions. Adequate allocation of resources both human and financial to laboratory services is essential to ensure availability of sufficient, adequately qualified and trained laboratory staff and a safe and functioning laboratory infrastructure with appropriate and well-maintained equipment and sufficient laboratory consumables. DR-TB control programs should have a rapid, reliable and safe means of collecting and transferring specimens, cultures and information from the patient and physician to appropriate levels of the laboratory service, and for returning the results. Specimens from patients suspected of having DR-TB as well as cultures of *M. tuberculosis* pose a significant public health risk if not properly transported. Cultures, in particular, constitute enriched infectious material containing large numbers of viable organisms, and the risk is compounded when cultures of resistant strains are transported. Transmission of TB including MDR-TB and XDR-TB is a well recognized risk for laboratory workers.[6,7] *M. tuberculosis* is classified as a Risk Group 3 laboratory pathogen by WHO, requiring specific laboratory containment measures.[7] Adequately equipped laboratory services to ensure safe handling of drug-resistant strains, especially during aerosol-producing procedures such as mycobacterial culture and DST, are, therefore, important. Appropriate engineering controls, maintenance of essential laboratory safety equipment, and laboratory staff training are equally important. Comprehensive systems for managing the quality of laboratory services are mandatory, including internal quality control and external quality assurance.

Organization of the Laboratory Network

Conventional TB laboratory networks have a pyramidal structure based on an appropriately large number of peripheral (Level I) laboratories accessible to all TB suspects and patients, a moderate number of intermediate (Level II) laboratories located in mid-sized population centers and health facilities, and a single (or more than one in large countries), central (Level III) laboratories at the provincial, state or national levels. Since 1994, the network of SRLs has been instrumental in supporting drug resistance surveys in all regions of the world, providing quality assurance through proficiency testing and validation of DST data. The SRL network is being expanded to meet the challenges of scaling up the response to DR-TB.

Central reference laboratories supporting DR-TB control programs should establish formal links with one of the SRLs to ensure adequate expert input on infrastructure development, budgeting and training. A sustained link with an SRL is also strongly recommended for DR-TB control programs in order to maintain external quality assurance and validation of DST results. Documented first-line DST proficiency of central laboratories, preferably by one of the SRLs, is a prerequisite for applications by DR-TB control program to the Green Light Committee (GLC). Implementation of laboratory services for culture and DST requires a reasonable balance between cost and turnaround time. Such services are most likely to be economically affordable and provide optimal results, if based on direct delivery of specimens to a central mycobacteriology laboratory that has large enough operational volume to ensure technical proficiency, has well trained personnel and is properly equipped. DST of isoniazid and rifampicin is needed as a minimum in any DR-TB control program; DST of other first-line antituberculosis drugs is also desirable, although less essential. In the initial phase of treatment for MDR-TB, DST of second-line drugs is best left to supranational or other TB reference laboratories with documented capacity, expertise and proficiency. Once DST of first-line drugs operates at a consistently high level of proficiency, laboratories serving populations and patients with significant previous exposure to second-line drugs may consider extending their services to DST of second-line drugs. Routine DST of second-line drugs is not recommended unless the required laboratory infrastructure and capacity have been established, rigorous quality assurance is in place and sustainable proficiency has been demonstrated to isoniazid and rifampicin.

Transport of Infectious Substances

Given the risks associated with transport of specimens and/or cultures from patients suspected of having DR-TB, programs should ensure appropriate systems for safe packaging and transportation of infectious materials. International organizations such as the Universal Postal Union, the International Civil Aviation Organization and the International Air Transport Association have developed strict guidelines and procedures to facilitate the safe and expeditious shipment of infectious substances.[8,9] Exchange of *M. tuberculosis* cultures between countries for diagnostic DST, retesting or proficiency testing is always subject to international regulations, including national import and export regulations specific to individual countries.

Microscopy, Culture and Identification of *M. tuberculosis* in DR-TB Control Programs

Microscopy

Microscopy for acid-fast bacilli (AFB) cannot distinguish viable from nonviable organisms, nor differentiate between drug-susceptible and drug-resistant *M. tuberculosis* or between different species of mycobacteria. The main uses of microscopy for DR-TB are, therefore, limited to assessing the initial infectiousness of patients, triaging specimens to different algorithms for culture and DST, and confirming that organisms growing on culture media are mycobacteria rather than contaminants. As AFB sputum smear microscopy is unable to distinguish between viable and nonviable bacilli, its utility for monitoring patient infectiousness and response to treatment is also limited. For example, even with adequate treatment, specimens from DR-TB patients may remain sputum smear-positive after they become culture-negative, suggesting that the bacilli are non-viable.

Culture

Quality of laboratory processing is of crucial importance. Delays in specimen transport, excessively harsh or insufficient decontamination, poor-quality culture media or incorrect incubation temperature can adversely affect the culture yield. Laboratory errors, such as mislabeling or cross-contamination between specimens during aerosol-producing procedures, may lead to false negative or false-positive results. In this context, laboratory findings should always be correlated with the patient's clinical condition and any diagnostic test should be repeated, if necessary. Low positive culture results on solid medium (<10 colonies) are not well correlated with clinical prognosis and should be interpreted with caution, especially if a single culture with low colony counts is reported. However, persistent positive cultures or any positive culture in the setting of clinical deterioration should be regarded as significant. The pros and cons of different culture media and techniques are described.[3,4]

Identification of *M. tuberculosis*

In countries with a high burden of TB, the vast majority of mycobacterial isolates will be *M. tuberculosis*. The prevalence of nontuberculous mycobacteria (NTM) varies from country to country and can be more common in patients living with HIV. Unless the species is confirmed as *M. tuberculosis*, mycobacterial isolates appearing phenotypically resistant to first-line drugs may represent infection with nontubercular mycobacteria (NTM) and not MDR-TB. Treatment of NTM is entirely different from treatment of MDR-TB. As a minimum, laboratories supporting DR-TB control programs should be able to identify *M. tuberculosis* by conventional biochemical identification tests or at least two other methods that follow international guidelines.

Drug Susceptibility Testing (DST)

In vitro DST plays a key role in identification and treatment of MDR-TB patients. These guidelines strongly recommend that countries should develop the capacity to provide access to DST for any patient in whom resistance is considered likely. This recommendation is consistent with international standards for TB care endorsed by WHO and other partners[10] and resolutions on TB endorsed by the World Health Assembly in 2007 calling for universal access to DST by 2015.[11] A number of different techniques are available for DST. Classic phenotypic methods involve culturing of *M. tuberculosis* in the presence of antituberculosis drugs to detect inhibition of growth. Phenotypic methods allow the detection of drug resistance regardless of mechanism or molecular basis. Phenotypic DST methods can be performed as direct or indirect tests on solid media. In the direct test, a set of drug-containing and drug-free media is inoculated directly with a concentrated specimen. An indirect test involves inoculation with pure culture grown from the specimen. Indirect phenotypic tests have been extensively validated and are currently regarded as the gold standard. Three methods are commonly used: proportion, absolute concentration and resistance ratio. Several rounds of proficiency testing in the SRL network have shown that DST results do not differ between the three methods for first-line antituberculosis drugs. For second-line DST, broth or liquid methods and the proportion method on solid medium have been studied; methods for the absolute concentration or resistance ratio on solid medium have not been validated. The current status of DST methodology, consensus on reliability and reproducibility, and critical concentrations for different methodologies can be found in a WHO policy guidance document on rational use of second-line DST.[1]

Genotypic approaches detect the genetic determinants of resistance rather than the resistance phenotype. Most genotypic methods involve two steps: first, a molecular nucleic amplification method such as polymerase chain reaction is used to amplify sections of the *M. tuberculosis* genome known to be altered in resistant strains. In the second step, amplification products (amplicons) are assessed for specific mutations correlated with resistance. Novel technologies for rapid detection of drug resistance are under development. Most are in early development phase, undergoing laboratory validation or in early stages of large-scale field studies to assess their feasibility, cost effectiveness and cost benefit. Technologies focused on rapid rifampicin resistance testing as a proxy for MDR-TB testing are most advanced. In the majority of settings, particularly where fixed-dose combination (FDC) first-line antituberculosis drugs are used, resistance to rifampicin is almost invariably associated with resistance to isoniazid. Detection of rifampicin resistance, therefore, serves as a reliable although not complete proxy for MDR-TB. The advantages of rapid rifampicin testing include earlier identification of patients on inappropriate first-line regimens; prompt screening of patients at risk of MDR-TB and early interruption of MDR-TB transmission. Several tests for rapid detection of rifampicin resistance have been validated in laboratory-based studies. The use of rapid rifampicin resistance testing is recommended in high-risk MDR-TB settings including high-burden HIV settings, however, confirmation of MDR-TB by conventional DST is still regarded as the gold standard, and adequate laboratory capacity to ensure a quality-assured diagnosis of MDR-TB, therefore, remains a fundamental requirement. No rapid molecular tests for detection of XDR-TB are currently available and conventional and the newer liquid DST techniques are considered the most reliable methods for determining XDR-TB. Some of the newer liquid and agar techniques can determine the presence of XDR-TB within 14 days.

Limitations of DST

The accuracy of DST varies with the drug tested. For the first-line antituberculosis drugs, DST is most accurate for rifampicin and isoniazid and it is less reliable and reproducible for streptomycin, ethambutol and pyrazinamide.[1] Testing of in vitro susceptibility of second-line anti-tuberculosis drugs is much more problematic, as outlined in WHO policy guidance on second-line DST.[1] Aminoglycosides, polypeptides and fluoroquinolones have been tested in different laboratory environments and shown to have relatively good reliability and reproducibility. Data on the reproducibility and reliability of DST for the other second-line drugs are much more limited, have not been established or the methodology for testing does not exist.[1] Susceptibility testing of second-line drugs is hampered by technical difficulties due to in vitro drug instability, drug loss due to protein-binding, heat inactivation, incomplete dissolution, filter sterilization and varying drug potency. Moreover, the critical concentration defining resistance is often very close to the minimal inhibitory concentration (MIC) required to achieve antimycobacterial activity, increasing the probability for misclassification of susceptibility or resistance and leading to poor reproducibility of DST results. In addition, laboratory technique, medium pH, incubation temperature and incubation time may also affect DST results. Cross-resistance and a lack of understanding of the molecular mechanisms underlying TB drug resistance further compound the problem. Emerging evidence shows a clear association between phenotypic drug resistance and specific molecular mutations, however, not all mutations conferring resistance to second-line drugs have been described, nor have the underlying molecular mechanisms for the detected mutations been elucidated. Cross resistance between the fluoroquinolones (ciprofloxacin, ofloxacin and levofloxacin) is almost complete. Limited evidence suggests that the third-generation fluoroquinolones, notably moxifloxacin, do not have complete cross-resistance with the older generations[12–15] and may have enhanced clinical benefit due to their low MICs, enhanced antimycobacterial activity, and improved biochemical structure providing metabolic stability and long half-life, theoretically reducing the selection of resistant mutants.[16] While the clinical benefit of newer-generation fluoroquinolones has been validated in one small retrospective study,[17] more clinical and laboratory research is needed to understand the extent of fluoroquinolone cross-resistance and its clinical relevance. Cross-resistance between the aminoglycosides and/or the polypeptides is complex and data are very limited. The aminoglycosides kanamycin and amikacin have very high cross-resistance. Cross-resistance between other aminoglycosides and polypeptides appears relatively low, but more studies are needed.[1]

Rational use of DST in DR-TB Control Programs

Complex, incomplete and even contradictory information on cross-resistance, limited knowledge of the genotypes conferring resistance in second-line drugs and the technical limitations of second-line DST have important implications for laboratory infrastructure and design of treatment modalities in DR-TB control programs. Proficiency in DST is a combination of laboratory technique and workload, requiring adequate number of specimens to be tested. In most settings, this implies centralization of laboratory services for DST and particularly for DR-TB programs with small number of patients. Current WHO policy guidance on DST is as follows:[7]

- Laboratory capacity to reliably detect MDR-TB through quality-assured DST of isoniazid and rifampicin resistance is a minimum prerequisite for DR-TB control programs.
- Formal links with one of the laboratories in the SRL network are preferable to ensure adequate expert input on laboratory design, specimen and process flow, biosafety, maintenance of equipment and external quality assurance of DST result.
- Strategies for laboratory services in support of DR-TB control programs should follow a systematic approach and take into account the constraints of DST outlined above. DST should be focused on those drugs for which a reliable and reproducible methodology is available.
- Routine DST of second-line drugs is not recommended unless the required laboratory infrastructure and capacity have been established, rigorous quality assurance is in place and sustainable proficiency has been demonstrated for isoniazid and rifampicin. In order to retain proficiency and expertise, it is recommended that second-line DST only be performed if at least 200 specimens from high-risk patients are expected per year.
- At this time, routine DST of drugs in groups 4 (ethionamide, protionamide, cycloserine, terizidone, *p*-aminosalicylic acid) and 5 drugs (clofazimine, linezolid, amoxicillin-clavulanate, thioacetazone, clarithromycin, imipenem) is not recommended as reliability and reproducibility of laboratory testing cannot be guaranteed.

Time for Testing and Reporting: Turnaround Time

Growth detection and identification of *M. tuberculosis* may take 3 to 8 weeks in solid media and 1 to 2 weeks in broth media. DST of an *M. tuberculosis* isolate takes an additional 2 to 4 weeks in solid media and 1 week in broth media. To ensure rapid diagnosis of *M. tuberculosis* and DR-TB, laboratories should define standard turnaround times, which should be strictly followed.

Infection Control and Biosafety in the Laboratory

The relative hazards of infective microorganisms handled in the laboratory are classified by WHO according to their risk of causing human disease, the potential for laboratory spread and whether effective treatment and prevention measures are available.[7] Related biosafety levels for laboratories have been defined, taking into account the pathogenic agent, the facilities available, and the equipment, practices and procedures required to ensure a safe laboratory working environment.[7] *M. tuberculosis* is classified by WHO as a Risk Group 3 laboratory pathogen.[7] Mycobacteriological culture and DST generate high concentration aerosols requiring biosafety level 3 containment precautions. Laboratory standards require the following essential measures to be in place and enforced:

- Appropriate and specific administrative controls including good laboratory practice, standard operating procedures and accident management plans
- Appropriate engineering controls functioning adequately as designed
- Personal protective equipment appropriate for the tasks being performed
- Proper waste management procedures
- Proper procedures for general laboratory safety including physical, electrical and chemical safety.

Biosafety level 3 containment requires the strengthening of laboratory operations and safety programs, specifically those related to laboratory design, the use of specialized equipment to prevent or contain aerosols and health surveillance of laboratory staff. Published guidelines on biosafety level 3 precautions should be rigorously followed and expert engineering consultation sought when establishing laboratory infrastructure for DST.[1,7] Health and medical surveillance of laboratory personnel involved in mycobacteriological culture and DST are strongly recommended. Surveillance should include a detailed medical history, targeted baseline health assessment, monitoring of respiratory signs and symptoms, and a proactive plan for appropriate medical investigations when indicated. Laboratory workers, who choose to disclose that they are living with HIV, should be offered safer work responsibilities and should be discouraged from working with MDR-TB specimens. Pregnant women should be reassigned until after childbirth and lactation.

Quality Control and Quality Assurance

A diagnosis of DR-TB has profound implications for the individual patient. Accuracy of the laboratory diagnosis is crucial, and a comprehensive laboratory quality assurance program must be in place to ensure the accuracy, reliability and reproducibility of DST results. Quality control or quality assurance procedures should be performed regularly as an integral part of laboratory operations. Microscopy, culture and DST are necessary as per laboratory manuals and technical documents. Central reference laboratories involved in DR-TB control programs should establish formal links with one of the laboratories in the SRL network to help ensure the quality of laboratory services and the validation of DST results.The SRL network ensures DST standards by a system of external quality assurance that should preferably be established before the implementation of DR-TB control programs. As a minimum, external quality assurance with an SRL should comprise: An initial assessment visit, proficiency testing with an adequate number of coded isolates and periodic rechecking of isolates obtained within the DR-TB control program. Proficiency testing by the SRL involves regular distribution to national TB reference laboratories of panels of coded *M. tuberculosis* strains with predefined drug resistance profiles. The test results by the reference laboratory are compared with the coded SRL results in blinded fashion and specific performance indicators like sensitivity, specificity, reproducibility are calculated for each drug and for the reference laboratory as a whole. As a minimum performance indicator, proficiency testing should correctly identify resistance to isoniazid and rifampicin in more than 90% in two out of three recent rounds of panels. The SRL network is in agreement that panels for second-line proficiency testing should not include XDR strains of *M. tuberculosis*; rather, panels with different permutations of monoresistance to second-line drugs are currently being developed, which will be compiled to allow reliable assessment of the overall capability of national reference laboratories to identify XDR-TB.

References

1. Drug susceptibility testing of second-line antituberculosis drugs: WHO policy guidance. Geneva, World Health Organization. 2008.
2. Guidelines for surveillance of drug resistance in tuberculosis. Geneva, World Health Organization, 2003 (WHO/CDS/TB/2003/320; WHO/CDS/CSR/RMD/2003.3).
3. Laboratory services in tuberculosis control. Parts I, II and III. Geneva, World Health Organization, 1998 (WHO/TB/98.258).
4. The public health service national tuberculosis reference laboratory and the national laboratory network: minimum requirements, roles, and operation in low-income countries. Paris, International Union Against Tuberculosis and Lung Disease. 1998.
5. http://www.who.int/tb/dots/laboratory/policy/en/index3.html.
6. Joshi Rajnish, Arthur L Reingold, Dick Menzies, Pai Madhukar. Tuberculosis among healthcare workers in low- and middle-income countries: a systematic review. PLoS Med. 2006; December 3:e494.
7. Laboratory biosafety manual, 3rd ed. Geneva, World Health Organization. 2004 (WHO/CDS/CSR/LYO/2004.11).
8. Recommendations on the transport of dangerous goods: model regulations, 12th rev. ed. New York, United Nations. 2002 (ST/SG/AC.10/1/Re.12).
9. Infectious substances shipping guidelines, 3rd ed. Montreal, International Air Transport Association, 2002.
10. International standards for tuberculosis care. The Hague, Tuberculosis Coalition for Technical Assistance, 2006 (available at http://www.who.int/tb/publications /2006/ istc_ report.pdf; accessed May 2008).
11. World Health Assembly (WHA) Resolution EB120.R3. Geneva: 2007.
12. Ben Yang Zhao, Richard Pine, John Domagala and Karl Drlica. Fluoroquinolone action against clinical isolates of *Mycobacterium tuberculosis*: effects of a C-8 methoxyl group on survival in liquid media and in human macrophages. Antimicrobial Agents and Chemotherapy. 1999;43:661-6.
13. Yuzhi Dong, Chen Xu, Xilin Zhao, John Domagala and Karl Drlica. Fluoroquinolone action against mycobacteria: effects of C-8 substituents on growth, survival and resistance. Antimicrobial Agents and Chemotherapy. 1998;42:2978-84.
14. N Lounis, B Ji, C Truffot-Pernot and J Grosset. Which aminoglycoside or fluoroquinolone is more active against *Mycobacterium tuberculosis* in mice? Antimicrobial Agents and Chemotherapy. 1997;41:607-10.

15. Alvirez-Freites EL, Carter JL, Cynamon MH. In vitro and in vivo activities of gatifloxacin against *Mycobacterium tuberculosis*. Antimicrobial Agents and Chemotherapy. 2002;46:1022-5.
16. Somasundaram S, Paramasivan NC. Susceptibility of *Mycobacterium tuberculosis* strains to gatifloxacin and moxifloxacin by different methods. Chemotherapy. 2002;46:1022-5.
17. Wing Wai Yew, Chi Kuen Chan, Chi Chiu Leung, Chi Hung Chau, Cheuk Ming Tam, Poon Chuen Wong, et al. Comparative roles of levofloxacin and ofloxacin in the treatment of multi-drug-resistant tuberculosis: preliminary results of a retrospective study from Hong Kong. Chest. 2003;124:1476-81.

Chapter 9

Multi-drug-resistant Tuberculosis: Diagnosis and Treatment

Introduction

Drug-resistant tuberculosis (DR-TB) has been reported since the early days of introduction of antitubercular chemotherapy, but recently multi-drug-resistant tuberculosis (MDR-TB) has been an area of growing concern, and is posing threat to global efforts of tuberculosis control. Prevalence of MDR-TB in a community mirrors the functional state and efficacy of tuberculosis control program and realistic attitude of the community towards implementation of such programs.[1] Management of DR-TB and MDR-TB is difficult, much expensive, challenging and quite often leads to treatment failure. This chapter aims to illustrate the diagnosis and treatment of drug-resistant and multi-drug-resistant tuberculosis.

Definition

Drug-resistant tuberculosis is defined as a case of tuberculosis excreting bacilli resistant to one or more antitubercular drugs. Multi-drug-resistant tuberculosis (MDR-TB) is defined as disease due to *M. tuberculosis* that is resistant to isoniazid and rifampicin with or without resistance to other drugs (the culture and drug susceptibility test result being from an RNTCP-accredited laboratory). Mono-resistance is defined as resistance to one antituberculosis drug whereas poly-resistance is defined as resistance to more than one antituberculosis drug, other than both isoniazid and rifampicin.

Mechanism of Drug Resistance

Drug resistance in tuberculosis occurs by random single-step spontaneous mutation at a low but predictable frequency in large bacterial populations. There is no convincing evidence for the role of plasmids or transposons as in other bacterial pathogens. The probability of drug-resistant mutants in the case of Rifampicin is 10^{-8}, for INH, Streptomycin and Ethambutol is 10^{-6} and for Ethionamide, Cycloserine, Capreomycin and Thiacetazone is 10^{-3}. The probability of resistance developing in a 2.5 cm cavity which harbors 10^8 to 10^9 bacilli is 10^6 for INH and 10^8 for Rifampicin and 10^{14} for INH and Rifampicin together. In reality, therefore, only one of the bacilli in 10^{14} organisms will be resistant to both isoniazid and rifampicin. This illustrates a very fundamental principle that multi-drug-resistant tuberculosis is a manmade problem.[3]

Genetic Basis of Drug Resistance

Dramatic discoveries in the field of molecular biology in the last few years have greatly increased our understanding of the mechanism of drug resistance. The findings of such discoveries led to the conclusion that the primary mechanism of multiple drug resistance in tuberculosis is due to alterations in individual drug target genes.[1] Isoniazid resistance has been found to be due to a defect in the Kat G gene which codes for the catalase peroxidase enzyme. Mutation in Kat G, Inh A and ahp C (alkyl hydroperoxide reductase) genes are found in upto 90% of isoniazid resistance. Rifampicin resistance (> 96%) has been associated with mutations in the rpo B gene,[2] Pyrazinamide resistance (72–97%) to pncA mutations, Ethambutol (47–65%) to mutations in emb AB gene, Streptomycin resistance with rrs or rpsL mutations and fluoroquinolone resistance (75–94%) with substitutions in gyr A gene. Apart from these 11 genes, additional genes and mechanisms may play a role particularly in association with lower levels of resistance.[3]

Virulence and Drug-resistant Strains

The traditionally received wisdom about drug-resistant strains of tuberculosis that they are less virulent was based substantially on the observation by Cohn, et al.[4] that virulent strains of *M. tuberculosis*, when selectively bred in the laboratory for high-level resistance to INH, became significantly less capable of producing progressive infection in animal models. This was associated with loss of catalase activity by bacilli. Snider, et al. observed that there is a no lesser risk of infection when contacts are exposed to tubercular bacilli resistant to high concentration of INH and SM.[5] Ordway, et al.[6] have observed that some MDR-TB strains that exhibit in vitro growth rates and animal virulence characteristics comparable to the most virulent, wild type drug susceptible strains. Frieden, et al.[7] in their report of multi-institutional spread of notorious 'Strain W' in New York City reported despite mutation in the Kat G locus, strain was catalase positive and grows rapidly in culture media and animals. Overall, evidences indicate that current drug-resistant strains have demonstrated the capacity to produce progressive disease in both normal and immunosuppressed contacts.

Impact of Drug Resistance on the Outcome of Chemotherapy

In early treatment era, it was recognized that the resistance with isoniazid (H) and streptomycin (S) was associated with increased risk of treatment failure[8] but in the current situation, the loss of single drug to resistance is potentially less significant because of the availability and use of potent agents such as rifampicin, pyrazinamide and ethambutol (E). The most reliable data on treatment outcome were derived from British Medical Research Council (BMRC) short-course chemotherapy trials performed in East Africa, Hong Kong and Singapore.[9] Failure rate of isoniazid (H), rifampicin (R), pyrazinamide (Z) and streptomycin (S) containing regimen among such cases was less than 5% in contrast to approximately 20% failure rate among cases assigned to less-potent regimens. Thus, it is possible to obtain good result with use of six months' short-course chemotherapy with isoniazid, rifampin, pyrazinamide and streptomycin or ethambutol when initial susceptibility test indicates resistance to isoniazid and/or streptomycin. It was also confirmed in Indian study that strains resistant to isonizid, streptomycin or both neither pose a major problem nor affect the result of treatment in a big way, provided proper regimens are used. On the contrary, patients infected with organisms resistant to rifampicin, isoniazid or both have a high rate of treatment failure[10-12] and this forms a major threat to tuberculosis control programs particularly for countries like India with poor resources.[13] Four separate studies from New York city between 1995 and 1996 on response to therapy for patient with MDR-TB[14-17] reported better outcome can be demonstrated with early recognization of resistance and administration of effective drugs.

Diagnosis of Multi-drug-resistant Tuberculosis

It is needless to emphasize that early diagnosis and treatment of drug-resistant and multi-drug-resistant tuberculosis is of paramount importance not only from the patient's perspective but also for the community at large. Failing this there will be propagation of the deadly drug-resistant bacilli, decreased chances of cure for the patient, increasing cost of therapy and unnecessary drug toxicity. The diagnosis of drug-resistant and multi-drug-resistant tuberculosis is based on—clinical, radiological and bacteriological evidences.

Clinical Evidence

This comprises of the signs and symptoms and past history of antitubercular therapy. History of prior treatment with antitubercular drugs is most important. The other important aspects of the history include contact with a known case of resistant tuberculosis and patient's place of residence, which may have a high prevalence of drug resistance. The salient points in the past treatment history should include the drugs and regimens followed, dosage of drugs and duration of each course of treatment, regularity in taking the drugs, response to treatment in terms of relief of symptoms and bacteriological indices, if available, and any adverse drug reactions suffered. The ICMR in its study has shown that longer duration of chemotherapy and single-drug therapy in the past was associated with greater degrees of resistance.[10] In the context of our country, where illiteracy is the main culprit, several difficulties may be encountered in eliciting reliable information. Some of the common problems faced by the physician include unawareness or forgetfulness of the patient so that he is unable to give a proper history, poor record-keeping of prescriptions, sputum examination reports and X-rays, drugs dispensed by private practitioners without a proper prescription and the practice of prescribing combipacks, making it impossible for the patient to remember the names. MDR-TB suspect is defined as a TB patient who fails an RNTCP Category I or III treatment regimen and any RNTCP Category II patient who is sputum-smear-positive at the end of the fourth month of treatment or later.[18] It must be remembered that clinical evidences are the least reliable for the diagnosis of drug-resistant and multi-drug-resistant tuberculosis. However, clinical deterioration in the presence of sputum-smear positivity and/or radiological worsening can be considered due to resistance.

Radiological Evidence

Though radiology is not a very reliable indicator for predicting drug resistance, yet it serves to complement the clinical and bacteriological evidence of the patient. The presence of multiple or giant cavities and destroyed lung increases the probability of drug resistance. Change in size of cavities, increase in size of existing lesions and appearance of new lesions are signs of disease progression and activity. Serial X-rays showing worsening in the forms as described above at the end of three months of regular and adequate chemotherapy can make one suspicious of drug resistance. These radiological findings at the end of three months in addition to positive sputum and/or clinical worsening can be diagnosed as resistant tuberculosis.[19] However, one should also realize that radiological worsening may be due to pneumonia, pulmonary embolism and supervening carcinoma.

Bacteriological Evidence

The bacteriological criteria serve as the gold standard in the detection of drug-resistant tuberculosis. This is based on sputum-smear microscopy and culture of *M. tuberculosis* and drug susceptibility testing (DST) to the various primary- and second-line antitubercular drugs. Sputum-smear microscopy, after starting standard chemotherapy, can show a positive, negative or suboptimal response. While positive response is characterized by sputum conversion at 2/3 months of chemotherapy, a negative response could mean persistent smear positivity at the end of three months of adequate chemotherapy and a suboptimal response by an initial fall in the sputum grade followed by a gradual rise—the so-called 'fall and rise' phenomenon[20] while the patient is on antitubercular therapy. The last two patterns increase the probability of drug-resistant tuberculosis. The confirmation of the presence of drug resistance is obtained by culture of *M. tuberculosis* and drug susceptibility testing. Even the definition of drug resistance is one that is based on susceptibility test results, i.e confirmed MDR-TB case is an MDR-TB suspect, who is sputum-culture positive and whose TB is due to *Mycobacterium tuberculosis* that are resistant in vitro to at least isoniazid and rifampicin[18] (the culture and DST result being from an accredited laboratory). Ideally DST should be done in all patients undergoing retreatment, but since this is not feasible in an Indian set-up, it is better to do DST for MDR-TB suspects. It is, however, noteworthy that culture and sensitivity, in spite of continuing to be the gold standard for diagnosis of tuberculosis and drug resistance, is not fool proof and one has to keep in mind the limitations of this highly specific test. This is because the technique is complex and it is difficult to perform sensitivity tests accurately even when skilled personnel are available and laboratory facilities are of a high standard. This is true even in highly industrialized nations such as the United Kingdom and the United States. In the United Kingdom, retesting of 234 strains of drug-resistant bacilli by a reference laboratory showed discordant reports in 50 to 70% of the results reported by local laboratories.[19] Additional limitations are the difficulty and unreliability of testing susceptibility to second-line drugs. In the United States, 43 laboratories, which were having above average laboratory standards, tested the results of a reference laboratory. The results obtained were as follows—consistently good in 23, adequate in 9 and poor in 11. The WHO, thus, concluded that the wide scale on which unreliable sensitivity tests are reported, even in technically advanced countries, gives a cause for concern.[21-23] However, recently due to setting up of supranational reference laboratory network, there is an improvement in quality susceptibility testing of national reference laboratories and surveys carried out within the WHO/IUATLD global project on drug resistance surveillance. These initiatives apply to surveillance and not to clinical practice.[24] Susceptibility testing for isoniazid, rifampicin, the fluoroquinolones, and the injectable agents is fairly reliable. For other agents, it is less reliable, and basing individualized treatments on DST for these agents should be avoided. The clinical effectiveness or ineffectiveness of a drug cannot be predicted by DST with 100% certainty.[25]

Laboratories performing culture/susceptibility testing are situated in only a few major cities in India. The WHO definition of resistance based on drug susceptibility reports, therefore, becomes only a theoretical exercise in our country in most occasions.[20] The laboratories vary in reliability; errors occur in labs, different sensitivity reports are obtained of the same patient from different laboratories due to sampling of different populations of bacilli and different techniques employed. Standardization, co-ordination and cross-checking facilities with reference laboratories do not exist in our country by and large, thus magnifying the problem. On this background, it is pertinent to reaffirm that drug susceptibility testing should not be accepted uncritically, they should be correlated with prior treatment history, smear result and X-ray and should be used as a guide for future therapies and not dictate treatment options. If sensitivity report does not fit with other available evidences, it should be discussed with a microbiologist and the test repeated.

Rapid Culture Technique

In this technique, culture time is reduced from an average 38.5 days to 18 days. Technique usually applied is BACTEC system and Mycobacterial Growth Indicator Tube (MGIT). In BACTEC, 7H12, and in MGIT, 7H9 middle Brooke media are used. In BACTEC method, the released radio-labeled carbon dioxide is detected that indicates growth of *Mycobacterium tuberculosis* whereas, in MGIT, the oxygen-sensitive fluorescent compound is used to detect growth of *M. tuberculosis*. The rapid culture technology takes much shorter time as compared to L-J media.[26,27] A higher degree of concordance has been documented between susceptibility data from the BACTEC system and those obtained by conventional solid media method.[28] In fact, the rapid radiometric system offers a substantially more quantitative approach to the determination of susceptibility than other method,[29] another major advantage of BACTEC system that it can also perform susceptibility test for pyrazinamide.[30]

Molecular Biological Technique

For identification of resistance-associated mutation molecular techniques, like DNA sequencing, Line Probe Assay (LiPA), DNA microarrays, molecular beacons, single-strand conformation polymorphism, fluorescent Resonance Energy Transfer probes, other PCR-based techniques or Mycobacteriophages-based assays like FAST Plaque TB and Luciferase receptor phages (LRPs) has been used. WHO with the Stop TB Partnership, UNITAID and the Foundation for Innovative New Diagnostics (FIND) together unveiled a new Policy endorsing use of Line Probe Assays in low-resource countries. There are two types, the Geno Type MTB-DR assay and INNO-LiPA Rif. TB assay. Advantages include rapid screening of patients with MDR-TB risk and results within 2 days as compared to 2–3 months for conventional cultures. At present, their use is limited to culture isolates and direct testing of sputum specimens. They are not recommended as a complete replacement to the conventional culture and DST.[31] Currently, LiPA is not useful for detecting mutations responsible for drug resistance in second-line drugs. The Xpert MTB/RIF assay enables simultaneous detection of Mycobacterium tuberculosis (MTB) and rifampicin resistance and it was endorsed by WHO in 2010. The Xpert MTB/RIF was found to be highly sensitive (98%) and specific (98%) in detecting tuberculosis and rifampicin resistance (a reliable proxy for MDR) directly from sputum, in less than two hours. The assay is robust enough to be performed outside of conventional laboratories, at district and subdistrict level of health system but requires uninterrupted power supply. Widespread implementation of Xpert MTB/RIF would greatly enhance the diagnostic capacity for TB and MDR TB; its accuracy and ease of use represents a major milestone for TB and MDR TB care and control.[31] Molecular techniques involve detection of resistant genes or DNA sequencing of *M. tuberculosis* by amplification of nucleic acid and its identification. The Polymerase Chain Reaction single strand conformational polymorphism (PCR SSCP)[32] and restriction fragment length polymorphism (RFLP)[33,34] analysis are usually applied. The PCR when compared with culture results, the sensitivity, specificity, and positive predictive value were found 83.5%, 99% and 94.2% respectively. RFLP gives fingerprint of strains which is specific for each strain of *M. tuberculosis*. So it has more valuable place for molecular epidemiology in differentiating the strains. Overall, RFLP analysis has immense potential as a tool to study transmission patterns and the natural histories of primary and reinfection tuberculosis specifically in HIV-infected patients,[34] while

Luciferase Reporter Assay rapid system based on enzyme Luciferase, involves the introduction of this enzyme into *Mycobacterium tuberculosis* via a reporter phage system. Exposure of Luminuous Mycobacterium to antimicrobial agents would block luminous activity in the sensitive bacilli but with no effect on resistant bacilli. This method requires substantial growth of mycobacterium population (about 10^6); yet, the potential of such methodology is intriguing, perhaps playing a role in industrial screening of large number of compounds for antimycobacterial activity.[35] The expectation that molecular techniques would surpass conventional methods has not yet been realized because most of the techniques still require detailed and systemic evaluation using standard techniques as references before their application in clinical setting. These techniques might be used as compliment to the standard methods.[36]

Treatment of Multi-drug-resistant Tuberculosis

The WHO recommends that treatment of drug-resistant and multi-drug-resistant tuberculosis should be ideally carried out in a hospital that has a specialized unit for dealing with such cases with trained doctors and laboratory personnel. There should be standard laboratory facilities for carrying out reliable drug susceptibility testing and uninterrupted supply of drugs. The management of multi-drug-resistant tuberculosis is an area that has been shrouded in a lot of myths and misconceptions, and, therefore, utterly chaotic. Though guidelines, in general, have been laid down by the WHO, which have been found cost-effective and feasible in resource-limited countries but they may not be applicable to every patient where individualized treatment regimens depending on reliable sensitivity report may be used. Use of standardized or individualized treatment regimens is currently subject of operational studies to assess the feasibility and cost effectiveness. In some countries, a standardized regimen for certain groups of patients may be more appropriate than an individualized regimen, while, in others, the converse may be the best. Most of the guidelines for the management of drug-resistant TB are primarily for high-income nations, where expert diagnostics and optimal care are available. Low-income nations will inevitably require different approaches than those of the more affluent, industrialized nations. Individualized regimens are based on individual DST and prior treatment history, require close follow-up by skilled professionals and incur high cost. Management issues in second-line drugs are complex, especially when individualized treatment regimens are used. Drugs are frequently changed as a result of adverse effects, delayed DST results and poor response to treatment. Standardized regimens for middle- to low-income nations are based on DRS data from representative patient populations. Such regimens reduce the number of specialist physicians needed and cost of tretment by 5 to 10 times. WHO has designed the DOTS-Plus regimen for managing MDR-TB in resource-poor nations like India. Even in countries where reliable DST is available, standardized regimens may be chosen as a strategy over individualized regimens for the following reasons: Interpretation of DST to some of the first- and second-line drugs is difficult and could mislead regimen design. Standardized regimens can give guidance to clinicians and prevent basing decisions on DST that is not reliable, turnaround time for many culture-based DST methods is long, the laboratory may not perform DST of certain drugs, or may perform them at different times. Results from rapid methods (molecular) may be available within days, but only for certain first-line drugs, such as isoniazid and rifampicin. Many laboratories perform second-line DST only after resistance to first-line drugs is confirmed. Accounting for the effectiveness of the five drug groups, it is a known fact that the first-line drugs are more powerful, cheaper and effective. Given the circumstances, it would be ideal to add one or more first-line drugs to any regimen based on the appropriate DST.

Second-line Drugs and their Dosage

The second-line drugs used for treatment of drug-resistant and multi-drug-resistant tuberculosis are given in Table 9.1 with their dosages in decreasing potency from top to bottom against *Mycobacterium tuberculosis*. It is generally thought that second-line drugs are frequently associated with very high rates of unacceptable adverse drug reactions, needing frequent interruption and change of regimen, but in clinical practice, it is observed that these drugs are

TABLE 9.1: Doses of antitubercular drugs used in previously treated patients of TB

Drugs	*Average daily dosage*	*Daily dosage (mg)*		*Type of anti-mycobacterial activity*
		Minimum	*Maximum*	
Group 1 First-line oral agents Pyrazinamide (Z) Ethambutol (E) Rifabutin (Rfb)	 25 mg/kg 15 mg/kg 5–10 mg/kg	 1200 800 150	 1500 1200 600	 Bactericidal Bacteriostatic
Group 2 Injectable agents Kanamycin (Km) Amikacin (Am) Streptomycin (S) Capreomycin (Cm)	 15 mg/kg 15 mg/kg 15 mg/kg 15 mg/kg	 750 750 750 750	 1000 1000 1000 1000	Bactericidal against actively multiplying organisms
Group 3 Flouroquinolone Moxifloxacin (Mfx) Levofloxacin (Lfx) Ofloxacin (Ofx)	 7.5–10 mg/kg 7.5–10 mg/kg 15–20 mg/kg	 400 800 500	 400 1000 1000	 Weakly bactericidal
Group 4 Oral Bacteriostatic second-line drugs Ethionamide (Eto) Prothionamide (Pto) Para-aminosalicyclic acid (PAS) Cycloserine (Cs) Terizidone (Trd)	 15–20 mg/kg 15–20 mg/kg 200–300 mg/kg 10–20 mg/kg 10–20 mg/kg	 500-750 500-750 10 g 500-750 500-750	 1000 1000 12 g 1000 1000	 Bacteriostatic

Contd...

Contd...

Drugs	*Average daily dosage*	*Daily dosage (mg)*		*Type of anti-mycobacterial activity*
		Minimum	*Maximum*	
Group 5 Agents with unclear role in treatment of Drug resistant TB				
Clofazimine (Cfz)	4–5 mg/kg	100	300	Bacteriostatic
Linezolid (Lzd)		600	1200	
Amoxicillin/clavulanate (Amx/Clv)	2 g/day	500/125 Twice a day	1000/250 Twice a day	Weakly bactericidal
Thioacetazone (Thz)	150 mg/day	-	-	
Imipenem/Cilastatin (Ipm/Cln)	500–1000 mg/IV every 6 hourly	500 every 6 hourly	1000 every 6 hourly	
High-dose isoniazid (high-dose H)	16–20 mg/kg	600	900	
Clarithromycin (Clr)	10–15 mg/kg	500 twice a day	500 twice a day	Bactericidal (pH-dependent)

fairly tolerated. The author himself in one of the studies reported that 41% patients experience some side effects but only 21.1% patients required stoppage or change of drug in their study of 39 patients of MDR-TB.[37] Thus, it is practically possible to treat the patients of MDR-TB with these drugs.

Cross Resistance

Cross resistance has been reported between thioamides and thioacetazone (one-way resistance—strains resitance to thioacetazone are susceptible to thioamides; the reverse is seldom the case), kanamycin/amikacin with streptomycin,[38] rifampicin with rifapentine, and rifabutin (> 70% strains) [39] and among various derivatives of fluoroquinolones.[40] Cross-resistance between the fluoroquinolones is almost complete. Limited evidence suggests that the third-generation fluoroquinolones (notably moxifloxacin) do not have complete cross-resistance with the older generations and may have enhanced clinical benefit due to their low MICs, enhanced antimycobacterial activity, and improved biochemical structure providing metabolic stability and long half-life, theoretically reducing the selection of resistant mutants. While the clinical benefit of newer-generation fluoroquinolones has been validated in one small retrospective study,[41] more clinical and laboratory research is needed to understand the extent of fluoroquinolone cross-resistance and its clinical relevance. Cross-resistance has also been reported between ethionamide and INH[42], amikacin and kanamycin,[38] amikacin and capreomycin.[38] Strains resistant to streptomycin/kanamycin/amikacin are still sensitive to capreomycin. It is ineffective to use two drugs of the same group or to use a drug potentially ineffective because of the cross-resistance.

General Principles for Designing Treatment Regimens for Multi-drug-resistant Tuberculosis

Early suspicion, diagnosis and appropriate treatment of MDR-TB is essential to prevent morbidity, mortality and transmission of MDR-TB. Treatment should be initiated in a specialized centre with standard laboratory facilities. Single drug should not be added to the failing regimen. Intermittent therapy is not effective in multi-drug-resistant tuberculosis and should be avoided. Past history of drugs taken by the patient and drugs commonly used in the country and prevalence of resistance to first-line and second-line drugs should be taken into consideration, when designing a standardized regimen. Regimens should consist of at least four drugs with either certain, or almost certain effectiveness. If the evidence about the effectiveness of a certain drug is unclear, the drug can be part of the regimen but it should not be depended upon for success. Often more than four drugs may be started if the susceptibility pattern is unknown, effectiveness is questionable for an/the agent(s) or if extensive, bilateral pulmonary disease is present. Design treatment regimens with a consistent approach based on the hierarchy of the five groups of antituberculosis drugs (see Table 9.2).

Use any first-line oral agent (Group-1) to which isolate is sensitive, use one injectable (Group-2), one fluoroquinolone (Group-3) and add as many second-line bacteriostatic agents (Group-4) to make up atleast four effective drugs. Group-5 drugs are not recommended for routine use except where an adequate regimen is impossible with Group 1 to 4. Do not use ciprofloxacin as an antituberculosis drug. When possible, pyrazinamide, ethambutol and fluoroquinolones should be given once per day as the high peaks attained in once-a-day dosing may be more efficacious. Once-a-day dosing is permitted for other second-line drugs depending on patient tolerance; however ethionamide/prothionamide, cycloserine and PAS have traditionally been given in split doses during the day to reduce adverse effects. The drug dosage should be determined by body weight. Most drugs should be started at full dose, except cycloserine, ethionamide and

TABLE 9.2: Grouping of antituberculosis drugs

Group	Drugs
Group 1 First-line oral agents	Ethambutol (E); Pyrazinamide (Z); Rifabutin (Rfb)
Group 2 Injectable agents	Kanamycin (Km); Amikacin (Am); Capreomycin (Cm); Streptomycin (S)
Group 3 Fluoroquinolones	Moxifloxacin (Mfx); Levofloxacin (Lfx); Ofloxacin (Ofx)
Group 4 Oral bacteriostatic second-line agents	Ethionamide (Eto); Protionamide (Pto); Cycloserine (Cs); Terizidone (Trd); P-aminosalicylic acid (PAS)
Group 5 (drugs with unclear efficacy or unclear role in MDR-TB treatment, not recommended by WHO for routine use in MDR-TB patients)	Clofazimine (Cfz); Linezolid (Lzd); Amoxicillin/clavulanate (Amx/Clv); Thioacetazone (Thz); Imipenem/cilastatin (Ipm/Cln); High-dose isoniazid (high-dose H); Clarithromycin (Clr)

PAS, in which case the dose of the drug can be increased over a two-week period (drug ramping).[42,43] The injectable agent should be continued for a minimum of 6 months, and for at least 4 months after the patient first becomes and remains smear- or culture-negative. Review of the patient's cultures, smears, X-rays and clinical status may also aid in deciding whether or not to continue an injectable agent longer than the above recommendation, particularly in the case of patients for whom the susceptibility pattern is unknown, effectiveness of one or more agents is questionable, or extensive or bilateral pulmonary disease is present.[25] Treatment of adverse drug effects should be immediate and adequate in order to minimize the risk of treatment interruptions and prevent increased morbidity and mortality due to serious adverse effects. The minimum duration of treatment is 18 months after culture conversion, preferably each dose is given as directly observed therapy (DOT) throughout the treatment. At least, the therapy should be under direct observation, preferably for 3 to 4 months or till the sputum conversion. If directly observed treatment is not possible, adherence to treatment must be ensured by intense health education to the patient and family member at the start of treatment and during each follow-up visits and other adherence measures like checking empty blister packs. No drug should be kept in reserve and the most powerful drugs (bactericidal) should be used initially and in maximum combination so as to ensure that the first battle is won and won permanently. DST of drugs with high reproducibility and reliability (and from a dependable laboratory) should be used to guide therapy. Do not depend on DST in regimen design for ethambutol, pyrazinamide, and Group 4 and 5 drugs. Pyrazinamide can be used for the entire treatment if it is judged to be effective. Many DR-TB patients have chronically inflamed lungs, which theoretically produce the acidic environment in which pyrazinamide is active. Alternatively, in patients doing well, Pyrazinamide can be stopped with the injectable phase if the patient can continue with at least three certain, or almost certain, effective drugs. Use adjunctive measures appropriately, including surgery, and nutritional and social support; all measures should be taken to persuade and encourage patients not to stop treatment despite all its discomforts as it is the last that stands between patient and death.[43-49]

DOTS-Plus

DOTS-Plus, now programmatic management of drug-resistant tuberculosis (PMDT), is an integral component of RNTCP to manage MDR-TB to be implemented through program infrastructure. The strategy is designed to manage MDR-TB using second-line anti-TB drugs within the DOTS strategy in low- and middle-income countries like India. Therefore, in every DOTS-implementing unit of the country, DOTS would be prioritized above DOTS-Plus with the view that DOTS reduces the emergence of MDR-TB, and, therefore, the need for DOTS-Plus overtime. The RNTCP under DOTS-PLUS will be using a standardized treatment regimen (STR) Category IV regimen, comprising of six drugs (kanamycin, levofloxacin, ethionamide, cycloserine, pyrazinamide and ethambutol) during 6–9 months of the intensive phase and four drugs (levofloxacin, ethionamide, cycloserine and ethambutol) during the 18 months of the Continuation Phase. *p*-aminosalicylic acid (PAS) is included in the regimen as a substitute drug, if any bactericidal drug (kanamycin, levofloxacin, pyrazinamide and ethionamide) or any 2 bacteriostatic (ethambutol and cycloserine) drugs are not tolerated. This Category IV regimen is highly suitable for high-TB prevalent nations as well as low- to middle-income countries like India. Injectable agent should be given atleast for six months and the whole treatment duration is minimum of 18 months beyond sputum conversion. Fully standardized second-line treatments have shown to be feasible and cost-effective in DR-TB treatment.[18,48] (For details of DOTS-Plus refer to chapter 25).

In our Indian set-up, most of the time, either DST results are not available or, if available, they are usually highly unreliable. Keeping this fact in mind, depending upon past history of anti-tuberculosis treatment, the author himself has used four groups of regimen in treating drug-resistant/multi-drug-resistant tuberculosis and found to be effective.[37] The suggested regimen by author is given in Table 9.3.

TABLE 9.3: Suggested regimen for drug-resistant/multi-drug-resistant tuberculosis before or without or unreliable DST reports

		Drug regimen	*Duration in months*	*Drugs given (Responders)*	*Duration in months*	*Drugs given (Nonresponders)*
I	Misused drugs like SHE and THZ	Rifampicin Isoniazid Ethambutol Pyrazinamide ± Streptomycin	2–3*	Rifampicin Isoniazid Ethambutol ± Pyrazinamide	9	Treat as Group II Or Take help of DST result
II	Misused drugs like SHREZ and THZ	Streptomycin Isoniazid Rifampicin Ethambutol Pyrazinamide	2–3*	Rifampicin Isoniazid Ethambutol ± Pyrazinamide	9	Treat as Group III Or Take help of DST result
III	Failed after adequate 5 drugs (SHREZ)	Kanamycin Fluoroquinolone (Levofloxacin/ Ofloxacin) Ethionamide Cycloserine Pyrazinamide Ethambutol	6	Ethionamide Fluoroquinolone (Levofloxacin/ Ofloxacin) Cycloserine Ethambutol	18	Treat as Group IV Or Take help of DST result and consider surgery
IV	Failed on group III treatment	Capreomycin PAS Moxifloxacin High-dose INH Clofazamine Linezolid Amoxycillin/ Clavulanate	6–12	PAS Moxifloxacin High-dose INH Clofazamine Linezolid Amoxycillin/ Clavulanate	18	Consider surgery

* Depending on sputum conversion can be used for 3–6 months, if toxicity does not intervene
R—rifampicin, H—isoniazid, E—ethambutol, Z—pyrazinamide, S—streptomycin, THZ—thiacetazone.

Duration of Treatment

The optimal duration of therapy for MDR-TB has not been clearly established and duration remains questionable. WHO guidelines recommend continuing therapy for a minimum of 18 months after culture conversion until there is conclusive evidence to support a shorter duration of treatment. Extension of therapy to 24 months may be indicated in chronic cases with extensive pulmonary damage. This is, however, a highly expensive approach that is difficult to implement in the majority of middle- and low-income countries like India which bear the high burden of MDR-TB. The duration of injectables is also controversial. The 2006 and 2008 WHO guidelines advice atleast 6 months or atleast 4 months after smear or culture conversion. WHO guidelines, 2011 advice atleast 8 months of injectable treatment. In addition, the duration has to be decided in correlation with other factors also like other drugs in the regimen, bacteriological status and drug toxicity.[43]

Monitoring of Treatment

Monitoring of treatment should be done with bacteriological, radiological and clinical methods. Sputum specimens should be obtained for semiquantitative smear and culture every month from third month onwards during the intensive phase of therapy. Sputum conversion is defined as two sets of consecutive negative smears and cultures, from samples collected at least 30 days apart. Both bacteriological techniques (smear and culture) should be used to monitor patients throughout the therapy. After sputum conversion, smear examination and culture are done once in three months till the end of therapy.[43] If such large number of smears and cultures for follow-up is not possible, then atleast five smears and cultures must be done for follow-up (4, 6, 12, 18 and 24 months), X-ray should be done every six months, whereas clinical monitoring preferably should be done every month.[37]

Adjuvant Therapies

In addition to the administration of antimicrobial drug therapy, various other treatment modalities may play a significant role in the management of patients. These include surgery, collapse therapy, laser therapy, immunomodulation therapy and gene therapy.

Surgery

The most common operative procedure is resection surgery. It is adjunct to chemotherapy and should not be considered as the last resort. Chemotherapy should be given atleast for two months prior to surgery and continued for 12 to 24 months after resection. It is indicated in patients who remain sputum-positive, with resistance to large number of drugs; and localized pulmonary disease.[43]

Collapse Therapy

It is a reversible surgical therapy, which involves collapse of lung by artificial pneumoperitonium or pneumothorax used for cavity containing diseased lung with the concept that compression of the cavity will change the local environment in the manner which will inhibit the mycobacteria. This therapy does not appear to be of general utility, although artificial pneumoperitoneum and pneumothorax may be helpful in highly selected cases.[50] However, controlled studies are lacking.

Laser Therapy

This has also been tried as an adjunct to chemotherapy in some countries such as Russia for the treatment of drug-resistant TB. This is effective in multicavitary disease with heavy bacterial loads particularly when there is an increased chance of failure of medical treatment. It is thought to have a role in the rapid killing of bacteria, increases and improves penetration of antitubercular drugs in walled off lesions and helps in early closure of cavities and is of proven benefit in tracheal and bronchial stenosis due to endobronchial growth. It also reduces the trauma of surgery and postoperative complications.

Immunotherapy or Immunomodulation

Therapeutic modulation of the immune system to enhance the host's immunity to control tuberculosis and to shorten the duration of chemotherapy required to 'cure' patients with drug-susceptible disease has been tried with some success. *Mycobacterium vaccae* have shown transiently favorable results when given to drug-resistant tuberculosis, who had failed chemotherapy.[51] Immune modulation can be affected by enhancing proinflammatory cytokines like IL-2, IL-12, IFN-γ, TNF-α, inhibiting the anti-inflammatory cytokines like IL-4, IL-5, IL-10, addition of serum to enhance humoral factors or diverting the harmful Th_2 immune pathway to the beneficial Th_1 response by vaccination utilizing *M. vaccae*. However, these therapies are adjuncts and have proved useful in selected cases of drug-resistant tuberculosis, and randomized control trials have failed to confirm the utility of this therapy.[52] Beneficial effect of parenterally used interferon gamma (IFN-γ) have been reported in disseminated disease attributable to mycobacteria other than tuberculosis that was refractory to chemotherapy.[53] Favorable results were reported following one-month use of inhaled IFN-γ, 500 microgram thrice weekly. Cytokine therapy has been shown to have clinical utility in modifying the inflammatory manifestation of the lepromatous type of disease.[54] Interleukin-2 (IL-2) was used to restore antigen responsiveness, presumably via enhancing IFN-γ production. Thalidomide has been shown to inhibit the in vitro release of TNF-α from peripheral blood monocytes. In patients with active tuberculosis, it induces a significant gain in weight.[55] However, the possibility that thalidomide agents may ameliorate tissue injury in tuberculosis needs further study.[56,57] The potential role of diverse agents such as transfer factor, indomethacin and levamisole is yet to be established.[58] Levamisole as adjunct to drug treatment has been reported to cause more rapid radiological clearing in the treated group. However, it did not significantly affect the clinical outcome.[59] *Mycobacterium w* (commercially available as Immuvac) has been extensively studied as an effective immunomodulator for treatment of leprosy. It enhances bacterial killing and lesion clearance when used as an adjuvant to multi-drug therapy for leprosy. *Mycobacterium w* shares antigens with *M. leprae* as well as *M. tuberculosis* suggesting its application in treatment of drug-resistant tuberculosis. A randomized control study has demonstrated that this drug may be responsible for overall reduction of the duration of therapy, with no change in sputum conversion rate compared with the traditional short-course chemotherapy in new as well as retreatment cases of tuberculosis.[60,61] Another advantage, though not proven, may be that Immuvac effect would be longer lasting and could take care of defaulters more meaningfully than chemotherapy alone, leading to a reduction in relapse rate and the emergence of MDR-TB. Recently, a randomized control trial has been initiated in 2007 and is under progress in order to establish its efficacy and safety as an adjunct therapy in New Pulmonary Tuberculosis (Category I) patients.

Gene Therapy

The decoding of the human genome provides another fascinating aspect in the future therapeutic intervention of tuberculosis. By identifying resistance genes, it will be possible to detect drug resistance before start of therapy and also to develop drugs that target these specific genes, enabling us to considerably reduce the duration of therapy.[62]

Role of Steroids

The adjuvant use of corticosteroids in DR-TB patients has been shown not to increase mortality and can be beneficial in conditions such as severe respiratory insufficiency, severe drug-induced rashes and central nervous system or pericardial involvement. Prednisolone is commonly used, starting at approximately 1 mg/kg and gradually decreasing the dose to 10 mg per week when a long course is indicated. Corticosteroids may also alleviate symptoms in patients with an exacerbation of obstructive pulmonary disease or when the patient is in a very low general condition. In these cases, prednisone may be given in a short course, tapering over 1 to 2 weeks, starting at approximately 1 mg/kg and decreasing the dose by 5 to 10 mg per day. Injectable corticosteroids are often used initially when a more immediate response is needed.[43]

Outcome of Treatment

The outcome of treatment of multi-drug-resistant tuberculosis is not very favorable and varied from 50 to 80% in different studies. In a retrospective analysis of 171 immunocompetent patients treated over a ten year-period (1973–83) at the National Jewish Hospital in Denver, the overall favorable outcome was only a little over 50%.[63] All patients were treated with individually tailored regimens in which they received at least 3 or 4 drugs which they had not received previously, or to which they were known to be susceptible. Of the 134 patients evaluated for efficacy, 65% became culture-negative and 35% failed to respond. Of those who became culture-negative, 14% eventually relapsed, giving an overall favorable outcome in 56% of patients. Of the patients who failed, 46% died of tuberculosis. In the Cape Province, South Africa, the five-year outcome of 240 MDR-TB patients was death in 48%, cure in 33%, 15% were having respiratory disability and 13% were still bacteriologically positive.[64] However, not all the reports are so grim. In a retrospective analysis reported from South Korea, of 107 patients with MDR-TB treated with at least four drugs to which they had not been exposed to before, or to which they were known to be susceptible, in 63 patients with sufficient follow-up data, 52 (82.5%) responded to chemotherapy. There was no subsequent relapse among the patients who responded, and there were no tuberculosis related deaths. The author concluded that MDR-TB responds relatively well to carefully selected regimens. However, the mean period of follow-up was only 17 months.[65] Experience of scientists of TRC, Chennai with MDR-TB has been equally discouraging. In about 170 patients with MDR-TB over a 12-year period (1986–1997), all but two of whom were HIV-negative, only one-third had a favorable outcome, and one-third died. These patients were treated with regimens which included at least three or four of the following drugs: ethionamide, ethambutol, pyrazinamide, cycloserine, streptomycin or kanamycin, PAS, thioacetazone and high-dose isoniazid (600 mg) with 10 mg of pyridoxine. Goble, et al. in a study on 171 patients, showed poor outcome after a mean follow-up period of 5 years, in which only 56% patients responded, and 20% of the mortality was attributed to TB.[63] Khanna, et al.[66] used Kanamycin (6 months), Cycloserine, Ethionamide and Sodium PAS for 18 months in hospitalized patients and observed bacteriological conversion in 10 out of 14 patients (71%). Purohit, et al.[67] used Kanamycin (6 months), Ethionamide, Sodium PAS and Isoniazid for 18 months on domiciliary basis and bacteriological conversion was achieved in 73% of the patients. In another study by Rupak Singla, et al.[68] bacteriological quiescence was achieved in 78% of the patients who completed the full therapy. Prasad, et al.[37] observed 75.5% sputum and culture conversion rate at the end of two years in 45 patients of MDR pulmonary tuberculosis patients by using kanamycin, ethionamide, PAS and cycloserine regimen. Out of 45 patients, 34 (75.5%) patients were decleared cured, these patients followed for average 17.4 months (3–60 months). Two patients relapsed (5.7%). So, long-term outcome was around 70%. This cohort had greater long-term success rates of 75% vs 56% and lower TB death rates, 12% vs 22% than the earlier one. Markers of response in order of reliability are bacteriology of sputum, radiology followed by the clinical picture. A systematic review and meta-analysis of the available therapeutic studies on the treatment of multi-drug-resistant tuberculosis showed that the overall treatment success estimate was 62% (95% CI 58–67%); however, the heterogeneity in study characteristics led to significant variation in reported treatment outcomes. Individualized treatment regimens had higher treatment success (64%, 95% CI 59–68%) than standardized regimens (54%, 95% CI 43–68%), although the difference was not significant. The proportion of patients treated successfully improved when treatment duration was at least 18 months, and if patients received directly observed therapy throughout the treatment. Studies that combined both factors had significantly higher pooled success proportions (69%, 95% CI 64–73%) than other studies of treatment outcomes (58%, 95% CI 52–64%).[69] The outcome for patients with MDR-TB is not very favorable in immunocompetent patients, the response in HIV-positive patients is even bleaker. In the outbreaks of MDR-TB in and around New York city, between 1988 and 1992, predominantly in HIV-infected individuals, mortality was in the order of 80% and the mean duration from diagnosis to death was 4 to 16 weeks. In a study of 173 patients hospitalized from 1983 to 1993 with MDR-TB, of whom 52% were known to be HIV-infected, 55% of the patients in the cohort died; mortality was significantly greater for HIV-positive than HIV-negative (72% vs 20%) patients. The median duration of survival of MDR-TB patients was 22 days to 1 month. In HIV-positive patients, only appropriate therapy was associated with prolonged survival.[63]

Conclusion

The subject of drug-resistant and multi-drug-resistant tuberculosis is a vast one and an area of growing concern among clinicians, epidemiologists and public health workers worldwide. New researches in the areas involving molecular biology and application of these in the field of epidemiology could help in better understanding of the mechanisms of drug resistance and development of newer diagnostic tools and effective drugs to control multi-drug-resistant tuberculosis. Till such time, multi-drug-resistant tuberculosis must be managed very effectively to reduce morbidity and mortality and transmission of multi-drug resistance tuberculosis. It must also be emphasized that even optimal treatment of multi-drug resistance tuberculosis will not alone curb the epidemic. Efforts must be focused on the effective use of first-line drugs in every new case so as to prevent the ultimate emergence of multi-drug-resistant tuberculosis.

References

1. Multi-drug-resistant tuberculosis. ICMR. 1999;29 (10 and 11):105-14.
2. Jin DT, Gross CA. Mapping and sequencing of mutations in the *E. coli* rpoB gene that lead to rifampicin resistance. J mol biol. 1988;202:45-58.
3. Multi-drug-resistant Tuberculosis. Chest. 1993;104(4)1194-8.
4. Cohn ML, Kovitz C, Oda U, Middlebrook G. Studies on isoniazid and tubercle bacilli, II: the growth requirements, catalase activities, and pathogenic properties of isoniazid-resistant mutants. Am Rev Tuberc. 1954;54:641-64.
5. Spider DE, Kelly GD, Cauthen GM, Thompson NJ, Kilburn JO. Infection and disease among contacts of tuberculosis cases with drug-resistant and drug-susceptible bacilli. Am Rev Respir Dis. 1985;132:125-32.
6. Ordway DJ, Sonnenberg MG, Donahue SA, Belisle JT, Orme IM. Drug-resistant strains of *Mycobacterium tuberculosis* exhibit a range of virulence for mice. Infect Immun. 1995;63:741-3.
7. Frieden TR, Sherman LF, Maw KL, et al. A multi-institutional outbreak of highly drug-resistant tuberculosis : epidemiology and clinical outcome. JAMA. 1996;276:1229-35.
8. Stewart SM, Crofton JW. The clinical significance of low degrees of drug resistance in pulmonary tuberculosis. Am Rev Respir Dis. 1964;89:811-29.
9. Mitchison DA, Nunn AJ. Influence of initial drug-resistance on the response to short-course chemotherapy of pulmonary tuberculosis. Am Rev Respir Dis. 1986;133:423-30.
10. Chandrasekaran S, Jagota P, Chaudhuri K. Initial drug resistance to antituberculosis drugs in urban and rural district tuberculosis program. Ind J Tub. 1992;39:171-5.

11. Paramasivan CN, Chandrasekaran V, Santha T, Sudarsanam NM, Prabhakar R. Bacteriological investigations for short-course chemotherapy under the tuberculosis program in two districts in India. Tuber Lung Dis. 1993;74:23-7.
12. Jain NK, Chopra KK, Prasad G. Initial and acquired isoniazid and rifampicin resistance to M. tuberculosis and its implications for treatment. Ind J Tub. 1992;39:121-4.
13. Mathew R, Santha T, Parthasarathy R, Rajaram K, Paramasivan CN, Janardhanam B, et al. Response of patients with initially drug-resistant organisms to treatment with short-course chemotherapy. Ind J Tuberc. 1993;40:119-23.
14. Salomon N, Perlman DC, Friedmann P, Buchstein S, Kreiswirth BN, Mildvan D. Predictors and outcome of multi-drug-resistant tuberculosis. Clin Infect Dis. 1995;21:1245-52.
15. Turett GS, Telzak EE, Torian LV. Improved outcomes for patients with multi-drug-resistant tuberculosis. Clin Infect Dis. 1995;21:1238-44.
16. Telzak EE, Sepkowitz K, Alpert P, et al. Multi-drug-resistant tuberculosis in patients without HIV infection. N Engl J Med. 1995;333:907-11.
17. Park MM, Davis AL, Schluger NW, Cohen H, Rom WN. Outcome of MDR-TB patients, 1983-1993 prolonged survival with appropriate therapy. Am J Respir Crit Care Med. 1996;153:317-24.
18. DOTS-Plus guidelines, Revised National Tuberculosis Control Program, Central TB Divison, Directorate General Health Services, Ministry of Health and Family Welfare, Nirman Bhawan, New Delhi. 2008.
19. National Consensus on MDR Tuberculosis Research Forum India. 1999.
20. Toman K. Tuberculosis case detection, treatment and monitoring. Jaypee Brothers Med. Pub. Pvt. Ltd. 2nd Ind. Ed. 2004; New Delhi.
21. Marks J. Cited in Fox, W. Bulletin of the international union against tuberculosis. 1972;47:49.
22. Wichelhausen RH and Robinson LB. American review of respiratory diseases. 1969;99:1.
23. Guidelines for the Management of Drug-resistant Tuberculosis, Global Tuberculosis Program. WHO/TB/96.210.
24. Laszlo A, et al. Quality assurance program for drugs susceptibility testing of mycobacterium tuberculosis in the WHO/IUATLD supranational laboratory network: first round of proficiency testing. Int J of Tuber Lung Dis. 1997;1:231-8.
25. Treatment of tuberculosis: Guidelines—4th ed. WHO/HTM/TB/2009.420.
26. Casal M, Gutierrez J, Vaquero M. Comparative evaluation of the mycobacteria growth indicator tube with the BACTEC 460 TB system and Löwenstein Jensen medium for isolation of mycobacteria from clinical specimens. Int J Tuberc Lung Dis. 1997;1:81-4.
27. Rivera AB, Tupasi TE, Grimaldo ER, Cardano RC, Co VM. Rapid and improved recovery rate of *Mycobacterium tuberculosis* in mycobacteria growth indicator. Int J Tuebrc Lung Dis. 1997;1:454-9.
28. Heifets LB. Clinical mycobacteriology. Philadelphia: WB Saunders. 1996.
29. Kiehn TE. The diagnostic mycobacteriology laboratory of the 1990s. Clin Infect Dis. 1993;17:S447-54.
30. WHO Press Release New Rapid Test for DR-TB for developing countries like Geneva, 2008.
31. Towards universal access to diagnosis and treatment of multi-drug-resistant and extensively drug-resistant tuberculosis by 2015. WHO progress report 2011. WHO/HTM/TB/2011.3.
32. Telenti A, Imboden P, Marchesi F, Schmidheini T, Bodmer T, et al. Direct automated detection of rifampicin-resistant *Mycobacterium tuberculosis* by polymerase chain reaction and single-strand conformation polymorphism. Antimicrob Agents Chemother. 1993a;37:2054-8.

33. Shoemaker SA, Fisher JH, Jones WE Jr, Scoggin CH. Restriction fragment analysis of chromosomal DNA defines different strains of *Mycobacterium tuberculosis* complex: analysis of restriction fragment heterogenicity using cloned DNA probes. Am Rev Respir Dis. 1986;133:1065-8.
34. Cohn DL, O'Brien RJ. The use of restriction fragment length polymorphism (RFLP) analysis for epidemiological studies of tuberculosis in developing countries. Int J Tuberc Lung Dis. 1998;2:16-26.
35. Dubow MS. Antituberculosis drug screening [commentary]. Lancet. 1993;342:448-9.
36. Hazbon MH. Recent advances in molecular methods for early diagnosis of tuberculosis and drug-resistant tuberculosis. Biomedica. 2004;24(Suppl):149-62.
37. Prasad R, Verma SK, Sahai S, Kumar, Jain A. Efficacy and safety of kanamycin, Ethionamide, PAS, and Cycloserine in Multi-drug-resistant Pulmonary Tuberculosis Patients. Ind J Chest Dis Allied Sci. 2006;48:183-6.
38. Tsukamura M, Mzumo. Cross-resistant relationships among the aminoglycoside antibiotics in *Mycobacterium tuberculosis*. J Gen Microbiol. 1995;98:611.
39. Venkataraman P, Paramsivan CN, Prabhakar R. In vitro activity of rifampicin, rifapentine and rifabutin against South Indian isolates *Mycobacteirum tuberculosis*. Ind J Tub. 1993;40:17.
40. Jain NK, Surpal BB, Khanna SP, Fatma T. In vitro activity of ofloxacin against clinical isolates of *Mycobacterium tuberculosis*. Ind J Tub. 1996;43:183-6.
41. Yew WW, Chan CK, Leung CC, et.al. Comparative roles of levofloxacin and ofloxacin in the treatment of Multi-drug-resistant Tuberculosis: Preliminary results of a retrospective study from Hong-Kong. Chest. 2003;124:1476-81.
42. Canetti G, Kreis B, Thibur R, Gay P, Oe-Lirzin M. Donnees actualles su la resistance primare deus la tuberculose pulmonaire de "L" adulte in France, deuxieme enquiete In Centre d'Etudes sur la resistance Primaire (1) aunees 1865-66. Rev Tuberc Pneumol. 1967;31:433-74.
43. Guidelines for the programmatic management of drug-resistant tuberculosis—WHO 2008.
44. Prasad R. Management of Multi-drug-resistant Tuberculosis practitioner's viewpoint. Ind J Tub. 2007;54:3-11.
45. Treatment of tuberculosis: Guidelines for National Programs. Geneva, WHO, 2003 (WHO CDS/TB/2003.313)
46. Crofton J, Chaulet P, Maher D, Guidelines for the Management of Drug-resistant Tuberculosis, Geneva, WHO, 1997 (Document WHO/TB/96: 210).
47. Mukerjee JS, Rich ML, Socci AR, et al. Programs and principles in the treatment of multi-drug-resistant tuberculosis. Lancet. 2004;363:474-81.
48. Suarez PG, et al. Feasibility and cost effectiveness of standardized second-line drug treatment for chronic tuberculosis patients; a national cohort study in Peru. Lancet. 2002;359:1980-9.
49. Mukherjee J, Socci A, Acha J, et al. The PIH guide to the management of multi-drug-resistant tuberculosis. International edition.
50. Nitta AT, Iseman MD, Newell JD, Madsen LA, Goble M. Ten-year experience with artificial pneumoperitoneum for end-stage, drug-resistant pulmonary tuberculosis. Clin Infect Dis. 1993;16:219-22.
51. Etemadi A, Farid R, Stanford JL. Immunotherapy for drug-resistant tuberculosis [Letter]. Lancet. 1992;340:1360-1.
52. Stanfort JL. Frontiers in mycobacteriology. Symposium sponsored by National Jewish Center for Immunology and Respiratory Medicine, Vail, Colorado. 1997.

53. Holland SN, Eisenstein EM, Kuhns DB, et al. Treatment of refractory disseminated nontuberculous mycobacterial infection with interferon gamma. N Engl J Med. 1994;330:1348-55.
54. Kaplan G. Recent advances in cytokine therapy in leprosy. J Infect Dis. 1993;167:S18-S22.
55. Moller DR, Wysocka M, Greenlee BM. Inhibition of IL-12 production by thalidomide. J Immunol. 1997;159:5157-17.
56. Tremontana JM, Utaipat U, Molloy A, Akarawesi P, Burroughs M, Makonkawkwykoon S, et al. Thalidomide treatment reduces tumor necrosis factor-alpha production and enhances weight gain in patients with pulmonary tuberculosis. Mol Med. 1995;1:384-97.
57. Klausner JD, Makonkawkeyoon S, Akarasewi P, Nataka K, Kasinerk W, Cooral L, et al. The effect of thalidomide on the pathogenesis of human immunodeficiency virus type 1 and *Mycobacterium tuberculosis* infection. J Acquir Immune Defic Syndr Hum Retroviral. 1996;11:247-57.
58. Edwards D, Kirkpatrick CH. The immunology of mycobacterial diseases. Am Rev Respir Dis. 1986;134:1062-71.
59. Singh MM, Kumar P, Malaviya AN, Kumar R. Levamisole as an adjunct in the treatment of pulmonary tuberculosis. Am Rev Respir Dis. 1981;123:277-9.
60. Patel N, Deshpande MM, Shah M. Effect of an immunomodulator containing Mycobacterium w on sputum conversion in pulmonary tuberculosis. J Indian Med Assoc. 2002;100:191-3.
61. Patel N, Tripathi SB. Improved cure rates in pulmonary tuberculosis category II (retreatment) with mycobacterium w. J Indian Med Assoc. 2003;101:680-2.
62. Ian Smith. Stop TB : Is DOTS the Answer? Ind J Tub. 1999;46:81-9.
63. Goble M, Iseman MD, Madson LA, Waite D, Ackerson L, Horsburg CR Jr. Treatment of 171 patients with pulmonary tuberculosis resistant to isoniazid and streptomycin. N Engl J Med. 1993;328:527.
64. Schaaf HS, Botha P, Beyers N, Gie RP, Vermeulen HA, Groenewald P, et al. The 5-year outcome of multi-drug-resistant tuberculosis patients in the Cape Province of South Africa. Trop Med Int Health. 1996;1:718.
65. Park SK, Kim CT, Song SD. Outcome of chemotherapy in 107 patients with pulmonary tuberculosis resistant to isoniazid and rifampicin. Int J Tuber Lung Dis. 1998;2:877.
66. Khanna BK. Treatment of long-term tuberculosis treatment failures. Ind J Tub. 1985;32:171.
67. Purohit SD, Gupta M, Agnihotri SP, Madan A, Gupta PR. Management of chemotherapy failures. Ind J Tub. 1991;38:3.
68. Singla R, Myneedu VP, Jaiswal A, Puri MM, Jain RC. Ethionamide, Cycloserine, Isoniazid, Sodium PAS and Kanamycin in retreatment of drug failure pulmonary tuberculosis patients. Ind J Tub. 1995;42:23.
69. Evan W, Orenstein BS, Basu S, Shah NS, et al. Treatment outcomes among patients with multi-drug-resistant tuberculosis: systematic review and meta-analysis.Lancet Infect Dis. 2009;9:153-61.

Chapter 10

Multi-drug-resistant Tuberculosis: Management in Special Situations

Introduction

Compared to drug-sensitive Tuberculosis, Drug-resistant Tuberculosis (DR-TB) is more demanding in terms of cost of treatment, duration of treatment, higher adverse reactions to second-line drugs, resources required by the treatment providers, and the prolonged adherence required by the patients. To add to these issues, certain associated special situations make the treatment of Multi-drug-resistant Tuberculosis and Extensively Drug-resistant Tuberculosis (M/XDR-TB) more difficult.[1,2] This chapter outlines the management of M/XDR-TB in special conditions and situations like pregnancy, breastfeeding, contraception, children, diabetes mellitus, renal insufficiency, liver disorders, seizure disorders, psychiatric disorders and substance dependence.

M/XDR-TB in Pregnancy

There is a lack of experience in treating pregnant women with M/XDR-TB. Although teratogenicity has been demonstrated in only a few of the drugs used to treat M/XDR-TB, all except ethambutol have uncertain safety information available. This all makes treating M/XDR-TB during pregnancy very challenging. It is prudent to solicit the opinion of an experienced gynecologist/obstetrician and chest physician while treating such patients.[3–7] All female patients of childbearing age should be tested for pregnancy upon initial evaluation. Pregnancy is not a contraindication for the treatment of M/XDR-TB, which poses great risks to the lives of both mother and fetus.[8,9] However, birth control is strongly recommended for all nonpregnant women receiving therapy for M/XDR-TB because of the potential consequences for both mother and fetus resulting from frequent and severe adverse drug reactions. M/XDR-TB patients found to be pregnant prior to treatment initiation or whilst on treatment are evaluated in consultation with a gynecologist/obstetrician taking into consideration the factors like: Risks and benefits of M/XDR-TB treatment, severity of the M/XDR-TB, gestational age and potential risk to the fetus. The risks and benefits of treatment should be carefully considered, with the primary goal of smear conversion to protect the health of the mother and child, both before and after birth. Since the majority of teratogenic effects occur in the first trimester, therapy may be delayed until the second trimester. The decision to postpone the start of treatment should be agreed by both patient and doctor after analysis of the risks and benefits. When the therapy is started, three or four oral drugs with demonstrated efficacy against the infecting strain should be used and then reinforced with an injectable agent and possibly other drugs immediately postpartum.[10] For the most part, aminoglycosides should not be used in the regimens of pregnant patients and can be particularly toxic to the developing fetal ear. Capreomycin may also carry a risk of ototoxicity but is the injectable drug of choice if an injectable agent cannot be avoided. Ethionamide can increase the risk of nausea and vomiting associated with pregnancy, and teratogenic effects have been observed in animal studies. If possible, ethionamide should be avoided in pregnant patients. Further management of M/XDR-TB patients, who are pregnant prior to initiation of M/XDR-TB treatment or whilst on M/XDR-TB treatment, are based on the duration of pregnancy. If the duration of pregnancy is < 20 weeks, the patient should be adviced to opt for a Medical Termination of Pregnancy (MTP) in view of the potential severe risk to both the mother and fetus. If the patient is willing, she should be referred to a gynecologist/obstetrician for MTP following which M/XDR-TB treatment can be initiated if the patient has not started M/XDR-TB treatment or continued if the patient is already on M/XDR-TB treatment. For patients who are unwilling for MTP or have pregnancy of > 20 weeks , the risk to the mother and fetus needs to be explained clearly and a modified M/XDR-TB should be started like: for patients in the first trimester (≤ 12 weeks), kanamycin and ethionamide are omitted from the M/XDR-TB regimen and PAS is added. For patients who have completed the first trimester (> 12 weeks), kanamycin is replaced with PAS. Postpartum, PAS may be replaced with kanamycin and continued until the end of the Intensive Phase. Pregnant M/XDR-TB patients need to be monitored carefully both in relation to the treatment and the progress of the pregnancy. This approach should lead to good results, since the patient should be smear negative at the time of parturition, and mother and infant do not need to be separated. Breastfeeding should be encouraged as long as the patient is sputum negative.

M/XDR-TB in Breastfeeding

Timely and properly applied chemotherapy is the best way to prevent transmission of tubercle bacilli to the baby. A woman, who is breastfeeding and has drug-resistant TB, should receive a full course of antituberculosis treatment. In lactating mothers on treatment, most antituberculosis drugs will be found in the breast milk in concentrations that would equal only a small fraction of the therapeutic dose used in an infant. However, any effect on infants of such exposure during the full course of M/XDR-TB treatment has not been established. Therefore, when resources are available, it is recommended to provide infant formula options as an alternative to breastfeeding. The mother and her baby should not be completely separated. However, if the mother is sputum smear-positive, the care of the infant should be left to family members until she becomes sputum smear-negative, if this is feasible. When the mother and infant are together, this common time should be spent in well-ventilated areas or outdoors. In some settings, the mother may be offered the option of using a surgical mask or an N-95 respirator until she becomes sputum smear-negative.

M/XDR-TB in Contraception

All women of childbearing age who are receiving M/XDR-TB therapy should be adviced to use birth control measures because of the potential risk to both mother and fetus. There is no contraindication to the use of oral contraceptives with the nonrifamycin-containing regimens. It should be remembered that oral contraceptives might have decreased efficacy due to vomiting and drug interactions with second-line drugs. These patients should be adviced to take their contraceptives apart from times when they may experience vomiting caused by the antituberculosis treatment. Patients who vomit at any time directly after, or within the first two hours after, taking the contraceptive tablet, should use a barrier method of contraception until a full month of the contraceptive tablets can be tolerated. Thus, for prevention of pregnancy, the use of barrier methods (condoms/diaphragm), IUDs (CuT) or depotmedrox-progesterone are recommended based on individual preference and eligibility. Similarly, all women of child-bearing age identified as DR-TB suspects should be advised to use a reliable and appropriate contraceptive method till the results of culture and Drug Susceptibility Test (DST) are available. For patients with mono- and poly-resistant TB that is susceptible to rifampicin, the use of rifampicin interacts with the contraceptive drugs resulting in decreased efficacy of protection against pregnancy. A woman on oral contraception while receiving rifampicin treatment may choose between two options: following consultation with a physician, use of an oral contraceptive pill containing a higher dose of estrogen (50 μg); or use of another form of contraception.

M/XDR-TB in Children

There is only limited reported experience with the use of second-line drugs for extended periods in children. Frank discussion with family members is critical, especially at the outset of therapy. The risks and benefits of each drug should be carefully considered in designing a regimen. Children with drug-resistant TB generally have primary resistance transmitted from an index case with drug-resistant TB. When DST is available, it should be used to guide therapy, although children with paucibacillary TB are often culture-negative. Nevertheless, every effort should be made to confirm drug-resistant TB bacteriologically by the use of DST and to avoid exposing children unnecessarily to toxic drugs. The treatment of culture-negative children with clinical evidence of active TB disease and contact with a documented case of drug-resistant TB should be guided by the results of DST and the history of the contact's exposure to antituberculosis drugs.[11] M/XDR-TB is life-threatening, and no antituberculosis drugs are absolutely contraindicated in children. Children who have received treatment for drug-resistant TB have generally tolerated the second-line drugs well.[11-12] Fluoroquinolones have been shown to retard cartilage development in beagle puppies,[13]experience with the use of fluoroquinolones in humans has not demonstrated similar effects.[14-15] It is considered that the benefit of fluoroquinolones in treating M/XDR-TB in children outweighs any risk. Additionally, ethionamide, PAS and cycloserine have been used effectively in children and are well tolerated. In general, dose of antituberculosis drugs should be according to the body weight as given below in tabulated form (Table 10.1). Monthly monitoring of body weight is, therefore, especially important in pediatric cases, with adjustment of doses as children gain weight.[16] Doses of all drugs, including the fluoroquinolones, should be given at the higher end of the recommended ranges whenever possible, except ethambutol.[11-17] Ethambutol should be dosed at 15 mg/kg, and not at 25 mg/kg as sometimes used in adults with M/XDR-TB, as it is more difficult to monitor for optic neuritis in children. In children who are not culture-positive initially, treatment failure is difficult to assess. Persistent abnormalities on chest radiograph do not necessarily signify a lack of improvement. In children, weight loss or, more commonly, failure to gain weight adequately, is of particular concern and often one of the first signs of treatment failure. This is another key reason to monitor weight carefully in children. Anecdotal evidence suggests that adolescents are at high risk for poor treatment outcomes. Early diagnosis, strong social support, individual and family counseling and a close relationship with the medical provider may help improve outcomes in this group.

M/XDR-TB in Diabetes Mellitus

Diabetes must be managed closely throughout the treatment of M/XDR-TB. The healthcare provider should be in close communication with the physician, who manages the patient's diabetes. Diabetic patients with M/XDR-TB are at risk for poor outcomes. In addition, the presence of diabetes mellitus may potentiate

TABLE 10.1: Pediatric dosing of second-line antituberculosis drugs

Drug	*Daily dose (mg/kg)*	*Frequency*	*Maximum daily dose*
Streptomycin	20–40	Once daily	1 g
Kanamycin	15–30	Once daily	1 g
Amikacin	15–22.5	Once daily	1 g
Capreomycin	15–30	Once daily	1 g
Ofloxacin	15–20	Once or twice daily	800 mg
Levofloxacin	7.5–10	Once daily	750 mg
Moxifloxacin	7.5–10	Once daily	400 mg
Ethionamide	15–20	Once or twice daily	1 g
Prothionamide	15–20	Once or twice daily	1 g
Cycloserine	10–20	Once or twice daily	1 g
P-aminosalicylic acid	150	Twice daily	12 g

the adverse effects of antitituberculosis drugs, especially renal dysfunction and peripheral neuropathy. Oral hypoglycemic agents are not contraindicated during the treatment of M/XDR-TB but may require the patient to increase the dosage. Use of ethionamide or protionamide may make it more difficult to control insulin levels. Creatinine and potassium levels should be monitored more frequently, often weekly for the first month and then at least monthly thereafter.

M/XDR-TB in Renal Insufficiency

Renal insufficiency due to longstanding TB disease itself, previous use of aminoglycosides or concurrent renal disease, is not uncommon. Great care should be taken in the administration of second-line drugs in patients with renal impairment. Consideration needs to be taken that M/XDR-TB patients require aminoglycosides for 6 months or more. Other drugs, which also might require dose or interval adjustment in presence of mild to moderate renal impairment are: Ethambutol, quinolones, cycloserine and PAS. In the presence of severe renal impairment, many other drugs may also require adjustments as given below in tabulated form (Table 10.2). In M/XDR-TB patients, blood urea and serum

TABLE 10.2: Adjustment of antituberculosis medication in renal insufficiency

Drug	*Change in frequency*	*Recommended dose and frequency for patients with creatinine clearance < 30 mL/min or for patients receiving hemodialysis*
Isoniazid	No change	300 mg once daily, or 900 mg three times per week
Pyrazinamide	Yes	25–35 mg/kg per dose three times per week (not daily)
Ethambutol	Yes	15–25 mg/kg per dose three times per week (not daily)
Ofloxacin	Yes	600–800 mg per dose three times per week (not daily)
Levofloxacin	Yes	750–1000 mg per dose three times per week (not daily)
Moxifloxacin	No change	400 mg once daily
Cycloserine	Yes	250 mg once daily, or 500 mg/dose three times per week
Terizidone	-	Recommendations not available
Prothionamide	No change	250–500 mg per dose daily
Ethionamide	No change	250–500 mg per dose daily
P-aminosalicylic acid[e]	No change	4 g/dose, twice daily
Capreomycin	Yes	12–15 mg/kg per dose two or three times per week (not daily)
Kanamycin	Yes	12–15 mg/kg per dose two or three times per week (not daily)
Amikacin	Yes	12–15 mg/kg per dose two or three times per week (not daily)
Clarithromycin	Yes	Usual dose 500 mg twice daily but can be reduced to 250 mg twice daily
Linezolid	No change needed	Usual adult dose is 600 mg twice daily
Clofazimine	Yes	Begin at 300 mg daily and decrease to 100 mg after 4 to 6 weeks
Amoxycillin and Clavulanic acid	Yes	Dose used is 625 mg twice daily, 1000 mg should not be administered

creatinine should be monitored prior to treatment initiation, monthly for three months after treatment initiation and then every three months whilst injection Kanamycin is being administered. In patients with mild renal impairment, the dose of aminoglycosides may be reduced. In the presence of severe renal failure, the aminoglycoside therapy should be discontinued and replaced with other potent non-nephrotoxic antituberculosis drugs.[18]

M/XDR-TB in Liver Disorders

Pyrazinamide is the most hepatotoxic of the three first-line drugs (Rifampicin, Isoniazid, Pyrazinamide). Among the second-line drugs, ethionamide, protionamide and PAS can also be hepatotoxic, although less than any of the first-line drugs. Hepatitis occurs rarely with the flouroquinolones. The potential for hepatotoxicity is increased in elderly, alcoholics and in patients with pre-existing liver disease. In general, most of the second-line drugs can be safely used in the presence of mild hepatic impairment, as they are relatively less hepatotoxic than the first-line drugs. However, pyrazinamide should be avoided in such patients. All other drugs can be used, but close monitoring of liver enzymes is advised. If significant aggravation of liver inflammation occurs, the drugs responsible may have to be stopped. Once a patient on second-line drugs develops hepatitis, other etiologies should also be excluded, such as viral hepatitis, alcoholic hepatitis and drug-induced hepatitis by non-TB drugs.[19]

M/XDR-TB in Seizure Disorders

TB might itself involve central nervous system and may cause seizures. However, when seizures are present for the first time during anti-TB therapy, they are likely to be the result of an adverse effect of one of the anti-TB drugs. Among the second-line drugs, cycloserine, ethionamide and fluoroquinolones have been associated with seizures. Some patients requiring treatment for M/XDR-TB will have a past or present medical history of a seizure disorder. The first step in evaluating such patients is to determine whether the seizure disorder is under control and whether the patient is taking antiseizure medication to control the disorder. If the seizures are not under control, initiation or adjustment of antiseizure medications will be needed prior to the start of M/XDR-TB therapy. In addition, if other underlying conditions or causes for seizures exist, they should be corrected. Pyridoxine should be given with cycloserine to prevent seizures. Cycloserine should, however, be avoided in patients with active seizure disorders that are not well-controlled with medication. In cases where no other drug is appropriate, cycloserine can be given and the antiseizure medication adjusted as needed to control the seizure disorder. The risk and benefits of using cycloserine should be discussed with the patient and the decision on whether to use cycloserine are made together with the patient. Antiepileptic drugs may have drug interactions with cycloserine and quinolones. Hence, close monitoring of serum levels of antiepileptic drugs should be done.[19,20]

M/XDR-TB in Substance Dependence

Patients with substance dependence disorders should be offered treatment for their addiction. Complete abstinence from alcohol or other substances should be strongly encouraged, although active consumption is not a contraindication for antituberculosis treatment. If the treatment is repeatedly interrupted because of the patient's dependence, therapy should be suspended until successful treatment or measures to ensure adherence have been established. Good DOT gives the patient contact with and support from healthcare providers, which often allows complete treatment even in patients with substance dependence. Cycloserine will have a higher incidence of adverse effects in patients dependent on alcohol or other substances, including higher incidence of seizures. However, if cycloserine is considered important to the regimen, it should be used and the patient closely observed for adverse effects, which are then adequately treated.

M/XDR-TB in Patients with Psychosis

There is a high baseline incidence of depression and anxiety in patients with M/XDR-TB, often connected with the chronicity and socioeconomic stress factors related to the disease. For M/XDR-TB patients with a concurrent psychiatric illness, it is advisable to have an evaluation carried out by a psychiatrist before the start of treatment for M/XDR-TB. The initial evaluation documents any pre-existing psychiatric condition and establishes a baseline for comparison if new psychiatric symptoms develop while the patient is on treatment. Any identified psychiatric illness at the start or during treatment should be fully addressed. If a healthcare worker with psychiatric training is not available, the treating healthcare provider should document any psychiatric conditions the patient may have at the initial evaluation. Treatment with psychiatric medication, individual counseling, and/or group therapy may be necessary to manage the patient suffering from a psychiatric condition or adverse psychiatric effect due to medication.[21,22] Fluoroquinolones and ethionamide have been associated with psychosis. Pyridoxine prophylaxis may minimize risk of neurologic and psychiatric adverse reactions. Cycloserine may cause severe psychosis and depression leading to suicidal tendencies. However, the use of cycloserine is not absolutely contraindicated for the psychiatric patient. Adverse effects of cycloserine may be more prevalent in the psychiatric patient, but the benefits of using this drug often outweigh the potential higher risk of adverse effects. Close monitoring is recommended if cycloserine is used in patients with psychiatric disorders. If patient on cycloserine therapy develops psychosis, antipsychotic treatment should be started and cycloserine therapy should be temporarily suspended. Once symptoms resolve and patient is stabilized, cycloserine therapy may be resumed. Such patients may require antipsychotic treatment till anti-TB treatment is completed. When any patient on M/XDR-TB treatment develops psychosis, other etiologies such as psychosocial stresses, depression, hypothyroidism, illicit drug and alcohol use, should also be looked for. All health-care workers treating drug-resistant TB should work closely with a mental health specialist and have an organized system for psychiatric emergencies.[21,22]

References

1. WHO/IUATLD. Global Project on Antituberculosis Drug Resistance Surveillance. Antituberculosis drug resistance in the world. Report No.2. HO/CDS/TB/2000.278.
2. World Health Organization. The WHO/IUATLD. Global Project on Antituberculosis Drug Resistance Surveillance: Antituberculosis drug resistance in the world. Report No.3.Geneva: Switzerland. WHO/CDS/TB/2004.
3. Drobac PC, del Castillo H, Sweetland A, Anca G, Joseph JK, Furin J, Shin S. Treatment of multidrug-resistant tuberculosis during pregnancy: long-term follow-up of 6 children with intrauterine exposure to second-line agents. Clin Infect Dis. 2005;40:1689-92.
4. Shin S, Guerra D, Rich M, Seung KJ, Mukherjee J, Joseph K, et al. Treatment of multidrug-resistant tuberculosis during pregnancy: a report of 7 cases. ClinInfect Dis. 2003;36:996-1003.
5. Duff P. Antibiotic selection in obstetric patients. Infect Dis Clin North Am. 1997;11:1-12.
6. Valleho JG, Surke Jr. Tuberculosis and Pregnancy Clinic Chest Med. 1992;13:693-707.
7. Hamadeh MA, Glassroth J. Tuberculosis and Pregnancy: Chest. 1992;101:1114-20.1.
8. Figueroa-Damián R, Arredondo-García JL. Neonatal outcome of children born to women with tuberculosis. Archives of Medical Research. 2001;32:66-9.
9. Brost BC, Newman RB. The maternal and fetal effects of tuberculosis therapy. Obstetrics and Gynecology Clinics of North America. 1997;24:659-73.
10. Duff P. Antibiotic selection in obstetric patients. Infectious Disease Clinics of North America. 1997;11:1-12.
11. Swanson DS, Starke JR. Drug-resistant tuberculosis in pediatrics. Pediatric Clinics of North America. 1995;42:553-81.
12. Mukherjee JS, Joseph JK, Rich ML, Shin SS, Furin JJ, Seung KJ, et al. Clinical and programmatic considerations in the treatment of MDR-TB in children: a series of 16 patients from Lima, Peru. Int J Tuber Lung Dis. 2003;7:637-44.
13. Takizawa T, Hashimoto K, Minami T, Yamashita S, Owen K. The comparative arthropathy of fluoroquinolones in dogs. Human and Experimental Toxicology. 1999;18:392-9.
14. Warren RW. Rheumatologic aspects of pediatric cystic fibrosis patients treated with fluoroquinolones. Pediatric Infectious Disease Journal. 1997;16:118-22.
15. Hampel B, Hullmann R, Schmidt H. Ciprofloxacin in pediatrics: Worldwide clinical experience based on compassionate use—safety report. Pediatric Infectious Disease Journal. 1997;16(1):127-9.
16. Loebstein R, Koren G. Clinical pharmacology and therapeutic drug monitoring in neonates and children. Pediatric Review. 1998;19:42-428.
17. Siberry GK, Iannone R, eds. The Harriet Lane Handbook, 15th ed. Baltimore, Mosby; 2000.
18. Ruckenstein MI. Vertigo and disequilibrium with associated hearing loss. Otolaryngeal Clin North Am. 2000;33:535-62.
19. Braunwald E. Harrison's Principal of Internal Medicine. 15th edition. New York: McGraw-Hill, 2001.
20. WHO. Treatment of tuberculosis: Guidelines for national programmes. WHO/CDS/TB 2003.313. Geneva: WHO 2003.
21. Lansdown FS, Beran M, Litwak T. Psychotoxic reaction during ethionamide therapy: Am Rev Resp Dis. 1967;95:1053-5.
22. Patel AM, McKeon J. Avoidance and management of adverse reactions to antituberculosis drugs. Drugs Saf. 1995;12:1-25.

Chapter 11

Multi-drug-resistant Tuberculosis: Monitoring of Treatment and Adverse Drug Reaction

Introduction

The initial evaluation serves to establish a baseline and may identify patients who are at increased risk for adverse effects or poor outcomes. The monitoring of treatment and the management of adverse effects may have to be more intensive in patients with pre-existing conditions or conditions identified at the initial evaluation (diabetes mellitus, renal insufficiency, acute or chronic liver disease, thyroid disease, mental illness, drug or alcohol dependence, HIV infection, pregnancy, lactation and others). This chapter aims to address the monitoring requirements for the treatment of Drug-resistant Tuberculosis (DR-TB), adverse effects associated with different second-line drugs, strategies for the early detection and treatment of adverse effects and also adverse effects in Human Immunodeficiency Virus (HIV) coinfected patients with DR-TB.

Pretreatment Screening and Evaluation

The required initial pretreatment clinical investigation includes a thorough medical history and physical examination. The recommended initial evaluation and monitoring during treatment of DR-TB are shown in Table 11.1.

TABLE 11.1: Pretreatment evaluation and monitoring during MDR-TB treatment

Monitoring evaluation	*Recommended frequency*
Evaluation by clinician	At baseline, and at least monthly until conversion, then every 2–3 months
Screening by DOT worker	At every DOT encounter
Sputum smears and cultures	For follow-up examination four sputum specimens will be collected and examined by smear and culture at least 30 days apart from the 3rd to 7th month of treatment (i.e. at the end of the months 3, 4, 5, 6 and 7) and at 3-monthly intervals from the 9th month onwards till the completion of treatment (i.e. at the end of the months 9, 12, 15, 18, 21 and 24)
Weight	At baseline and then monthly
Drug susceptibility	At baseline in programs doing individualized treatment or in programs doing standardized treatments that need to confirm MDR-TB. For patients who remain culture-positive, it is not necessary to repeat DST within less than 3 months of treatment

Contd...

Contd...

Monitoring evaluation	*Recommended frequency*
Chest radiograph	At baseline, and then every 6 months
Serum creatinine	At baseline, then monthly, if possible while receiving an injectable drug. Every 1–3 weeks in HIV-infected patients, diabetes and other high-risk patients
Serum potassium	Monthly while receiving an injectable agent. Every 1–3 weeks in HIV-infected patients, diabetics and other high-risk patients
Thyroid stimulating hormone (TSH)	Every 6 months, if receiving ethionamide/protionamide and/or PAS; and monitor monthly for signs/symptoms of hypothyroidism. TSH is sufficient for screening for hypothyroidism; it is not necessary to measure hormone thyroid levels
Liver serum enzymes	Periodic monitoring (every 1–3 months) in patients receiving pyrazinamide for extended periods or for patients at risk for or with symptoms of hepatitis. For HIV-infected patients, do monthly monitoring
HIV screening	At baseline, and repeat, if clinically indicated
Pregnancy tests	At baseline for women of childbearing age, and repeat if indicated
Hemoglobin and white blood count	If on linezolid, monitor weekly at first, then monthly or as needed based on symptoms; there is little clinical experience with prolonged use. For HIV-positive patients on an ART regime that includes AZT, monitor monthly initially and then as needed based on symptoms.
Lipase	Indicated for work-up of abdominal pain to rule out pancreatitis in patients on linezolid, stavudine, didanosine and zalcitabine
Lactic acidosis	Indicated for work-up of lactic acidosis in patients on linezolid or antiretroviral treatment
Serum glucose	If receiving gatifloxacin, monitor glucose frequently (weekly) and educate patient on signs and symptoms of hypoglycemia and hyperglycemia

Monitoring Progress of Treatment

Clinically, the most important way to monitor response to treatment is through regular history taking and physical examination. The classic symptoms of TB like cough, sputum production, fever and weight loss generally improve within first few months of treatment and should be monitored frequently by healthcare providers. Patients should be monitored closely for signs of treatment failure. The recurrence of TB symptoms after sputum conversion, for example, may be the first sign of treatment failure. For children, height and weight should be measured regularly to ensure that they are growing normally. A normal growth rate should resume after a few months of successful treatment. Objective laboratory evidence of improvement often lags behind clinical improvement. The chest radiograph may be unchanged or show only slight improvement, especially in retreatment patients with chronic pulmonary lesions. Chest radiographs should be taken at least every six months, when a surgical intervention is being considered, or whenever the patient's clinical situation has worsened. The most important objective evidence of improvement is conversion of the sputum smear and culture to negative. While sputum smear is still useful clinically because of its much shorter turnaround time, sputum culture is much more sensitive and is necessary to monitor the progress of treatment. Sputum examinations are also dependent on the quality of the sputum produced. So care should be taken to obtain adequate specimens. Persistently positive sputums and cultures for *Mycobacterium tuberculosis* bacilli should be assessed for Nontuberculous Mycobacteria (NTM), as overgrowth with NTM in lung damage secondary to TB is not uncommon. In such cases, although DR-TB may be adequately treated, treatment may need to be directed towards the NTM as well. Sputum conversion is slower in DR-TB than in drug-susceptible TB. Paucibacillary culture results should not be automatically regarded as negative when treating DR-TB. Acquired drug resistance and treatment failure often begin with the growth of one or two colonies on a sputum culture. Culture conversion should not be considered to be equivalent to cure. A certain proportion of patients may initially convert and later revert to positive sputum culture. Sputum smears and cultures should be monitored closely throughout treatment. These guidelines recommend that the tests be performed monthly before smear and culture conversion, with conversion defined as two consecutive negative smears and cultures taken 30 days apart. After conversion, the minimum period recommended for bacteriological monitoring is monthly for smears and quarterly for cultures. Programs with adequate culture capacity may choose to do cultures more frequently, every 1 to 2 months, after conversion. Specimens for monitoring do not need to be examined in duplicate, but doing so can increase the sensitivity of monitoring. For patients who remain smear- and culture-positive during treatment or who are suspects for treatment failure, DST can be repeated. It is usually not necessary to repeat Drug Susceptibility Testing (DST) within less than three months of the completion of treatment.

Monitoring for Adverse Effects During Treatment

Close monitoring of patients is necessary to ensure that the adverse effects of second-line drugs are recognized quickly by healthcare personnel. The ability to monitor patients for adverse effects daily is one of the major advantages of Directly Observed Therapy (DOT) over self-administration of DR-TB treatment. The majority of adverse effects are easy to recognize. Commonly, patients will volunteer that they are experiencing adverse effects. However, it is important to have a systematic method of patient interviewing since some patients may not reveal even severe adverse effects. Other patients may be distracted by one adverse effect and forget to tell the healthcare provider about others. Laboratory screening is invaluable for detecting certain adverse effects that are more occult. The recommendations based on the experience of several DOTS-Plus projects[1] for the minimal frequency of essential laboratory screening is given above in tabulated form. More frequent screening may be advisable, particularly for high-risk patients. Nephrotoxicity is a known complication of the injectable drugs, both of the aminoglycosides and of capreomycin. This adverse effect is occult in onset and can be fatal. The optimal timing for checking serum creatinine is unknown, but most current treatment programs for DR-TB check serum creatinine at least monthly. In addition, patients with a history of renal disease (including comorbidities such as HIV and diabetes), advanced age or any renal symptoms should be monitored more closely, particularly at the start of treatment. An estimate of the glomerular filtration rate may help to further stratify the risk of nephrotoxicity in these patients. Electrolyte imbalance is a known complication of the antituberculosis injectable drugs, most frequently with capreomycin. It is generally a late effect occurring after months of treatment, and is reversible once the injectable drug is suspended. Since electrolyte imbalance is often occult in the early stages and can be easily managed with electrolyte replacement, serum potassium should be checked at least monthly in high-risk patients, and in all those taking capreomycin.[2] Hypothyroidism is a late effect provoked by PAS and ethionamide. It is suspected by clinical assessment and confirmed by testing the serum level of thyroid stimulating hormone (TSH). The use of these agents together can produce hypothyroidism in up to 10% of patients.[3] Since the symptoms can be subtle, it is recommended that patients are screened for hypothyroidism with a serum TSH at 6 to 9 months, and then tested again every 6 months or sooner if symptoms arise. The dosing of thyroid replacement therapy should be guided using serum levels of TSH. Goiter can develop due to the toxic effects of PAS, ethionamide or protionamide.

Management of Adverse Effects

Second-line drugs have many more adverse effects than the first-line anti-tuberculosis drugs. Proper management of adverse effects begins with patient education. Before starting treatment, the patient should be instructed in detail about the potential adverse effects that could be produced by the prescribed drug regimen. Prompt evaluation, diagnosis and treatment of adverse effects are extremely important, even if the adverse effect is not particularly dangerous. Patients may have significant fear and anxiety about an adverse effect if they do not understand why it is happening. These emotions, in turn, may augment the severity of the adverse effect, as in the case of nausea and vomiting. If the adverse effect is mild and not dangerous, continuing the treatment regimen, with the help of ancillary drugs if needed, is often the best option. In patients with highly resistant TB, a satisfactory replacement drug may not be available, so that suspending a drug will make the treatment regimen less potent. Some adverse effects may disappear or diminish with time, and patients may be able to continue receiving the drug if sufficiently motivated. The adverse effects of a number of second-line drugs are highly dose-dependent. Reducing the dosage of the offending drug is another method of managing adverse effects, but only in cases where the reduced dose is still expected to produce adequate serum levels and not compromise the regimen. With cycloserine and ethionamide, for example, a patient may be completely intolerant at one dose and completely tolerant at a slightly lower dose. Unfortunately, given the narrow therapeutic margins of these drugs, lowering the dose may also affect efficacy, so every effort should be made to maintain an adequate dose of the drug according to body weight.

Pyridoxine (vitamin B6) should be given to all patients receiving cycloserine or terizidone to help prevent neurological adverse effects. The recommended dose is 50 mg for every 250 mg of cycloserine (or terizidone) prescribed. Psychosocial support is an important component of the management of adverse effects. The common adverse effects, the likely responsible antituberculosis agents and the suggested management strategies are given below in a tabulated form (Table 11.2).

TABLE 11.2: Common adverse effects, suspected agent(s) and management strategies of antituberculous drugs used in drug-resistant patients of TB

Adverse effect	*Suspected agent*	*Suggested management strategies*
Seizures	**Cs** H Fq	• Suspend suspected agent pending resolution of seizures • Initiate anticonvulsant therapy (e.g. phenytoin, valproic acid) • Increase pyridoxine to maximum daily dose (200 mg per day) • Restart suspected agent or reinitiate suspected agent at lower dose, if essential to the regimen • Discontinue suspected agent if this can be done without compromising regimen • Anticonvulsant is generally continued until MDR-TB treatment is completed or suspected agent discontinued • History of previous seizure disorder is not a contraindication to the use of agents listed here if a patient's seizures are well controlled and/or the patient is receiving anticonvulsant • Patients with history of previous seizures may be at increased risk for development of seizures during MDR-TB.
Peripheral neuropathy	**Cs** **Lzd** **H** S Km Am Cm Eto/Pto Fq	• Increase pyridoxine to maximum daily dose (200 mg per day) • Change injectable to capreomycin if patient has documented susceptibility to capreomycin • Initiate therapy with tricyclic antidepressants such as amitriptyline. Non-steroidal anti-inflammatory drugs or acetaminophen may help alleviate symptoms • Lower dose of suspected agent, if this can be done without compromising regimen • Discontinue suspected agent if this can be done without compromising regimen. • Patients with co-morbid disease (e.g. diabetes, HIV, alcoholneuropathy (dependence) may be more likely to develop peripheral neuropathy, but these conditions are not contraindications to the use of the agents listed here • Neuropathy may be irreversible; however, some patients may experience improvement when offending agents are suspended.
Hearing loss	**S** **Km** **Am** **Cm** Clr	• Document hearing loss and compare with baseline audiometry if available • Change parenteral treatment to capreomycin if patient has documented susceptibility to capreomycin • Decrease frequency and/or lower dose of suspected agent if this can be done without compromising the regimen (consider administration three times per week) • Discontinue suspected agent if this can be done without compromising the regimen • Patients with previous exposure to aminoglycosides may have baseline hearing loss. In such patients, audiometry may be helpful at the start of MDR-TB therapy • Hearing loss is generally not reversible • The risk of further hearing loss must be weighed against the risks of stopping the injectable in the treatment regimen • While the benefit of hearing aids is minimal to moderate in auditory toxicity, consider a trial use to determine if a patient with hearing loss can benefit from their use

Contd...

Contd...

Adverse effect	*Suspected agent*	*Suggested management strategies*
Psychotic Symptoms	**Cs** **H** Fq Eto/Pto	• Stop suspected agent for a short period of time (1–4 weeks) while psychotic symptoms are brought under control • Initiate antipsychotic therapy • Lower dose of suspected agent if this can be done without compromising regimen • Discontinue suspected agent if this can be done without compromising regimen • Some patients will need to continue antipsychotic treatment throughout MDR-TB therapy • Previous history of psychiatric disease is not a contraindication to the use of agents listed here but may increase the likelihood of psychotic symptoms developing during treatment • Psychotic symptoms are generally reversible upon completion of MDR-TB treatment or cessation of the offending agent.
Depression	**Cs** Fq Eto/Pto H	• Offer group or individual counseling • Initiate antidepressant therapy • Lower dose of suspected agent if this can be done without compromising regimen • Discontinue suspected agent if this can be done without compromising regimen • Socioeconomic conditions and chronic illness should not be underestimated as contributing factors to depression • Depressive symptoms may fluctuate during therapy and may improve as illness is successfully treated • History of previous depression is not a contraindication to the use of the agents listed but may increase the likelihood of depression developing during treatment.
Hypo-thyroidism	**PAS** **Eto/Pto**	• Initiate thyroxine therapy • Completely reversible upon discontinuation of PAS or ethionamide/ protionamide • The combination of ethionamide/protionamide with PAS is more frequently associated with hypothyroidism than the individual use of each drug.
Nausea and vomiting	**Eto/Pto** **PAS** H E Z	• Assess for dehydration; initiate rehydration if indicated • Initiate antiemetic therapy • Lower dose of suspected agent if this can be done without compromising regimen • Discontinue suspected agent if this can be done without compromising regimen rarely necessary • Nausea and vomiting universal in early weeks of therapy and and usually abate with time on treatment and adjunctive therapy • Electrolytes should be monitored if vomiting is severe • Reversible upon discontinuation of suspected agent • Severe abdominal distress and acute abdomen have been reported with the use of clofazimine. Although these reports are rare, if this effect occurs, clofazimine should be suspended.
Gastritis	**PAS** **Eto/Pto**	• H2-blockers, proton-pump inhibitors, or antacids • Stop suspected agent(s) for short periods of time (e.g. 1–7 days) • Lower dose of suspected agent, if this can be done without compromising regimen • Discontinue suspected agent if this can be done without compromising regimen • Severe gastritis, as manifested by hematemesis, melena or haematechezia, is rare • Dosing of antacids should be carefully timed so as to not interfere with the absorption of antituberculosis drugs (take 2 hours before or 3 hours after antituberculosis medications) • Reversible upon discontinuation of suspected agent(s).

Contd...

Contd...

Adverse effect	*Suspected agent*	*Suggested management strategies*
Hepatitis	**Z** **H** **R** Eto/Pto PASE Fq	• Stop all therapy pending resolution of hepatitis • Eliminate other potential causes of hepatitis • Consider suspending most likely agent permanently • Re-introduce remaining drugs, one at a time while monitoring liver function • History of previous hepatitis should be carefully analysed to determine most likely causative agent(s); these should be avoided in future regimens • Generally reversible upon discontinuation of suspected agent.
Renal toxicity	**S** **Km** **Am** **Cm**	• Discontinue suspected agent • Consider using capreomycin if an aminoglycoside had been the prior injectable in regimen • Consider dosing 2–3 times a week if drug is essential to the regimen and patient can tolerate (close monitoring of creatinine) • Adjust all anti-tuberculosis medications according to the creatinine clearance • History of diabetes or renal disease is not a contraindication to the use of the agents listed here, although patients with these co-morbidities may be at increased risk for developing renal failure • Renal impairment may be permanent.
Electrolyte disturbances (hypokalemia and hypomagnesemia)	**Cm** **Km** **Am** S	• Check potassium • If potassium is low, also check magnesium (and calcium if hypocalcemia is suspected) • Replace electrolytes as needed • If severe hypokalaemia is present, consider hospitalization • Amiloride 5 to 10 mg QD or spironolactone 25 mg QD may decrease potassium and magnesium wasting and is useful in refractory cases • Oral potassium replacements can cause significant nausea and vomiting. Oral magnesium may cause diarrhea.
Optic neuritis	**E** Eto/Pto	• Stop E • Refer patient to an ophthalmologist • Usually reverses with cessation of E • Rare case reports of optic neuritis have been attributed to streptomycin.
Arthralgias	**Z** Fq	• Initiate therapy with non-steroidal anti-inflammatory drugs • Lower dose of suspected agent if this can be done without compromising regimen • Discontinue suspected agent if this can be done without compromising regimen • Uric acid levels may be elevated in patients on pyrazinamide. Allopurinol appears not to correct the uric acid levels in such cases • Symptoms of arthralgia generally diminish over time, even without intervention

Antitubercular agent: Isoniazid (H), Rifampicin (R), Ethambutol (E), Pyrazinamide (Z), Streptomycin (S), Kanamycin (Km), Amikacin (Am), Capreomycin (Cm), Flouroquinolones (Fq), Ethionamide (Eto), Protionamide(Pto), P-aminosalicylic acid (PAS), Cycloserine (Cs), Clofazimine (Cfz), Linezolid (Lzd), Clarithromycin (Clr).
Drugs that the strongly associated with adverse effects shown in bold.

Conclusion

The initial evaluation, timely and intensive monitoring for, and management of, adverse effects caused by second-line drugs are essential components of DR-TB control programs. Poor management of adverse effects increases the risk of default or irregular adherence to treatment, and may result in death or permanent morbidity.The physicians should be familiar with the common adverse effects of MDR-TB therapy. Patients experiencing adverse effects should be referred to specialists who have experience in treating the adverse effects. It is rarely necessary to suspend antituberculosis drugs completely. Ancillary drugs for the management of adverse effects should be available to the patient and without charge.

References

1. Nathanson E, Gupta R, Huamani P, Leimane V, Pasechnikov AD, Tupasi TE, et al. Adverse events in the treatment of multidrug-resistant tuberculosis: results from the DOTS-Plus initiative. Int J of Tuber Lung Dis. 2004;8:1382-4.
2. Shin S, Furin J, Alcantara F, et al. Hypokalemia among patients receiving treatment for multidrug-resistant tuberculosis. Chest. 2004;125:974-80.
3. Furin JJ, Mitnick CD, Shin SS, Bayona J, Becerra MC, Singler JM, et al. Occurrence of serious adverse effects in patients receiving community-based therapy for multidrug-resistant tuberculosis. Int J Tuber Lung Dis. 2001;5:648-55.

Chapter 12

Multi-drug-resistant Tuberculosis: Case-based Approach

Case I

TS, a 18-year-old female diagnosed as pulmonary tuberculosis in 1995 was prescribed rifampicin, isoniazid and ethambutol, which she stopped herself after four months due to improvement. After five months of asymptomatic period, she again developed symptoms and prescribed Rifampicin, Isoniazid and ethambutol, which she stopped after one month due to drug intolerance. Next time she received Rifampicin, Isoniazid, Ethambutol and Pyrazinamide in fix dose combination of controversial quality for the next three months without any improvement. Thereafter treatment was changed to Streptomycin, Rifampicin, Isoniazid, Ethambutol and Pyrazinamide for the next two months, without any response. Then she received Category II treatment under RNTCP for nine months and still her sputum remained positive for AFB. In June 1997, she was hospitalized and her sputum was sent for culture and sensitivity for *Mycobacterium tuberculosis* and was treated with daily Streptomycin, Rifampicin, Isoniazid, Ethambutol and Pyrazinamide in adequate doses under supervision. After four months of regular treatment, her sputum remained positive for AFB. Her sputum culture and sensitivity report revealed resistance to Rifampicin, Isoniazid and Streptomycin. Considering the past history of treatment, radiological, symptomatic deterioration and sensitivity report, she was diagnosed as MDR-TB. She was treated with injection Kanamycin 0.75 g, PAS 10 g (in two divided doses), ethionamide 500 mg and cycloserine 500 mg daily, 300 mg of Isoniazid was also given. Her sputum smear was examined every month for AFB. Kanamycin was stopped after four months when her sputum smear became negative for AFB. Rest of the treatment was continued for a period of 18 months. At the end of the treatment, sputum smear and culture were negative for MTB. On subsequent follow-up for the next five years, there was no relapse.

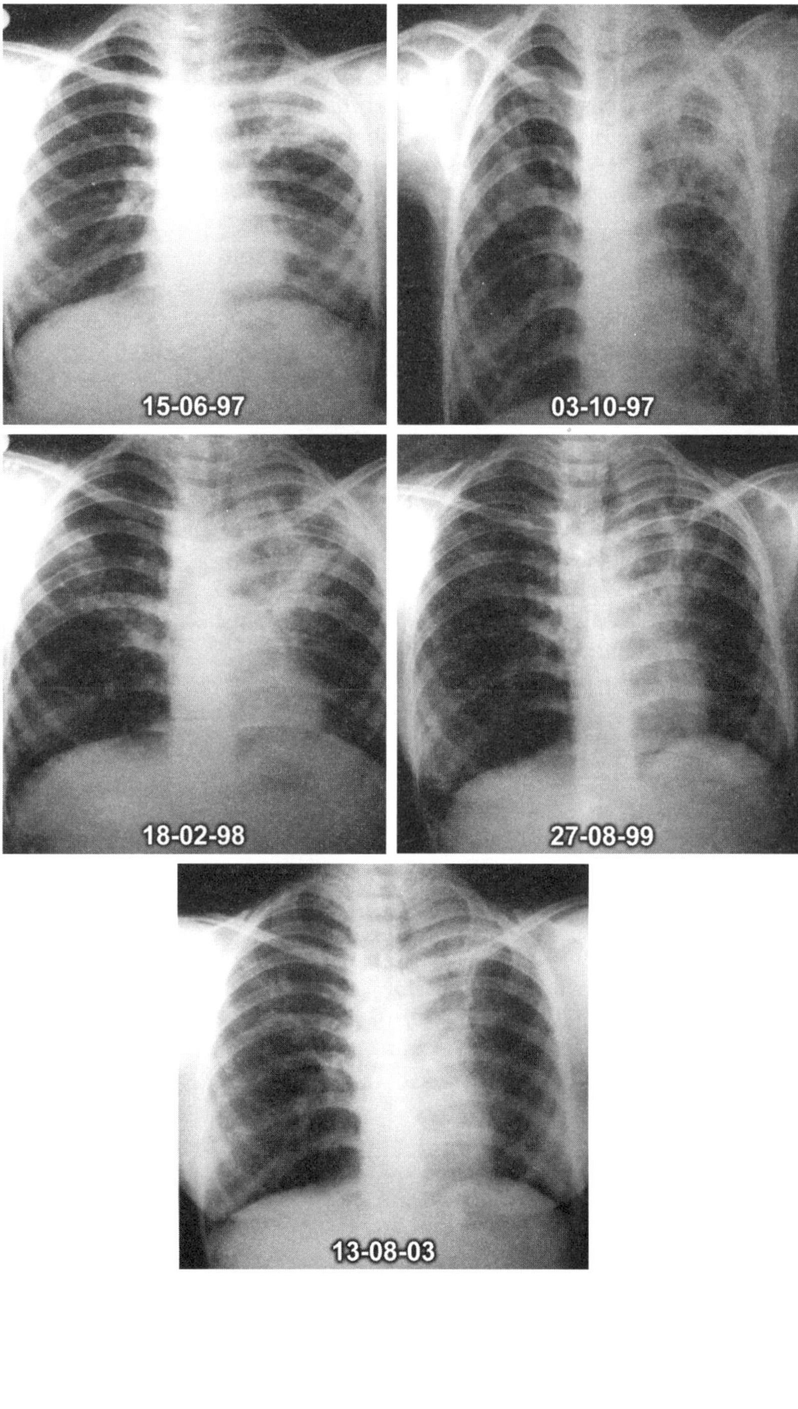
15-06-97
03-10-97
18-02-98
27-08-99
13-08-03

Case II

SS, a 15-year-old female, weighing 35 kg, was diagnosed as a sputum positive new case of pulmonary tuberculosis in February 1998, with bad family history of her brother, who died of pulmonary tuberculosis after prolonged treatment

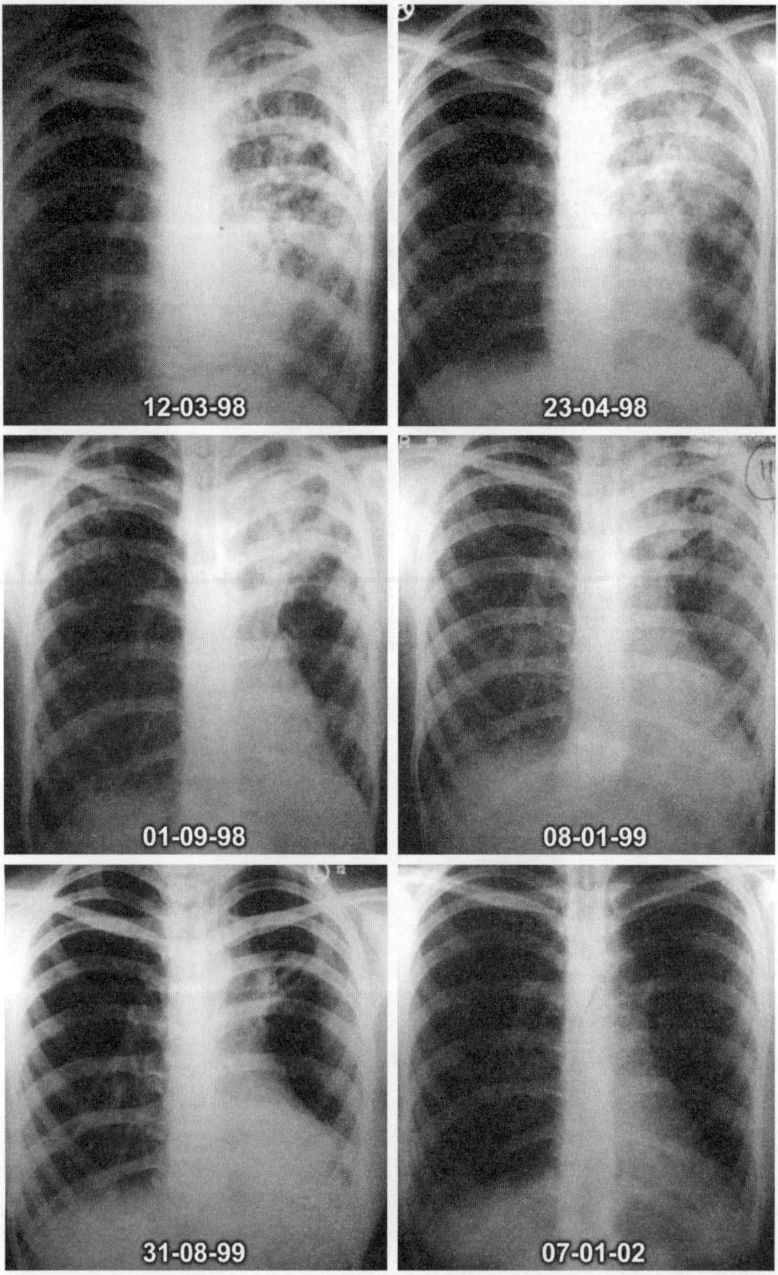

for four years. She was prescribed four drug regimen comprising rifampicin, isoniazid, ethambutol and pyrazinamide in adequate doses, which she took regularly for two months, without any significant improvement clinically, radiologically as well as bacteriologically. Then she sought advice from another physician who added streptomycin and sparfloxacin to her previous regimen of four drugs. She took six drug regimen regularly for six months with negligible response clinically and radiologically. Subsequently, she consulted us, when her sputum was positive for AFB and was also sent for culture and sensitivity for *Mycobacterium tuberculosis*. In light of her previous treatment experiences and outcomes, she was suspected as a case of primary MDR-TB. Pending sensitivity report, she was started on kanamycin 0.75 g, isoniazid 300 mg, PAS 8 g (in two divided doses), ethionamide 500 mg and cycloserine 500 mg daily in single dose, in September 1998. With the passage of time, she showed improvement clinically and radiologically, when her sputum became negative after four months. At the same time, her sputum culture and sensitivity report from four different laboratories (sent at the beginning of treatment) showed lots of discrepancies, with two of them labeling her as a case of MDR-TB while the other labeling her as polydrug resistance other than MDR. Regardless of conflicting sensitivity reports, we adhered to our regimen. Kanamycin was stopped after she became sputum negative, and rest of the treatment was continued for another 20 months. At the end of two years of treatment, she was smear and culture negative with dramatic clearing of chest radiograph and weight gain of about seven kg. She was followed for five years (till 2002), without any relapse.

Case III

MR, a 32-year-old male weighing 43 kg, was diagnosed as a case of pulmonary tuberculosis in 1992 and was treated with 2RHEZ/4RHE and declared cured. He has relapsed in 1994 and was again treated by different doctors for two years with different inadequate regimens with drug-including streptomycin, rifampicin, isoniazid, ethambutol and pyrazinamide without any response. He consulted another physician and took kanamycin (two months), ethionamide (two months), isoniazid and thiacetazone for one year without any response. He came to us in September 1997 with complaints of cough, fever, loss of appetite and weight. His serial chest X-rays showed progressive deterioration and his sputum was positive for AFB. Sputum was sent for culture and sensitivity for MTB. Pending the culture and sensitivity report, he was prescribed Streptomycin, Rifampicin, Isoniazid, Ethambutol and Pyrazinamide in adequate doses with intensive health education. At the end of three months of regular treatment, he did not respond clinically and his sputum remained positive for AFB. Sputum culture (sent at the time of starting five drugs) and sensitivity showed resistance to Streptomycin, Pyrazinamide, PAS and Ethionamide with susceptibility to rifampicin, isoniazid, ethambutol, thiacetazone and cycloserine. However, in view of past history of ATT, his sensitivity report was ignored and was assumed as a case of MDR-TB and treatment was changed to injection kanamycin 0.75 g, PAS 10 g (in two divided doses), ethionamide 500 mg, pyrazinamide 1500 mg and ofloxacin 600 mg

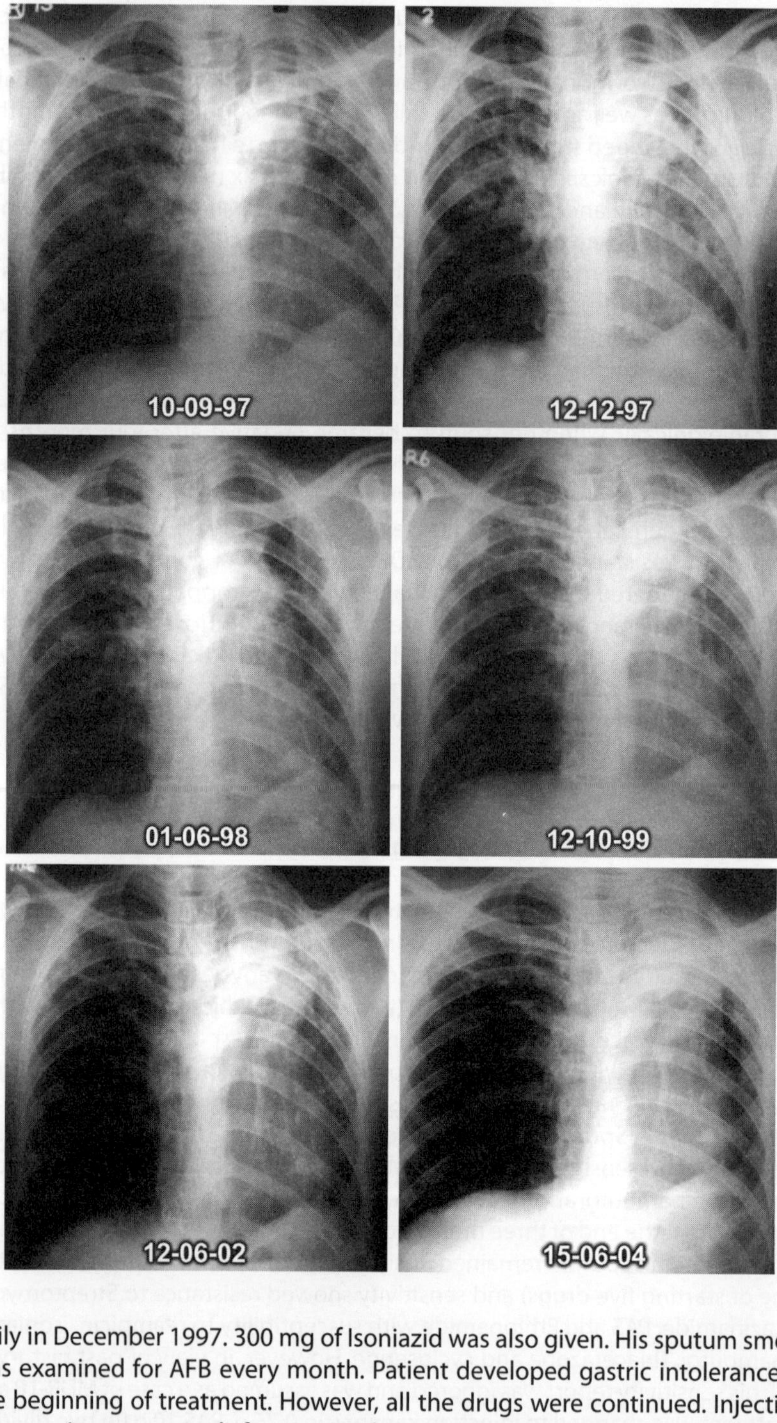

daily in December 1997. 300 mg of Isoniazid was also given. His sputum smear was examined for AFB every month. Patient developed gastric intolerance in the beginning of treatment. However, all the drugs were continued. Injection Kanamycin was stopped after six months in June 1998 when his sputum became negative for AFB and rest of the drugs were continued for another 18 months.

Patient responded clinically, radiologically and bacteriologically. Sputum smears for AFB and cultures were negative for MTB at the end of the treatment. Till now, after five years of regular follow-up, he has not relapsed.

Case IV

NK, a 27-year-old-male weighing 40 kg, presented with bilateral pulmonary tuberculosis with previous antitubercular treatment. Different doctors treated him for four years for pulmonary tuberculosis with different regimens in various combinations with drugs including streptomycin, isoniazid, rifampicin, ethambutol and pyrazinamide. His sputum was positive for AFB, which was sent for culture and sensitivity for *M. tuberculosis*. Pending culture report, treatment was started with five-drug regimen of Streptomycin 0.75 g, Isoniazid 300 mg, Rifampicin 450 mg, Ethambutol 800 mg and Pyrazinamide 1000 mg, daily in single dose, which he took regularly for two months without any clinical, radiological or bacteriological response. Sputum culture and sensitivity sent earlier revealed drug resistance to streptomycin, isoniazid and rifampicin. On the basis of this report, and previous history of treatment, he was kept on kanamycin 0.75 g, ethionamide 500 mg, ofloxacin 600 mg, ethambutol 800 mg

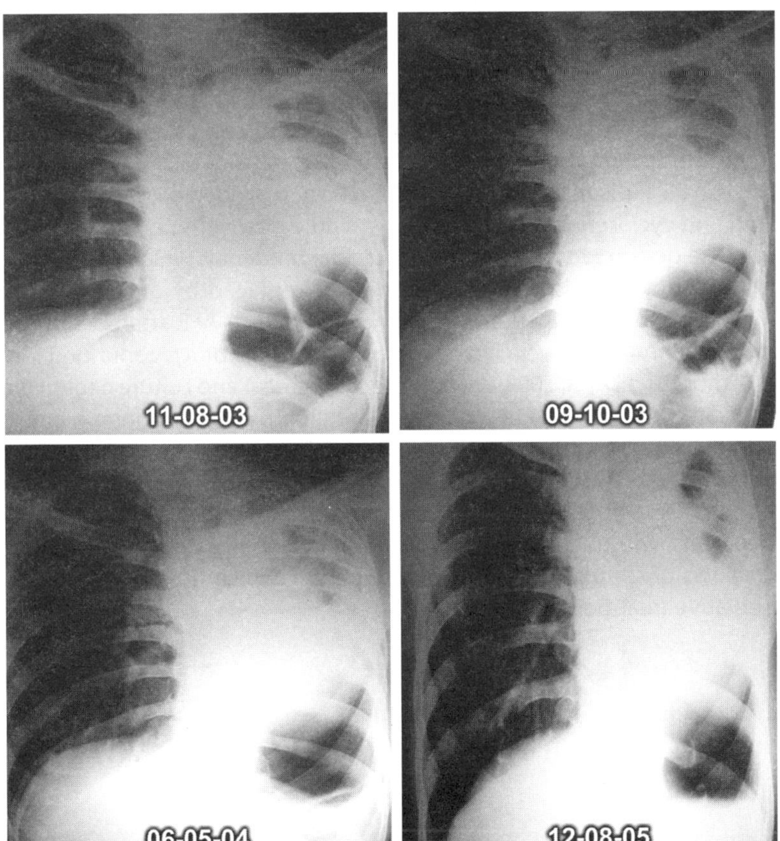

and pyrazinamide 1000 mg daily in single dose. Isoniazid in single dose of 300 mg daily was also added. He responded clinically and bacteriologically, but his chest radiograph revealed no change on left side (which was destroyed), with some clearing of shadows in right lung. Sputum conversion occurred after six months of treatment, when kanamycin was stopped, and rest of drugs were continued for the next 18 months. At the end of treatment, his sputum was negative for AFB and he has gained weight of six kg, but radiographical shadows persisted without much change, which in all likelihood will persist throughout his life and may be the source of infection and hemoptysis in future.

Case V

NR, a 35-year-old-male, weighing 40 kg, presented with bilateral pulmonary tuberculosis, with previous history of antitubercular treatment, from different doctors in various inadequate regimens, using streptomycin, isoniazid, rifampicin, ethambutol and pyrazinamide. At the time of presentation to us in January 2001, his sputum was positive for AFB, which was also sent for culture and sensitivity for *M. tuberculosis*. Pending sensitivity report, he was kept on regimen containing streptomycin 0.75 g, isoniazid 300 mg, rifampicin 450 mg, ethambutol 800 mg and pyrazinamide 1000 mg. Despite four months of regular treatment, there was no response on clinical, radiological and bacteriological parameters. Sputum sensitivity sent at the beginning of treatment reported resistance to streptomycin, isoniazid, ethambutol and rifampicin. In light of this sensitivity report, previous inadequate treatment and lack of response to four months' treatment of five drugs, he was diagnosed as a case of MDR-TB, and kept on kanamycin 0.75 g, isoniazid 300 mg, PAS 8 g (in two divided doses), ethionamide 500 mg and cycloserine 500 mg daily in a single dose. After one month of this therapy, he developed psychosis with suicidal tendency, which was managed by antipsychotic drugs, and cycloserine was replaced by ofloxacin 600 mg daily in a single dose. His sputum became negative for AFB after six months of treatment, when kanamycin was stopped, and rest of drugs continued for the next 18 months till April 2003, when he became smear and culture negative, and was declared cured. While he was on this regimen, chest radiographic picture deteriorated, but sputum smear always remained negative. Considering this radiological deterioration as intercurrent pyogenic infection, we adhered to our antitubercular regimen with some appropriate antibiotics. He was followed up for two years, without any relapse, although he experienced occasional bouts of streaking of sputum during follow-up period, which used to improve with conservative treatment.

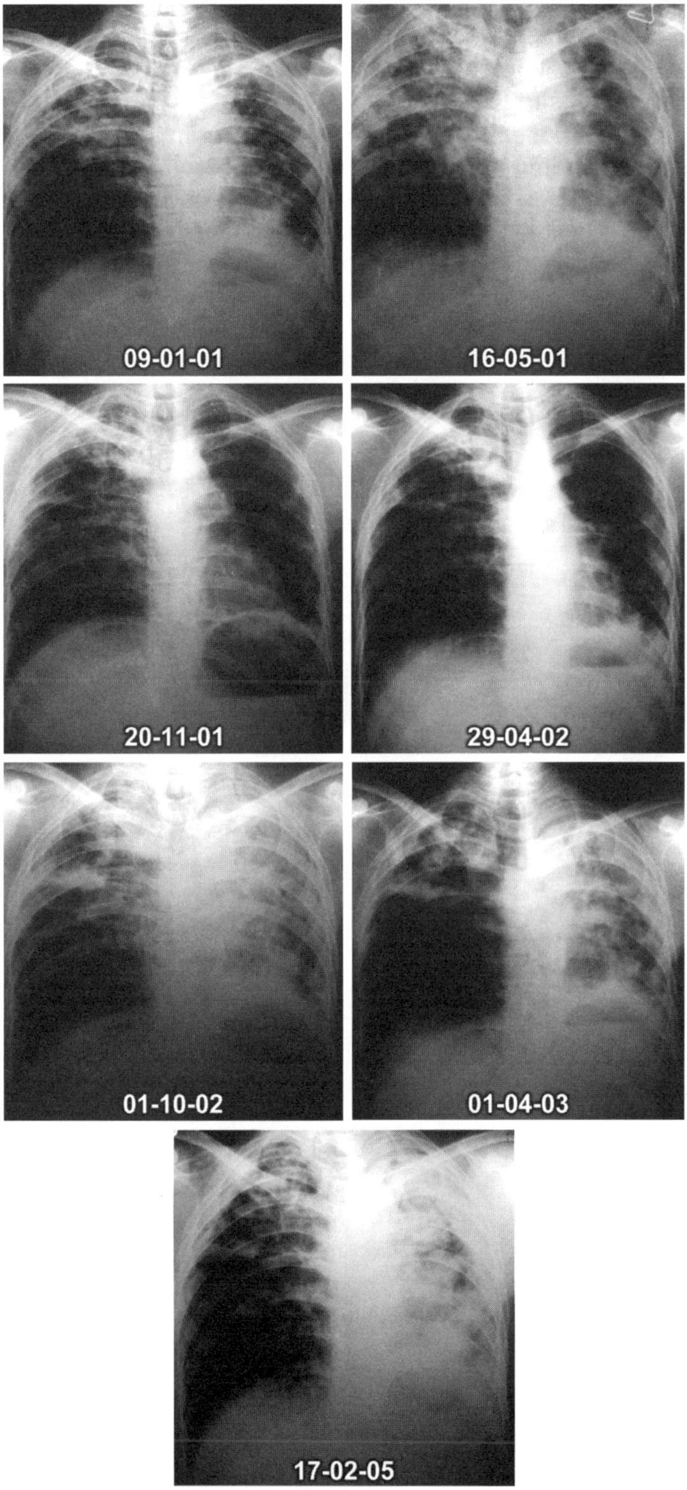
09-01-01
16-05-01
20-11-01
29-04-02
01-10-02
01-04-03
17-02-05

CASE VI

A 22-year-old female AV was diagnosed as a new case of sputum positive pulmonary tuberculosis in 2006. She was started on a regimen based on rifampicin, isoniazid, ethambutol, pyrazinamide from a private practitioner. She developed vomiting and gastritis and after which she stopped her antituberculosis drugs. She then consulted multiple private practitioners taking the prescribed treatment consisting of primary line of anti-TB drugs for 1–2 months, then stopping at her own with partial relief of symptoms each time. In May 2008, she presented to us. Her sputum was found to be positive for AFB.

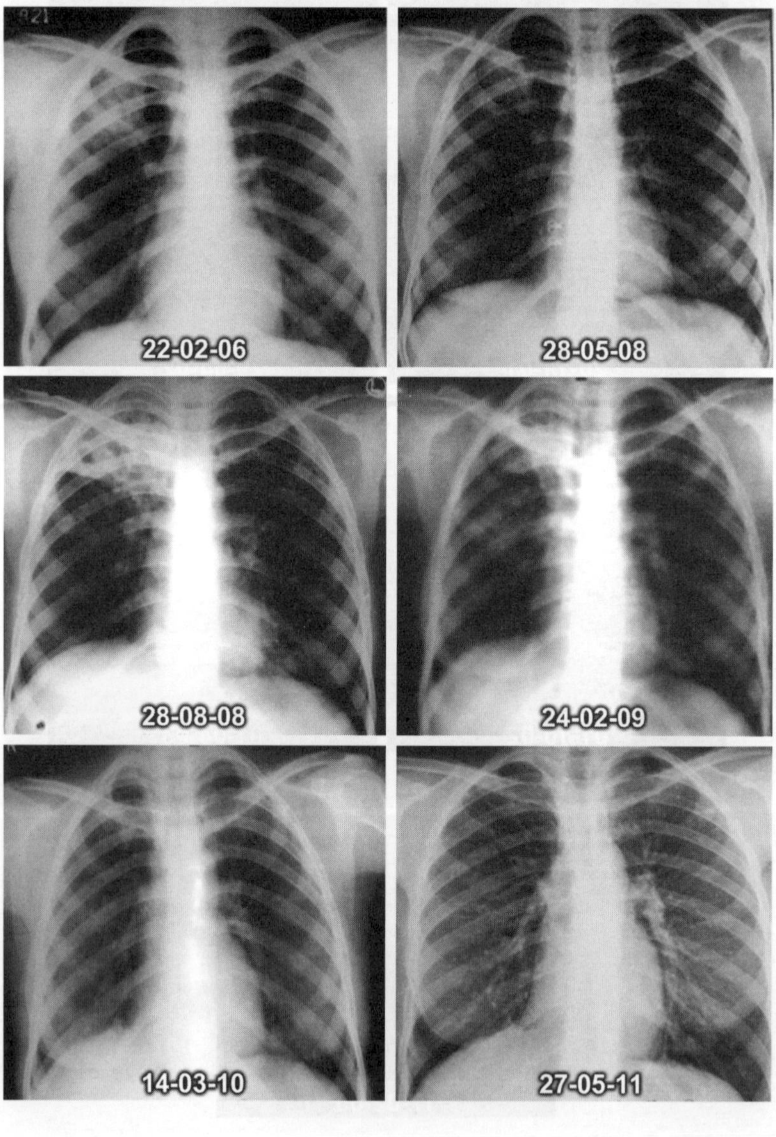

Sputum was sent for culture and sensitivity for mycobacterial tuberculosis and she was started on a five-drug regimen consisting of rifampicin, isoniazid, ethambutol, pyrazinamide and streptomycin. Her sputum culture sensitivity received in August 2008 showed growth of *Mycobacterium tuberculosis*, which was resistant to rifampicin and isoniazid. She was started on regimen for MDR-TB consisting of injection kanamycin, pyrizinamide, ethambutol, Ethionamide, cycloserine and ofloxacin. Her clinical condition improved, sputum for AFB and culture for *Mycobacterium* became negative fourth month onwards. Kanamycin and pyrizinamide were stopped after six months. Rest of the treatment was continued for eighteen months. Patient responded clinically, radiologically and bacteriologically. Sputum and culture were negative for *Mycobactertium tuberculosis* at the end of treatment in 2010. On subsequent follow-up for one year, she was asymptomatic.

Chapter 13

Multi-drug-resistant Tuberculosis: Adherence to Therapy

Introduction

Any practitioner treating a patient for tuberculosis is assuming an important public health responsibility to prevent ongoing transmission of the infection and the development of drug resistance. To fulfil this responsibility, the practitioner must not only prescribe an appropriate regimen, but also utilize local public health services and other agencies when necessary, to assess the adherence of the patient and to address poor adherence when it occurs. Treatment of Multi-drug-Resistant Tuberculosis (MDR-TB) involves second-line drugs, which are much more expensive, less effective and have more side effects than standard tuberculosis drugs. Treating MDR-TB requires experience, special expertise and multiple strategies. This chapter aims to outline the various strategies for treatment delivery that will improve adherence among patients receiving treatment for MDR-TB.

Education of Patients and Their Families

All patients and their families should receive health education and information about MDR-TB, its treatment, potential adverse drug reactions and the need for adherence with therapy. Educational interventions should commence at the start of therapy and continue throughout the course of treatment. Education can be provided by the attending doctors, nurses, community health workers, and other healthcare workers. Materials need to be appropriate to the literacy levels of the population and should be culturally sensitive.

Treatment Delivery Settings

Hospitalization, clinic-based treatment and community-based care are the various strategies employed by DOTS-Plus projects in various countries.[1,2] Regardless of the mode of delivery, the management of MDR-TB depends on a steady supply of medicines provided to patients free of charge through a reliable network of educated providers. Although early in the history of MDR-TB treatment, strict hospitalization of patients was considered necessary. Home-based care provided by trained lay and community health workers can achieve comparable results and, in theory, may result in decreased nosocomial spread of the disease. In each setting, care should be delivered by a multidisciplinary team of providers, including physicians, nurses, social workers and community health workers or volunteers. The roles and responsibilities of each of these groups of providers will vary depending on the needs and resources available in specific settings. Hospitals should provide acceptable living conditions, sufficient activities so that patients avoid boredom, adequate food, a proper heating system in cool areas, fans or cooling systems in hot climates and proper infection control measures. Prisons require specific measures to improve adherence.[3]

Adherence to Therapy

Patients with MDR-TB are more likely to have had problems with nonadherence in the past.[4] Adherence to MDR-TB therapy is particularly difficult because of its prolonged treatment regimens with larger number of drugs that have more serious adverse effect profiles.[5] Thus, MDR-TB patients are at increased risk of nonadherence to treatment. Adherence is an essential element to prevent the generation of pan-resistant strains with the potential for community-wide spread and virtually no possibility of cure for the patient.[6] MDR-TB treatment can be successful, with high overall rates of adherence, when adequate support measures are provided.[1] These measures include enablers and incentives for delivery of DOT to ensure adherence to treatment and may include nutritional supplementation, emotional support, education of patients, family and peers on MDR-TB treatment, reimbursement of travel expenses to patient and attendants and effective management of adverse effects.

Directly Observed Therapy (DOT)

Because MDR-TB treatment is the last therapeutic option for many patients and because there is a serious public health consequence if therapy fails in a patient with MDR-TB, it is recommended that all patients receiving treatment for MDR-TB receive DOT either in the community, at health centres or within the hospital setting. DOT should be provided in such a way that it does not place undue burden on patients and their families. Long transportation times and distances, short clinic operation hours and difficulty in accessing services may all reduce the efficacy of DOT.

Who can Deliver DOT for MDR-TB Patients?

The first choice is to use healthcare workers (HCW), where possible, as DOT providers. If this is not possible, trained community members can serve as effective DOT workers. With appropriate training and support, they can visit patients in their homes or workplaces. Receiving DOT from a community member is often a convenient alternative to the health center and can result in excellent treatment adherence.[7] However, community members need more intensive training, ongoing supervision by health professionals and support to deliver DOT for MDR-TB than those that deliver DOT for drug-susceptible TB. A family member should not deliver DOT.

Alternative to DOT for MDR-TB Patients

Default rate in DOTS regimens in India ranges from 5 to 20%, being highest in Category-II regimen, which is an 8- to 9-month therapy. With 24 months or more therapy duration, the default rates is going to be higher significantly and the patient's previous habit of defaulting may be the reason for his current status of being MDR-TB. DOT has shown to be highly efficacious in ensuring patient adherence. DOT, which is practiced under revised national control programme (RNTCP), also incurs huge toll on exchequer in terms of human resource and logistical requirements. So, providing drugs free of cost for four weeks, to be consumed at home ensuring adherence to treatment by intense health education to patient and family members at the start of treatment and during follow-up each month and other adherence measures like checking empty blister packs should be considered as an alternative to DOT in treating MDR-TB patients.

Maintaining Confidentiality

The health worker should explore the need to maintain strict confidentiality regarding the patient's disease. In some cases, this may entail working out a system, whereby the patient can receive medication without the knowledge of others.

Socioeconomic Interventions

Socioeconomic problems, including hunger, homelessness and unemployment, should be addressed to enable patients and their families to adhere to MDR-TB treatment. These problems have been successfully tackled through the provision of "incentives" and "enablers". Enablers are goods or services that make it easier for patients to adhere to treatment, such as the provision of transportation vouchers. Incentives are goods or services that are used to encourage patients to adhere to therapy, such as the provision of clothing. Maximal interventions should be given to patients who need it the most. Programs should benefit from professional social workers, who can assess the need for such socioeconomic interventions and monitor their delivery.

Social and Emotional Support

Having MDR-TB can be an emotionally devastating experience for patients and their families. Considerable stigma is attached to the disease and this may interfere with adherence to therapy. In addition, the long nature of MDR-TB therapy combined with the adverse effects of the drugs may contribute to depression, anxiety and further difficulty with treatment adherence. The provision of emotional support to patients may increase the likelihood of adherence to therapy. This support may be organized in the form of support groups or one-to-one counseling by trained providers. Informal support can also be provided by physicians, nurses, DOT workers and family members. Ideally a multidisciplinary team, comprising of a social worker, nurse, health educator, companion and doctor, should be set up to act as a "support to adherence" team to the patient.

Follow-up of the Nonadherent Patient

When a patient fails to take drugs regularly, a system should be in place that allows prompt patient follow-up. Most commonly this involves a DOT worker visiting the patient's home the same day to find out why the patient has defaulted and to ensure that treatment is resumed promptly and effectively. The situation should be addressed in a sympathetic, friendly and nonjudgmental manner. Every effort should be made to listen to reasons for the patient missing a dose(s) and to work with patient and family to ensure continuation of treatment. The transportation problems of the patient should be addressed.

Early and Effective Management of Adverse Drug Effects

Although rarely life-threatening, the adverse effects of second-line drugs can be debilitating for patients. Patients experiencing high rates of adverse effects may be at an increased risk of nonadherence. Therefore, early and effective management of adverse effects should be part of adherence-promotion strategies in the management of MDR-TB. In most cases, management of adverse effects can be accomplished using relatively simple and low-cost interventions without compromising the integrity of the MDR-TB treatment regimen.[8]

References

1. Mitnick C, Bayona J, Palacios E, Shin S, Furin J, Alcantara FE, et al. Community-based therapy for multi-drug-resistant tuberculosis in Lima, Peru. N Engl. J Med. 2003;348:119-28.
2. Leimane V, Riekstina V, Holtz TH, Zarovska E, Skripconoka V, Thorpe LE, et al. Clinical outcome of individualized treatment of multi-drug-resistant tuberculosis in Latvia: A retrospective cohort study. Lancet. 2005;365:318-26.
3. Tuberculosis control in prisons: A manual for programme managers. Geneva, World Health Organization, 2001 (WHO/CDS/TB/2001/281).
4. Mitchison DA. How drug resistance emerges as a result of poor compliance during short course chemotherapy for tuberculosis. Int J of Tuber Lung Dis. 1998;2:10-5.
5. Chaulk CP, Chaisson RE, Lewis JN, Rizzo RT. Treating multi-drug-resistant tuberculosis: Compliance and side effects. JAMA. 1994;271:103-4.

6. Espinal MA, Dye C, Raviglione M, Kochi A. Rational DOTS-Plus for the control of MDR-TB. Int J Tuberc Lung Dis. 1999;3:561-3.
7. Kim JY, Mukherjee JS, Rich ML, Mate K, Bayona J, Becerra MC. From multi-drug-resistant tuberculosis to DOTS expansion and beyond: Making the most of a paradigm shift. Tuberculosis. 2003;83:59-65.
8. Furin JJ, Mitnick CD, Shin SS, Bayona J, Becerra MC, Singler JM, et al. Occurrence of serious adverse effects in patients receiving community-based therapy for multi-drug-resistant tuberculosis. Int J Tuberc Lung Dis. 2001;5:648-55.

Chapter 14

Multi-drug-resistant Tuberculosis Contacts: Management

Introduction

Opportunities to halt the transmission of resistant mycobacteria in communities and to treat Drug-resistant Tuberculosis (DR-TB) in a timely fashion are often squandered. The main reasons are lack of investigation of contacts of MDR-TB patients, failure to ask patients presenting with active TB disease about any history of exposure to DR-TB, and lack of access by national treatment programs to second-line regimens and/or drug susceptibility testing (DST).

Close contacts of DR-TB patients are defined as people living in the same household, or spending many hours a day together with the patient in the same indoor living space. The available data indicate that close contacts of DR-TB patients, who develop active tuberculosis (TB), most commonly have drug-resistant disease.[1–5] While all contacts of TB require investigation, contacts of DR-TB require the priority. Because of the severe risk of morbidity and mortality of Extensively Drug Resistant Tuberculosis (XDR-TB), contact tracing of cases of XDR-TB should be given the highest priority. This chapter aims to outline the management of symptomatic adults and children who have or have had a known contact with a DR-TB patient.

Management of Symptomatic Adult Contacts of Patients with MDR-TB

All close contacts of DR-TB cases should be identified through contact tracing and evaluated for active TB by a physician. If the contact appears to have active TB disease, culture and DST should be performed. If DST is not available, or while DST results are awaited, an empirical regimen based either on the resistance pattern of the index case or on the most common resistance pattern in the community may be started. Delay in the diagnosis of MDR-TB and start of appropriate treatment can lead to increased morbidity and mortality as well as unchecked amplification and transmission of drug-resistant strains of TB. When investigation of a symptomatic adult contact yields no evidence of TB, a trial of a broad-spectrum antibiotic, particularly one that is not active against TB can be used. If the patient continues to have symptoms, chest computed tomography and bronchoscopy for smear and culture should be considered if available.Where these diagnostic tools are not available or the results are not conclusive, a diagnosis should be based on the clinical information at hand. If the initial investigation is not suggestive of active TB but the contact remains symptomatic, repeat physical examinations, smears and cultures should be performed monthly with repeat chest X-ray as needed.

Management of Symptomatic Pediatric Contacts of Patients with MDR-TB

DR-TB should be suspected in children with active TB in the following situations: A child who is a close contact of an DR-TB patient, a child who is a contact of a TB patient who died while on treatment when there are reasons to suspect that the disease was DR-TB and children with bacteriologically proven TB who are not responding to first-line drugs given with direct observation. The diagnosis of TB is more difficult in children than in adults. Symptoms of TB in young children can be non-specific, e.g. chronic cough or wheeze, failure to thrive and recurrent fevers. Bacteriological confirmation may be difficult to obtain because of the inability of children to produce a sputum sample, as well as the paucibacillary nature of pediatric TB and the increased likelihood of extra pulmonary TB in children. While every effort should be made to establish a bacteriological diagnosis in a child with suspected DR-TB, in practice, pediatric cases are often not confirmed bacteriologically. Use of scoring systems that have been produced to aid screening and diagnosis of active TB is strongly recommended.[6] Symptomatic pediatric household contacts should receive an evaluation by a physician, including history and physical examination, Tuberculin skin testing with purified protein derivative (PPD), radiological examination (chest X-ray examination and computerized tomography (CT), sputum smear, culture and DST: Every effort should be made to establish a bacteriological diagnosis in a child with suspected DR-TB. Bacteriological confirmation may include more aggressive measures such as induced sputum, gastric aspirate, lymph node aspirate or other relevant sample, plus culture and DST[6] and HIV counseling and testing in areas of high HIV prevalence or if parent(s) known, or suspected to be, HIV-infected. When the tuberculin (PPD) skin test result is >5 mm but the chest radiograph and gastric aspirate or sputum smear are negative, the symptomatic child can be treated with a broad spectrum antibiotic that is not active against TB. The child should be followed closely, with evaluations including smear test and culture on samples from induced sputum or gastric aspirates, or sputum samples whenever possible, as well as chest X-rays. The optimal frequency of these evaluations has not yet been determined. It is not clear whether the frequency of evaluation recommended for adults can be applied to children. If a child's clinical condition is highly suggestive of TB, or progressively deteriorates, empirical therapy designed according to the DST pattern of the strain from the index case can be started. Children with DR-TB who are incorrectly entered in Short Course Chemotherapy (SCC) may suffer significant and protracted morbidity as a result of the ongoing active disease, with the possibility of lifelong disability or even death. Because children with TB may never become sputum smear-positive, it is reasonable to initiate empirical DR-TB therapy based on the DST pattern of the contact. If DST of the contact is not available, therapy can be on the common DST patterns of resistance in the community.

Chemoprophylaxis of Contacts of DR-TB Index Cases

The only chemoprophylaxis regimens to have been studied are based on isoniazid and, to a lesser extent, rifampicin. Since by definition MDR-TB is resistant to both of these drugs, it is unlikely that use of these drugs to treat latent infection caused by an MDR-TB strain will prevent the development of active TB disease. Contacts of MDR-TB patients in whom latent infection is diagnosed may not be infected with the same strain; some may be infected with Isoniazid-susceptible strains, particularly in high-burden areas where many different strains of TB may circulate in homes, schools, workplaces, etc. Studies from high-burden TB areas have shown that approximately one-half to two-thirds of household members had the same strain of TB, as determined by genetic testing.[7–9] Close contacts of DR-TB patients should receive careful clinical follow-up for a period of at least two years. If active disease develops, prompt initiation of treatment with a regimen designed to treat DR-TB is recommended. On the basis of the currently available evidence, WHO does not recommend the universal use of second-line drugs for chemoprophylaxis in DR-TB contacts.

References

1. Kritski AL, Marques MJO, Rabahi MF, Viera MA, Werneck-Barroso E, Carvalho CE, et al. Transmission of tuberculosis to close contacts of patients with multi-drug-resistant tuberculosis. Am J Resp Crit Car Med. 1996;153:331-5.
2. Schaaf HS, Van Rie A, Gie RP, Beyers N, Victor TC, Van Helden PD, et al. Transmission of multi-drug-resistant tuberculosis. Pedia Infectious Dis J. 2000;19:695-9.
3. Teixeira L, Perkins MD, Johnson JL, Keller R, Palaci M, do Valle Dettoni V, et al. Infection and disease among household contacts of patients with multi-drug-resistant tuberculosis. Int J of Tuberc Lung Dis. 2001;5:321-8.
4. Schaaf HS, Gie RP, Kennedy M, Beyers N, Hesseling PB, Donald PR. Evaluation of young children in contact with adult multi-drug-resistant pulmonary tuberculosis: a 30-month follow-up. Pediatrics. 2002;109:765-71.
5. Bayona J, Chavez-Pachas AM, Palacios E, Llaro K, Sapag R, et al. Contact investigations as a means of detection and timely treatment of persons with infectious multi-drug-resistant tuberculosis. Int J Tuberc Lung Dis. 2003;7:501-9.
6. Guidance for national tuberculosis programmes on the management of tuberculosis in children. Geneva, World Health Organization 2006(WHO/HTM/TB/2006.371; WHO/FCH/CAH/2006.7).

7. Verver S, Warren RM, Munch Z, Richardson M, Van der Spuy GD, Borgdorff MW. Proportion of tuberculosis transmission that takes place in households in a high-incidence area. Lancet. 2004;363:212-4.
8. Schaaf HS, Vermeulen HAS, Gie RP, Beyers N, Donald PR. Evaluation of young children in household contact with adult multi-drug-resistant pulmonary tuberculosis cases. Pediatric Infectious Disease Journal. 1999;18:494-500.
9. Steiner P, Rao M. Drug-resistant tuberculosis in children. Seminars in Pediatric Infectious Diseases. 1993;4:275-82.

Chapter 15

Extensively Drug-resistant Tuberculosis: Current Status

Introduction

Drug resistance in tuberculosis is a growing global problem. The emergence of multi-drug resistant tuberculosis cases, particularly in the 1990s, has become an important health problem and threatens tuberculosis control worldwide. Mistreatment of multi drug resistant tuberculosis cases by physicians, the use of anti-tuberculosis drugs with low quality, poor experience in management, lack of laboratories to perform second-line anti-tuberculosis drug susceptibility testing and problems in adherence of patients to treatment lead to the development of extensively drug resistant tuberculosis (XDR). XDR-TB is a man made problem and its emergence can be prevented by prompt diagnosis and effective treatment with second-line drugs in multi-drug resistant tuberculosis (MDR-TB) cases. This chapter aims to review the present scenario of Extensively Drug-resistant tuberculosis.

Definition

The term XDR-Tuberculosis (XDR-TB) was used for the first time in November 2005[1,2] and provisionally defined as TB cases in persons harbouring *Mycobacterium tuberculosis* strains resistant in vitro to at least isoniazid (H) and rifampicin (R) (MDR definition) among first-line drugs, and to at least three or more of the six main classes of second-line drugs (aminoglycosides, polypeptides, fluoroquinolones, thioamides, cycloserine, and *p*-aminosalicyclic acid). Subsequent reports suggested different definitions for XDR-TB.[3] In October 2006 the WHO, also in consideration of the difficulty to test some second line drugs[4] and the fact that some forms of drug resistance are less treatable than others, revised the definition. XDR- TB was defined as resistance to at least isoniazid and rifampicin in addition to resistant to any fluoroquinolone, and to at least one of the three injectable second-line drugs (amikacin, capreomycin, or kanamycin).[3]

Prevalence of XDR-TB: Global Scenario

Extensively drug-resistant tuberculosis strains have been recognized for over a decade, surveillance data on the worldwide prevalence of XDR-TB were only first published in March 2006.[5] Between 2000 and 2004, XDR-TB was found in 17 countries. Data from most African and Asian countries were limited. Of 17,690 TB isolates, 20% were MDR-TB and 2% were XDR-TB, using an earlier definition of XDR-TB. These isolates were sampled from supranational reference laboratories, where MDR-TB isolates were probably over-represented. Nevertheless, the proportion of XDR-TB among MDR-TB isolates was astoundingly high in some nations, 15% in Latvia and 19% in Korea.[5] More recent surveillance data from the WHO indicate that XDR-TB is now found in 45 countries.[6] Among approximately 4000 MDR-TB isolates collected throughout the world and tested for susceptibility to SLDs, 7% were XDR-TB. The proportion of XDR isolates among MDR isolates varied among nations, from 0 to 30%, with Japan, the Republic of Korea and countries of the former Soviet Union reporting the highest proportions. The nations with the greatest absolute number of reported XDR-TB cases include countries of the former Soviet Union and South Africa.[6] In the USA, between 1993 and 2006, 49 patients (3% of the evaluated MDR-TB cases) have been reported with XDR-TB, mostly in areas with high TB morbidity and large immigrant populations, such as New York City and California.[7] In California alone, 18 XDR-TB cases, comprising nearly 4% of the evaluated MDR cases, were reported between 1993 and 2006.[8] In addition, there are increasing surveillance data regarding MDR-TB isolates that are resistant to fluroquinolones or an injectable agent, but not both (pre-XDR isolates). These strains are essentially one mutation away from becoming XDR. Among the evaluated MDR isolates, pre-XDR prevalence was found to be 14% in a South African convenience sample,[9] 18% in California,[8] 25% in Uzbekistan,[10] 42% in Russia[11] and 3.2 % in India (Gujarat).[12] In the fourth WHO/IUATLD anti-TB drug resistance surveillance report, thirty-five countries and two SARs have reported data on XDR-TB. The quality assurance for laboratory testing was variable among the countries reported. Data for XDR-TB from 46 countries that have reported continuous surveillance or representative surveys of second-line drug resistance among MDR-TB cases. Combining data from these countries, 5.4% of MDR-TB cases were found to have XDR-TB. Eight countries reported XDR-TB in more than 10% of MDR-TB cases; six of these countries were located in Eastern Europe and Central Asia. To date, a cumulative total of 84 countries have confirmed at least one case of XDR-TB.[13] Although our understanding of the magnitude and distribution of XDR-TB is increasing, currently available reports of XDR-TB prevalence are underestimated because drug-susceptibility testing (DST) is incomplete and surveillance data are lacking from many nations. In many low-income, high-TB-burden countries, poor laboratory capacity prevents culture and DST of *Mycobacterium tuberculosis*. Even in high-income nations that primarily contributed surveillance data for the WHO report on anti-TB drug resistance,[6] a large proportion of MDR cases did not have SLD-susceptibility testing and could not be assessed for XDR-TB. The second-line drug resistance data for countries with high burden of MDR tuberculosis is given in Table 15.1.

TABLE 15.1: Second-line drug resistance data for countries with high burden of MDR tuberculosis[13]

Country	*Year*	*Method*	*MDR-TB cases tested for second-line drug resistance*	*XDR cases among MDR-TB cases treated*	*Proportion of MDR cases that were XDR%*
Armenia	2007	Survey	199	8	4% (1.8–7.8)
Azerbaijan, Baku	2007	Survey	431	55	12·8% (9·8–16·3)
Bangladesh	2008	Surveillance	168	1	0·6%
China	2008	Survey	270	30	11·1% (7·6–15·5)
Estonia	2008	Surveillance	72	9	12·5%
Georgia	2006	Survey	70	3	4·3% (0·9–12·0)
India, Gujarat state	2006	Survey	216	7	3·2% (1·2–6·6)
Kazakhstan	2008	Surveillance	373	16	4·3%
Latvia	2008	Surveillance	128	19	14·8%
Lithuania	2003–06	Surveillance	173	25	14·5%
Moldova	2006	Survey	47	3	6·4% (1·3–17·5)
Russia, Tomsk Oblast	2003–05	Surveillance	458	30	6·6%
South Africa	2008	Surveillance	5451	573	10·5%
Tajikistan, Dushanbe and Rudaki	2009	Survey	100	21	21·0% (13·5–30·3)
Ukraine, Donetsk Oblast	2006	Survey	20	3	15·0% (3·2–37·9)

XDR-TB: India

Although isolated reports, both published and unpublished, indicate the existence of XDR-TB in the country, it is not possible as yet to estimate its magnitude and distribution from the available data. Drug Susceptibility Test (DST) results of Second-line antituberculous drugs should be interpreted with great caution due to limited capacity of laboratories, absence of quality-assurance and lack of standardized methodology. According to the data reported on XDR-TB from India, it varied from 1.5% to 11%[14-17] of MDR-TB. Multi-drug and extensively drug-resistant TB (M/XDR-TB) 2010 Global Report on Surveillance and Response estimated prevalence of XDR among MDR-TB patients as 3.2% (95% CI, 1.2–6.6%).[13] In a recent study XDR-TB was found is 8.5% of MDR-TB cases. Furthermore, 42.3% of MDR-TB cases were resistant to either ofloxacin or kanamicin (pre-XDR-TB) which in studies have shown to be an independent prognostic factor of poor outcome and survival in patients with MDR-TB.[16]

Mechanisms of Resistance in XDR-TB

The basis of drug resistance in tuberculosis is the selection of bacterial mutants with innate resistance to chemotherapy.[18,19] Epidemics of drug-resistant disease can be generated by three interrelated mechanisms: (1) Conversion of wild type pan-susceptible strains to drug-resistant strains during treatment (acquired resistance); (2) Increasing development of resistance in drug-resistant strains because of inappropriate chemotherapy (amplified resistance); and (3) Transmission of drug-resistant cases (transmitted resistance). Acquired and amplified drug resistance are the primary means by which tuberculosis drug-resistant strains have been generated. However, the key determinant that has led to the exponential rise in XDR-TB cases is likely to have been transmitted resistance. The role of transmitted resistance can be elucidated by noting the clonal strains evident in tuberculosis outbreaks. The MDR-TB outbreak in the early 1990s in New York City, fuelled by the HIV epidemic and urban settings, was primarily associated with a clinically virulent strain of Beijing/W genotype.[20,21] Moreover, 39 (85%) of 46 isolated XDR-TB strains in the Tugela Ferry outbreak in South Africa belonged to the KwaZulu-Natal (KZN) genotypic family of strains.[22] The Broad Institute (Cambridge, Massachusetts, USA) has sequenced three KZN clinical isolates from Tugela Ferry: (1) Drug-susceptible tuberculosis; (2) MDR-TB; and (3) XDR-TB.[23] The KZN family was first described to have resistance to first-line tuberculosis treatments in 1996.[24] It is suspected that this strain has accumulated resistance to several second-line drugs within just 5 years.[25,26] However, a countrywide study in South Africa (which notably excluded the KwaZulu-Natal Province) isolated seven different XDR-TB genotype families, of which the Beijing genotype was the most common.[27]

The transmission of drug-resistant tuberculosis largely depends on the virulence of the mutated organism.[28-30] Mutations may alter gene products that affect the organism's virulence and therein its reproductive fitness.[31] Mathematical modeling has allowed for theoretical assessment of the contribution of microbial fitness to the transmission of drug-resistant strains. Blower and Chou analyzed the evolution of "hot zones" (areas that have an MDR-TB prevalence of more than 5%) and showed a high rate of drug-resistant tuberculosis can occur even if the MDR strains are less fit than the wild type strains.[32] The study inferred that prediction of future drug-resistant tuberculosis transmission requires equal measurement of not only fitness, but also amplification probability, case-finding, and cure rates. These factors are more dependent on tuberculosis control strategies and less a function of biological potential. Cohen and Murray [33] also developed a mathematical model of the emergence of MDR-TB based on the assumption that drug-resistant strains have heterogenous fitness. The model showed that even when the average microbial fitness is low and a properly functioning tuberculosis control program is in place, a small population of drug-resistant strains might emerge from the background of drug-susceptible and less fit MDR-TB strains. The difference in the fitness between the circulating strains becomes the primary determinant of the future burden of transmitted MDR-TB. Ultimately, the only definitive way of determining bacterial fitness would be to observe its effects.[34,35] In animal modeling studies, certain endemic clinical isolates and related recombinant *M. tuberculosis* strains have shown a variety of phenotypic outcomes including that of hypervirulence.[36-38] Hence, the issue of the degree to which drug resistance alters the fitness of *M. tuberculosis* remains an open research question.

Resistance Determinants

Antibiotic resistance in *M. tuberculosis* develops primarily through mutations in chromosomal genes. *M. tuberculosis* lacks plasmids, has a low recombination rate and contains a unique, impermeable cell wall that prevents horizontal transfer of resistance genes.[39,40] The genes mediating resistance to many first- and second-line anti-TB drugs are listed in Table 15.2 below.[41] Rifampin resistance occurs in 95% of cases through nucleotide substitutions in an 81-bp core region of rpoB, the β-subunit of DNA-dependent RNA polymerase.[42,43] Isoniazid resistance is more complicated and can be mediated by mutations in several genes, including katG (40–60% of the time), inhA, ahpC, oxyR, kasA, furA and ndh. The mechanism of INH resistance is unknown in 10 to 15% of cases. Resistance determinants to many SLDs have also been elucidated. High-level fluroquinolones (FQ) resistance occurs in more than 90% of cases via mutations in the quinolone resistance-determining region of the gyrA gene that encodes a DNA gyrase. Mutations in a similar gene, gyrB, can also confer FQ resistance. Low-level FQ resistance in the absence of gyrA/B mutations occurs rarely but has been observed.[44,45] Resistance to aminoglycosides, such as streptomycin, amikacin and kanamycin, occurs approximately 70% of the time in the rrs gene that encodes 16S ribosomal RNA.[46] Streptomycin resistance is also associated with mutations in the rpsL gene[47,48] and gidB.[49] A substitution at a single position in rrs generally confers high-level resistance to both amikacin and kanamycin.[50] However, mutations outside of this gene also cause aminoglycoside resistance without complete cross-resistance. Half of MDR isolates in Estonia that lacked

TABLE 15.2: Classes of anti-TB drugs and genes mutated in drug resistance

Anti-TB drug	*Genes mutated in drug resistance*
First-line drugs	
Isoniazid	katG, inhA, ahpC, oxyR, kasA, furA, ndh
Rifampin	rpoB
Ethambutol	embCAB
Pyrazinamide	pncA
Streptomycin	rrs, rpsL, gidB
Second-line drugs	
Fluoroquinolones	gyrA, gyrB
Injectables:	
• Kanamycin and amikacin	rrs
• Capreomycin	rrs, tlyA
Cycloserine	alrA, ddl
Ethionamide	inhA, etaA/ethA
P-aminosalicylic acid	Unknown

rrs mutations were kanamycin-resistant and amikacin-sensitive.[51] Capreomycin resistance in *M. tuberculosis* is due to mutations in rrs and tylA.[52]

Recently, the genomes of three related *M. Tuberculosis* strains from Kwazulu-Natal (XDR, MDR and drug-sensitive) have been sequenced using high-throughout DNA sequencing. These strains have a different genetic background from the F15/LAM4/KZN strain causing the majority of cases in South Africa. While the data are not yet published, they are publicly available on the website of the Broad Institute.[53] The genomes differ from one another through a surprisingly small number of single-nucleotide polymorphisms (SNPs). The XDR and drug-sensitive strain differ by 33 SNPs and one insertion/deletion. The XDR and MDR strains share a number of identical mutations conferring INH, streptomycin and ethambutol resistance. However, they differ by 22 SNPs and one insertion/deletion. Some mutations unique to the XDR strain are in genes known to mediate antibiotic resistance, including substitutions in the rpoB and gyrA genes and a deletion in the pncA gene. Other SNPs occur in genes without proven roles in drug resistance, such as mmpL13a that encodes a protein involved in fatty acid transport and cell wall synthesis. Additional SNPs in the XDR strain are in uncharacterized genes (Rv2000 and Rv3471c). It is possible that some SNPs are compensatory mutations that permit bacterial survival despite the loss of fitness that accompanies drug resistance.

Factors Responsible for XDR-TB

Drug resistance in *M. tuberculosis* is due to the accumulation of mutations in the genome. Mismanagement of MDR-TB cases primarily results in XDR-TB, mainly by faulty or improper treatment, nonadherence to treatment guidelines, inappropriate, incomplete or erratic use of second-line drugs and use of poor quality second-line drugs. A report from South Korea revealed that XDR-TB was significantly associated with the cumulative duration of previous TB treatment received with second-line drugs.[53,54] Little or no access to reliable laboratory for drug susceptibility testing against first- and second-line drugs, lack of experience, poor training and skills to manage drug-resistant TB and factors linked to poor control practices like lack of measures to ensure adherence to treatment and treatment of tuberculosis in unmonitored private sectors played a major role in the development of XDR-TB. The two strongest risk factors for XDR-TB are: Failure of an anti-TB regimen that contains second-line drugs including an injectable agent and a fluoroquinolone and close contact with an individual with documented XDR-TB or with an individual for whom treatment with a regimen including second-line drugs is failing or has failed.[55]

XDR-TB and HIV

The association between HIV/AIDS and drug-resistant tuberculosis is complex and multifaceted.[56] HIV coinfection is not believed to increase the rate at which spontaneous resistance-conferring mutations occur, although it might increase the number of mutants that arise overall by enlarging the pool of individuals with active tuberculosis disease.[57] Additionally, HIV coinfection might increase selection for spontaneous mutations in several ways. Without proper management, individuals with HIV-associated tuberculosis could have diminished adherence due to increased pill burden, overlapping toxic effects, or fragmentation of care between separate tuberculosis and HIV/AIDS programs.[58,59] They are also prone to having subtherapeutic concentrations of antituberculosis drugs because of malabsorption [60,61] or drug interactions.[62,63] Patients with tuberculosis, with and without HIV coinfection, can be infected with drug-resistant tuberculosis strains, but those coinfected with HIV are much more likely than are their counterparts to progress to active tuberculosis disease after initial infection. Thus, patients coinfected with HIV are more likely and are often the first to show active drug-resistant tuberculosis after transmission in an outbreak,[64,65] whereas HIV-negative individuals may become latently infected and manifest disease years later, if at all. Finally, the risk factors for both drug-resistant tuberculosis and HIV/AIDS (e.g. injection drug use) could be similar,[66] creating the appearance that drug-resistant tuberculosis has increased prevalence in patients coinfected with HIV, such as in eastern Europe. In summary, although HIV infection might not itself be causing an increase in the rate of drug-resistance mutations, it certainly has the potential to increase the number of individuals who select for drug resistance or manifest active disease from resistant organisms, thereby potentially accelerating the propagation and spread of drug-resistant disease.

References

1. Shah NS, Wright A, Drobniewski F. Extreme drug resistance in tuberculosis (XDR-TB): Global survey of supranational reference laboratories for *Mycobacterium tuberculosis* with resistance to second-line drugs. Int J Tuberc Lung Dis. 2005;9:77.
2. Holtz TH, Riekstina V, Zarovska E, Laserson KF, Wells CD, Leimane V. XDR-TB: Extreme drug-resistance and treatment outcome under DOTS-Plus, Latvia, 2000-2002. Int J Tuberc Lung Dis. 2005;9:258.
3. Centers for Disease Control and Prevention (CDC). Extensively drug-resistant tuberculosis—United States, 1993–2006. MMWR. 2007;56:250-3.
4. Kim SJ, Espinal MA, Abe C, Bai GH, Boulahbal F, Fattorini L. Is second-line anti-tuberculosis drug susceptibility testing reliable? Int J Tuberc Lung Dis. 2004;8:1157-8.
5. Emergence of *Mycobacterium tuberculosis* with extensive resistance to second-line drugs wordwide, 2000–2004. MMWR. 2006;55:301-5.
6. The WHO/IUATLD Global Project on Anti-tuberculosis Drug Resistance Surveillance 2002–2007: fourth global report. WHO/HTM/TB/2008.394. Geneva, Switzerland: WHO, 2008.
7. Extensively drug-resistant tuberculosis—United States, 1993–2006. MMWR. 2007;56:250-3.
8. Banerjee R, Allen J, Westenhouse J. Extensively drug-resistant tuberculosis (XDR-TB) in California, 1993–2006.Clin. Infec. Dis. 2008;47:450-7.
9. Mlambo CK, Warren RM, Poswa X,Victor TC, Duse AG, Marais E. Genotypic diversity of extensively drug-resistant tuberculosis (XDR-TB) in South Africa. Epidemiological modelling study. Int J Tuberc Lung Dis 2008;12:99-104.
10. Cox HS, Kalon S, Allamuratova S. Multidrug-resistant tuberculosis treatment outcomes in Karakalpakstan, Uzbekistan: treatment complexity and XDR-TB among treatment failures. PLoS ONE. 2007;2:1126.

11. Toungoussova OS, Mariandyshev AO, Bjune G, Caugant DA, Sandven P. Resistance of multidrug-resistant strains of *Mycobacterium tuberculosis* from the Archangel Oblast, Russia, to second-line anti-tuberculosis drugs. Eur J Clin Microbiol Infect Dis 2005;24:202-6.
12. Ramachandran. R, Nalini S, Chandrasekar V, Dave PV, Sanghvi AS, Wares F. Surveillance of drug-resistant tuberculosis in the state of Gujarat, India. Int J Tuberc Lung Dis. 2009;13:1154-60.
13. Multidrug and Extensively Drug-resistant TB (M/XDR-TB) Global Report on Surveillance and Response. 2010, 2012.
14. Jain A, Dixit P, Prasad R. Pre-XDR and XDR in MDR and Ofloxacin and Kanamycin resistance in non-MDR Mycobacterium tuberculosis isolates. Tuberculosis. 2012; 92: 404-06.
15. Udwadia Z, Jain S, Rodrigues C, Mehta A. XDR-TB in India: What's in a name? The Lancet Infectious diseases. 2007;7:441-2.
16. Mondal R, Jain A. XDR *Mycobacterium tuberculosis* isolates, India (letter). Emerg Infect Dis 2007. available from http:/www.cdc.gov/EID/content/13/9/ 1429.htm.
17. Thomas A, Ramachandran R, Rehman F, et al. Management of Multi-drug Resistant Tuberculosis in the field: Tuberculosis Research Centre Experience. Indian J Tuberc 2007;54:117-24.
18. Gillespie SH. Evolution of drug resistance in *Mycobacterium tuberculosis*: Clinical and molecular perspective. Antimicrob Agents Chemother. 2002;46:267-74.
19. Dorman SE, Chaisson RE. From magic bullets back to the Magic Mountain: The rise of extensively drug-resistant tuberculosis.Nat Med. 2007;13:295-8.
20. Frieden TR, Sterling T, Pablos-Mendez A, Kilburn JO, Cauthen GM, Dooley SW. The emergence of drug-resistant tuberculosis in New York City. N Engl J Med. 1993;328:521-6.
21. Frieden TR, Woodley CL, Crawford JT, Lew D, Dooley SM. The molecular epidemiology of tuberculosis in New York City: The importance of nosocomial transmission and laboratory error. Tuber Lung Dis. 1996;5:407-13.
22. Gandhi NR, Moll A, Sturm AW. Extensively drug-resistant tuberculosis as a cause of death in patients coinfected with tuberculosis and HIV in a rural area of South Africa. Lancet. 2006;368:1575-80.
23. Broad Institute *Mycobacterium tuberculosis* Database. http://www.broad.mit.edu/annotation/genome/mycobacterium_tuberculosis_spp/MultiHome.html (accessed March 3, 2011).
24. Davies GT, Pillay M, Sturm AW, Wilkinson D. Emergence of multidrug-resistant tuberculosis in a community-based directly observed treatment programme in rural South Africa. Int J Tuberc Lung Dis. 1999;3:799-804.
25. Sturm AW. The UKZN "outbreak". Expert consultation on drug-resistant tuberculosis. Johannesburg: MRC Unit for TB epidemiology and Interventions Branch, 2006.
26. Pillay M, Sturm AW. Evolution of the extensively drug-resistant F15/LAM4/KZN strain of *Mycobacterium tuberculosis* in KwaZulu-Natal, South Africa. Clin Infect Dis. 2007;45:1409-14.
27. Mlambo CK, Warren RM, Poswa X, Victor TC, Duse AG, Marais E. Genotypic diversity of extensively drug-resistant tuberculosis (XDR-TB) in South Africa. Int J Tuberc Lung Dis. 2008;12:99-104.
28. Blower SM, Gerberding JL. Understanding, predicting and controlling the emergence of drug-resistant tuberculosis: A theoretical framework. J Mol Med. 1998;76:624-36.
29. Dye C, Williams BG. Criteria for the control of drug-resistant tuberculosis. Proc Natl Acad Sci USA. 2000;97:8180-5.

30. Dye C, Espinal MA. Will tuberculosis become resistant to all antibiotics? Proc Biol Sci. 2001;268:45-52.
31. Gillespie SH. Tuberculosis: Evolution in millennia and minutes. Biochem Soc Trans. 2007;35:1317-20.
32. Blower SM, Chou T. Modeling the emergence of the "hotzones": Tuberculosis and the amplification dynamics of drug resistance. Nat Med. 2004;10:1111-6.
33. Cohen T, Murray MB. Modeling epidemics of multidrug-resistant *M. tuberculosis* of heterogeneous fitness. Nat Med. 2004;10:1117-21.
34. Chiang SL, Mekalonos JJ, Holden DW. In vivo genetic analysis of bacterial virulence. Annu Rev Microbiol. 1999;53:129-54.
35. Gandotra S, Schnappinger D, Monteleone M, Hillen W, Ehrt S. In vivo gene silencing identifies the *Mycobacterium tuberculosis* proteasome as essential for the bacteria to persist in mice. Nat Med. 2007;13:1515-20.
36. Reed MB, Domenech P, Manca C. A glycolipid of hypervirulent tuberculosis strains that inhibits the innate immune response. Nature. 2004;431:84-7.
37. Constant P, Perez E, Malaga W. Role of the pks 15/1 gene in the biosynthesis of phenolglycolipids in the *Mycobacterium tuberculosis* complex. Evidence that all strains synthesize glycosylated p-hydroxybenzoic methyl esters and that strains devoid of phenolglycolipids harbor a frameshift mutation in the pks 5/1 gene. J Biol Chem. 2002;277:38148-58.
38. Maartens G, Wilkinson RJ. Tuberculosis. Lancet. 2007;370:2030-43.
39. Gillespie SH. Evolution of drug resistance in *Mycobacterium tuberculosis*: clinical and molecular perspective. Antimicrob. Agents. Chemother. 2002;46:267-74.
40. Warner DF, Mizrahi V. Tuberculosis chemotherapy: the influence of bacillary stress and damage response pathways on drug efficacy. Clin. Micro. Rev. 2006;19:558-70.
41. Riska PF, Jacobs WR, Alland D. Molecular determinants of drug resistance in tuberculosis. Int. J. Tuberc. Lung Dis. 2000;4:S4-10.
42. Telenti A, Imboden P, Marchesi F. Detection of rifampicin-resistance mutations in Mycobacterium tuberculosis. Lancet. 1993;13:647-50.
43. Williams DL, Waguespack C, Eisenach K. Characterization of rifampin resistance in pathogenic mycobacteria. Antimicrob. Agents Chemother. 1994;38:2380-6.
44. Cheng AFB, Yew WW, Chan EWC, ChinML, Hui MMM, Chan RCY. Multiplex PCR amplimer conformation analysis for rapid detection of gyrA mutations in fluoroquinolone-resistant *Mycobacterium tuberculosis* clinical isolates. Antimicrob. Agents Chemother. 2004;48:596-601.
45. Wang J-Y, Lee L-N, Lai H-C. Fluoroquinolone resistance in *Mycobacterium tuberculosis* isolates: associated genetic mutations and relationship to antimicrobial exposure. Antimicrob. Chemother. 2007;59:860-5.
46. Maus C, Plikaytis B, Shinnick T. Molecular analysis of cross-resistance to capreomycin, kanamycin, amikacin and viomycin in *Mycobacterium tuberculosis*. Antimicrob Agents Chemother. 2005;49:3192-7.
47. Cooksey RC, Morlock GP, McQueen A, Glickman SE, Crawford JT. Characterization of streptomycin resistance mechanisms among *Mycobacterium tuberculosis* isolates from patients in New York City. Antimicrob. Agents Chemother. 1996;40:1186-8.
48. Gegia M, Mdivani N, Mendes RE. Prevalence of and molecular basis for tuberculosis drug resistance in the republic of Georgia: validation of a QIAplex system for detection of drug resistance-related mutations. Antimicrob. Agents Chemother. 2008;52:725-9.
49. Okamoto S, Tamaru A, Nakajima C. Loss of a conserved 7-methylguanosine modification in 16S rRNA confers low-level streptomycin resistance in bacteria. Mol. Microb. 2007;63:1096-106.

50. Alangaden G, Kreiswirth B, Aouad A. Mechanism of resistance to amikacin and kanamycin in *Mycobacterium tuberculosis*. Antimicrob Agents Chemother. 1995;42:1295-7.
51. Kruuner A, Jureen P, Levina K, Ghebremichael S, Hoffner S. Discordant resistance to kanamycin and amikacin in drug-resistant *Mycobacterium tuberculosis*. Antimicrob Agents Chemother. 2003;47:2971-3.
52. Maus CE, Plikaytis BB, Shinnick TM. Mutation of the tlyA confers capreomycin resistance in *Mycobacterium tuberculosis*. Antimicrob. Agents. Chemother. 2005;49:571-7.
53. BROAD Institute—comparative analysis www.broad.mit.edu/annotation/genome/mycobacterium_tuberculosis_spp/.ToolsIndex.html J. Respir. Crit. Care Med. 2003;168:1342-5.
54. Jeon CY, Hwang SH, Min JH. Extensively drug resistant tuberculosis in South Korea: risk factors and treatment outcomes among patients at a tertiary referral hospital. Clin. Infect. Dis. 2008;46:42-9.
55. Prasad R, Garg R. XDR-TB: An emerging threat. Chest. India. 2007;8:3-4.
56. Guidelines for the programmatic management of drug-resistant tuberculosis—WHO 2008.
57. Soeters M, de Vries A, Kimpen J, Donald P, Schaaf H. Clinical features and outcome in children admitted to a TB hospital in the Western Cape—the influence of HIV infection and drug resistance. S Afr Med J. 2005;95:602-6.
58. Dye C, Williams BG, Espinal MA, Raviglione MC. Erasing the world's slow stain: strategies to beat multidrug-resistant tuberculosis. Science. 2002;295:2042-6.
59. Tsiouris SJ, Gandhi NR, El-Sadr WM, Friedland G. Tuberculosis and HIV-needed: a new paradigm for the control and management of linked epidemics. J Int AIDS Soc. 2007;9:62.
60. Havlir DV, Getahun H, Sanne I, Nunn P. Opportunities and challenges for HIV care in overlapping HIV and TB epidemics. JAMA. 2008;300:423-30.
61. Chideya S, Winston CA, Peloquin CA, et al. Isoniazid, rifampin, ethambutol and pyrazinamide pharmacokinetics and treatment outcomes among a predominantly HIV-infected cohort of adults with tuberculosis from Botswana. Clin Infect Dis. 2009;48:1685-94.
62. Sahai J, Gallicano K, Swick L, et al. Reduced plasma concentrations of antituberculosis drugs in patients with HIV infection. Ann Intern Med. 1997;127:289-93.
63. Cato A 3rd, Cavanaugh J, Shi H, Hsu A, Leonard J, Granneman R. The effect of multiple doses of ritonavir on the pharmacokinetics of rifabutin. Clin Pharmacol Ther. 1998;63:414-21.
64. Weiner M, Benator D, Peloquin CA, et al. Evaluation of the drug interaction between rifabutin and efavirenz in patients with HIV infection and tuberculosis. Clin Infect Dis. 2005;41:1343-9.
65. Alland D, Kalkut GE, Moss AR, et al. Transmission of tuberculosis in New York City. An analysis by DNA fingerprinting and conventional epidemiologic methods. N Engl J Med. 1994;330:1710-6.
66. Small PM, Hopewell PC, Singh SP. The epidemiology of tuberculosis in San Francisco. A population-based study using conventional and molecular methods. N Engl J Med. 1994;330:1703-9.

Chapter 16

Extensively Drug-resistant Tuberculosis: Diagnosis

Introduction

Preventing transmission of *Mycobacterium tuberculosis* relies on an accurate and rapid diagnosis. A key barrier to tuberculosis control is that current case detection rates are low. With the global rise in Extensively Drug-Resistant Tuberculosis (XDR), a key aspect of its initial containment will be the identification of the disease itself. Drug-Resistant Tuberculosis (DR-TB) often goes undetected and untreated in many countries. With the exception of a few developed countries, most national tuberculosis programs worldwide do not routinely provide diagnostic services based on culture and drug susceptibility testing (DST). The laboratory is an essential component in Tuberculosis (TB) control programs, and broader access to DST is a priority for most countries. Early choice of appropriate treatment is an essential determinant of favorable outcome, and rapid determination of drug resistance can allow a customized approach to treatment early in the course of the disease and can potentially reduce morbidity, mortality and infectiousness.[1] The diagnosis of XDR-TB is hampered by the absence of effective and affordable rapid diagnostic techniques for drug sensitivity. Several approaches, phenotypic and molecular, have been explored to develop rapid, reliable and accurate methods for the rapid detection of drug resistance in *M. tuberculosis*. This chapter aims to describe the phenotypic and genotypic methods as well as the new methodologies recently proposed for drug resistance detection in TB.

Conventional Phenotypic Methods for the Diagnosis in Solid Media

Phenotypic methods assess inhibition of *M. tuberculosis* growth in the presence of antibiotics to distinguish between susceptible and resistant strains. This is possible since *M. tuberculosis* isolates from patients never treated before are very uniform in their level of susceptibility, as shown by the narrow ranges of minimal inhibitory concentrations (MIC) of the main anti-tuberculosis drugs.[2] Phenotypic methods based on cultivation of *M. tuberculosis* in the presence of antibiotics have been most commonly performed on egg-based or agar-based solid media, and can also be performed as:

- **Direct method:** In this method, antibiotic-containing and control media are inoculated with a decontaminated and concentrated clinical specimen.
- **Indirect method:** In the indirect method, the antibiotic- containing and control media are inoculated with a bacterial suspension of the isolated strain.

There are three conventional phenotypic methods for drug susceptibility testing based on solid media: the proportion method, the resistance ratio method and the absolute concentration method. More recent methods are based on liquid media including the BACTEC radiometric and the Mycobacterial Growth Indicator Tube methods.

The Proportion Method

The proportion method is the most commonly used method worldwide and the recommended method for the diagnosis of DR-TB in India. It allows the precise determination of the proportion of resistant mutants to a certain drug. In this method, several 100-fold serial bacilli dilutions are inoculated into drug-containing and drug-free (control) media. One of those dilutions should produce a number of colonies that is easy to be counted. The number of colonies obtained in the drug-containing and control media are enumerated and the proportion of resistant mutants is then calculated. When performed in Löwenstein-Jensen medium tubes, the test is first read after 28 days of incubation at 37°C. If the proportion of resistant bacteria is higher than 1% for isoniazid, rifampicin and para-aminosalicylic acid, or 10% for the other drugs, the strain is considered resistant and the results are final; otherwise, the test is read again at 42 days of incubation to assess if the strain is susceptible to a certain drug. If the test is performed on agar, a Middlebrook 7H10/11 is used and the medium is incubated in a 10% CO_2 atmosphere. Results are interpreted after 21 days of incubation or even earlier if they show the strain to be resistant.[3]

The Resistance Ratio Method

This method is based on the resistance ratio, which corresponds to the MIC of a test strain divided by the MIC of the drug-susceptible reference strain H37Rv tested at the same time. Thus, it compares the resistance of an unknown strain with that of a standard laboratory strain. An isolate with a resistance ratio value of 2 or less is considered susceptible, while a resistance ratio value of 8 or more defines the isolate as resistant.[4]

The Absolute Concentration Method

This method uses a standardized inoculum grown on drug-free media and media containing graded concentrations of the drug(s) to be tested. Several concentrations of each drug are tested, and resistance is expressed in terms of the lowest concentration of the drug that inhibits growth, i.e. minimal inhibitory concentration (MIC). This method is greatly affected by inoculum size and the viability of the organisms. A strain is considered to be susceptible if the number of colonies on the drug containing medium is less than 20 with a 3+ or 4+ (confluent) growth on the drug-free control.

While these conventional phenotypic methods in solid media are relatively inexpensive and undemanding of sophisticated equipment, results usually take 12 to 16 weeks. Delayed identification of drug resistance results in inadequate treatment, which may generate additional drug resistance and continued transmission in the community.

Phenotypic Methods for the Diagnosis in Liquid Media

Automated liquid culture systems are more sensitive than solid media cultures, and they significantly reduce the turnaround time. However, even with liquid cultures, two to four weeks are still needed to obtain results, and their substantially higher cost is an issue for resource-limited countries.

The BACTEC Radiometric Method

The radiometric method is based on the commercial system BACTEC TB-460 (Becton Dickinson, Sparks, MD), which uses an enriched Middlebrook 7H9 liquid medium containing 14C-labeled palmitic acid as the sole carbon source (12B vial). Growth of the mycobacteria and consumption of the labeled fatty acid will produce 14 CO_2 that is detected inside the 12B vial by the BACTEC apparatus and expressed as a growth index. In the presence of a certain drug, susceptibility can be measured by inhibition of the daily increases in the growth index. The major advantage of the BACTEC radiometric method is the capacity to detect drug resistance faster than with the solid media-based methods; the major disadvantage is the cost of the system and the need for disposal of the radioactive waste from used vials.

The Mycobacterial Growth Indicator Tube

Several published studies have shown the excellent performance of the Mycobacterial Growth Indicator Tube system for the rapid detection of resistance to first- and second-line anti-TB drugs.[5] The Mycobacteria Growth Indicator Tube (MGIT) (Becton Dickinson, Sparks, MD) is part of the 'new generation' of TB diagnostic tools both in its manual version as well as in its more recently introduced automated format (Pfyffer 1997, Idigoras 2000). It is based on fluorescence detection of mycobacterial growth in a tube containing a modified Middlebrook 7H9 medium together with a fluorescence quenching-based oxygen sensor embedded at the bottom of the tube. Consumption of oxygen in the medium produces fluorescence when illuminated by an UV lamp.

New Phenotypic Methods

The laboriousness and long time required by conventional methods to give results and, on the other hand, the requirement for expensive equipment and the need for skilled technical personnel for most molecular techniques, continue to stimulate the search for alternative and affordable methods for drug resistance detection in TB.

Phage-based Methods

There are currently two formats of phage-based assays that have been described for the rapid detection of drug resistance in *M. tuberculosis*. The first one, also known as phage-amplified biologically, was originally described by Wilson, et al. in *M. tuberculosis* isolates[6] and the second format is based on reporter mycobacteriophages expressing luciferase.[7]

Phage-amplification method: This method relies on the biological amplification of mycobacteriophages and has gained wider application in the last decade. They are based on the ability of *M. tuberculosis* to support the growth of an infecting mycobacteriophage. The number of endogenous phages, representing the original number of viable *M. tuberculosis* bacilli, is then determined in a rapidly-growing mycobacterium, such as *M. smegmatis*.[8] The inhouse phage amplification test and the commercially available FastPlaque TB assay have been tested for the detection of rifampicin resistance both in *M. tuberculosis* isolates and directly on clinical specimens. The FastPlaque TB has been evaluated in a comparative study with the proportion method on Middlebrook 7H11 agar for determining rifampicin resistance directly in smear-positive sputum samples.[9] The study showed 100% sensitivity and specificity with results available within two days. A recent meta-analysis of the accuracy of phage-based methods for detecting rifampicin resistance in *M. tuberculosis* concluded that these assays performed on *M. tuberculosis* culture isolates have high sensitivity, but variable and slightly lower specificity.[10] Not enough evidence is available on the accuracy of these assays when performed directly on sputum samples. Safety and quality control issues related to the use of this technique should also be addressed carefully.

Luciferase reporter phage method: It is based on the efficient production of a light signal by viable mycobacteria infected with specific reporter phages expressing the firefly luciferase gene. Light production is dependent on phage infection, expression of the luciferase gene, and the level of cellular ATP.[7] Signals can be detected within minutes after the infection. *M. tuberculosis* isolates, susceptible to isoniazid or rifampicin, result in extinction of light production, while drug-resistant strains continue to produce light. Luciferase reporter tests have now been evaluated against the four first-line antibiotics with an overall agreement of 98.6% compared with the BACTEC TB-460 system.[11] Furthermore, in a recent study, two detection methods, photographic and luminometric were compared and the sensitivity for detecting isoniazid or rifampicin resistance was 100% concluding that both methods were appropriate as screening tests for MDR-TB surveillance.[12]

Colorimetric Methods

Several colorimetric methods have been proposed in the last few years for the rapid detection of drug resistance in *M. tuberculosis*. TK medium is a novel colorimetric system that indicates growth of mycobacteria by changing the color of the growth medium. These calorimetric methods use redox indicators or tetrazolium salts to detect mycobacterial growth. The tests are based on the reduction of the colored redox indicator added to the culture medium after *M. tuberculosis* has been exposed in vitro to different antibiotics. Resistance is detected by a change in color of the indicator, which is directly proportional to the number of viable mycobacteria in the medium.[13] A recent systematic review and meta-analysis of colorimetric redox indicator methods to detect multi-drug resistance in *M. tuberculosis* found evidence of a high sensitivity and specificity for the rapid detection of MDR-TB.[14] Colorimetric methods represent a good alternative for the rapid detection of drug resistance in laboratories with limited resources. TK Medium also permits susceptibility testing for drug resistance, and can allow for differentiation between *M. tuberculosis* and nontuberculous mycobacteria. Unfortunately, there is insufficient published evidence on the field performance of this test in developing countries.[15]

The Nitrate Reductase Assay

The nitrate reductase assay (NRA) is a quite simple technique based on the capacity of *M. tuberculosis* to reduce nitrate to nitrite, which is detected by adding a chemical reagent to the culture medium. *M. tuberculosis* is cultivated on Löwenstein-Jensen medium in the presence of an antibiotic and its ability to reduce nitrate is measured after 10 days of incubation. Resistant strains will reduce the nitrate, which is revealed by a pink-red color in the medium, while susceptible strains will lose this capacity as they are inhibited by the antibiotic.[16] Two recent studies applied the nitrate reductase assay directly on sputum samples and produced variable results for sensitivity and specificity and the best results were obtained for isoniazid or rifampicin resistance detection.[17,18]

Microscopic Observation Broth-drug Susceptibility Assay (MODS)

The MODS assay is based on the observation of the characteristic cord formation of M tuberculosis that is visualized microscopically in liquid medium with the use of an inverted microscope.[19] MODS uses simple light microscopy to detect early growth of *M. tuberculosis* as 'strings and tangles' of bacterial cells in the broth medium with or without antimicrobial drugs.[20] The agreement between MODS and the reference standard for drug susceptibility testing is 97% for isoniazid, 100% for rifampicin, and 99% for isoniazid and rifampicin combined (MDR). Lower values of agreement were obtained for ethambutol (95%) and streptomycin (92%). One minor disadvantage of MODS is the requirement for an inverted microscope for observation of the mycobacterial growth.

The Thin-layer Agar Method

Among novel, rapid phenotypic methods, the Thin Layer 7H11 agar (TL7H11) method or microcolony method is of relatively low cost. It has been adapted for the rapid detection of drug resistance directly from sputum samples, and has been shown in early studies to be accurate for the detection of MDR-TB compared with the reference proportion method, with results available in one week.[21]

Overall, large multicentric studies defining the accuracy of phenotypic DST methods are still unavailable. Practical issues, such as quality controls and training requirements, have not been adequately addressed under field conditions. The application of these approaches to support individualized treatment through determination of second-line drug susceptibility profiles remains largely unexplored, implying that their application in support of individualized treatment of MDR-TB and especially for XDR-TB remains uncertain.

Genotypic Methods

Genotypic methods for drug resistance in TB look for the genetic determinants of resistance rather than the resistance phenotype and involve two basic steps: Nucleic acid amplification such as polymerase chain reaction (PCR) to amplify the sections of the *M. tuberculosis* genome known to be altered in resistant strains and a second step of assessing the amplified products for specific mutations correlating with drug resistance.[22]

Deoxyribonucleic Acid (DNA) Sequencing and Pyrosequencing

Sequencing DNA of PCR-amplified products has become the most widely used genotypic method for detecting drug resistance in *M. tuberculosis*. It is accurate and reliable and it has become the reference standard for mutation detection. DNA sequencing has been widely used for characterizing mutations in the rpoB gene in rifampicin-resistant strains and to detect mutations responsible for resistance to other antituberculosis drugs.[23] Drug resistance detection in *M. tuberculosis* has also been described by pyrosequencing technology.[24] This technology is a short-read (30–50 bp) sequencing technique, which is based on the quantitative detection of pyrophosphate released following nucleotide incorporation into a growing DNA chain. Although this method is less cumbersome and expensive than traditional sequencing, the shorter sequences are not as discriminating. By using automated sequencers and well-trained staff, sequencing assays can be completed and identification results can be reported within 1 to 3 days. However, the installation, maintenance, and running of automated DNA sequencing on a daily basis are currently too expensive and labor-intensive for use in resource-poor settings. One study reported high specificity (100%) and sensitivity (94.6%) for detection of multidrug-resistant *M. tuberculosis* as well as high specificity (99.3%) and sensitivity (86.9%) for detection of extensively drug-resistant *M. tuberculosis* by pyrosequencing when compared to phenotypic DST.[25] The short turnaround time combined with multilocus sequencing of several isolates in parallel makes pyrosequencing an attractive method for drug resistance screening in *M. tuberculosis*.

Solid-phase Hybridization Techniques

There are currently two commercially available solid-phase hybridization techniques for the rapid detection of drug resistance in TB:

Line Probe Assay

Several commercial line probe assays are available for the detection of *M. tuberculosis* and mutations associated with drug resistance. WHO endorsed line probe assays in the year 2008. There are currently two types of line probe assays that are used frequently.

INNO-LiPA Rif. TB Assay

The Commercially available kit is known as the INNO-LiPA Rif. TB kit (Innogenetics, Gent, Belgium). This assay is used for the detection of resistance to rifampicin. The LiPA assay is based on reverse hybridization of amplified DNA from cultured strains or clinical samples to ten probes covering the core region of the rpoB gene of *M. tuberculosis*, immobilized on a nitrocellulose strip.[25] From the pattern of hybridization obtained, the presence or absence of mutated or wild regions is visualized by a colorimetric reaction and the strain can be considered as resistant or susceptible to rifampicin. A recent meta-analysis summarized the results obtained for the INNO-LiPA Rif. TB test, and showed that this line probe assay has high sensitivity and specificity when culture isolates are used.[26] The majority of studies had sensitivities of 95% or greater, and nearly all were 100% specific. The results, however, are less accurate when the test is directly applied to clinical specimens like sputum. There is a paucity of data on the application of this test directly to clinical specimens.

In 2009, Government of India planned to set up a network of 43 quality-assured laboratories under RNTCP which will be capable of undertaking rapid tests like LPA (Line Probe Assay) and liquid culture besides the conventional solid culture. These labs, supported by identified existing laboratories in the public and private sector, will be able to perform at least 220,000 cultures and DSTs essential for diagnosing and following up 30,000 MDR patients annually. As a part of the RNTCP-FIND collaborative projects in India, molecular Line Probe Assay (LPA) were validated in intermediate reference laboratories. In states like Andhra Pradesh, Gujarat and Maharashtra, patients detected as having rifampicin resistance by LPA would be immediately offered Category IV treatment.

GenoType MTBDR Assay

The GenoType MTBDR test is able to detect mutations in the rpoB gene for rifampicin resistance, and the most frequent mutation at codon 315 of the katG gene for Isoniazid resistance, either in isolates or clinical specimens. The specificity and sensitivity of the assay for rifampicin resistance were nearly 100%; for isoniazid-resistance, despite a 100% specificity, the sensitivity of the test ranged from 70% to 90%, depending on the prevalence of the particular mutation at the katG locus.[27,28]

GenoType MTBDRplus

This line probe assay is commercially available as Kit GenoType MTBDRplus assay (Hain Lifescience, Nehren, Germany). This is an advanced version of the

GenoType MTBDR assay, includes probes for the identification of other mutations in the hotspot region of the rpoB gene for rifampicin resistance, and probes to detect mutations in the promoter region of the inhA gene involved in isoniazid resistance. These improvements facilitate the detection of another 10% to 20% of isoniazid-resistant cases, with an enhancement in rapid MDR-TB diagnosis.

GenoType MTBDRsl Assay: GenoType *M. tuberculosis* drug-resistant second-line assay (MTBDRsl; Hain Lifescience), was developed to detect resistance to ethambutol, fluoroquinolones, and injectable aminoglycosides/cyclic peptides, i.e. to detect XDR strains among MDR strains. In a very recent report, Hillemann, et al. presented the first evaluation of the MTBDRsl test.[29,30] In this study, the MTBDRsl test detected mutations in 91% of strains resistant to fluoroquinolones 85% resistant to amikacin, 87% resistant to cyclic peptide capreomycin, and 69% of the strains resistant to ethambutol.[29] Thus, the combined use of GenoType MTBDRplus and GenoType MTBDRsl allows the rapid detection of XDR-TB.

Rifoligotyping: It is a solid-phase reverse hybridization test for rapid detection of rifampicin resistance. This is an inhouse low-cost assay for the detection of rifampicin resistance-associated mutations in the rpoB gene of *M. tuberculosis*. This test was developed in Netherlands. It also involves a combination of DNA amplification and reverse-line blot hybridization. DNA of the rpoB gene of *M. tuberculosis* is amplified by PCR with specific primers and the PCR products are hybridized to oligonucleotides on a DNA membrane, encoding the wild type rpoB sequence, and the most frequent mutations in rifampicin-resistant strains. Amplified products from rifampicin-resistant strains will fail to hybridize to one or more of the wild type oligonucleotides, and in most cases, will hybridize to one of the mutant oligonucleotides bound to the membrane.

Real-time PCR Techniques

Real-time PCR techniques have also been introduced recently for the rapid detection of drug resistance in TB. Different probes have been used for detection, such as the TaqMan probe, Fluorescence Resonance Energy Transfer probes, molecular beacons and biprobes.[31] Real-time PCR methods are based on hybridization of amplified nucleic acids with fluorescent-labeled probes spanning DNA regions of interest and monitored inside thermal cycles. The fluorescent signal increases in direct proportion to the amount of amplified product inside the reaction tube. The main advantages of real-time PCR techniques are the speed of the test and a lower risk of contamination. The main disadvantages would be the requirement for expensive equipment and reagents, and the need for skilled technical personnel. Real-time PCR techniques have been applied to *M. tuberculosis* strains and, more recently, directly to clinical samples.[32] Results are generally obtained in an average of 1.5 to 2.0 hours after DNA extraction. Real-time PCR could eventually be implemented in reference laboratories with the required capacity to properly set up the technique and in settings where it can contribute to the management of TB patients.

Microarrays

Microarrays, also known as biochips or DNA chips, have been proposed as genotypic methods for detecting drug resistance in *M. tuberculosis*. They are based on the hybridization of DNA obtained from clinical samples to oligonucleotides immobilized on a solid support, such as miniaturized glass slides. They have been tested to detect resistance to isoniazid and rifampicin.[33] The recently described CombiChip Mycobacteria Drug-Resistance detection DNA chip is an oligonucleotide microchip coupled with PCR for the detection of resistance to isoniazid and rifampicin. The overall specificity was 100% and 95.3% for detecting isoniazid and rifampicin resistance respectively. For the time being, and due to the high cost involved, the use of microarrays for detecting drug resistance in *M. tuberculosis* is still beyond the reach of most clinical mycobacteriology laboratories, especially in high-burden countries.

TB GeneXpert/Xpert MTB/RIF Assay

It is a fully automated nucleic acid amplification test (NAAT) platform that can detect TB and rifampin resistance.[34,35] It was developed through a partnership between Cepheid and Foundation for Innovative New Diagnostics (FIND), the University of Medicine and Dentistry of New Jersey, and funded by the National Institute of Allergy & Infectious Diseases. WHO endorsed TB GeneXpert/Xpert MTB/RIF assay for diagnosis of TB and rifampicin resistance in December 2010. It has unprecedented sensitivity for detecting MTB—even in smear negative, culture positive specimens. It was observed that the pooled sensitivity was 98% (95% CI 97%-99%) for smear-positive, culture-positive TB and 68% (95% CI 59%-75%) for smear-negative, culture-positive TB; the pooled sensitivity was 80% (95% CI 67%-88%) in people living with HIV and 89% (95% CI 81%-94%) in people without HIV infection. For rifampicin resistance detection, Xpert achieved a pooled sensitivity of 94% (95% CI 87%-97%) and pooled specificity of 98% (95% CI 97%-99%).[36] Results are obtained in two hours and it requires no instrumentation other than the GeneXpert System. Xpert test is currently recommended as the initial diagnostic test in individuals suspected of MDR-TB or HIV-associated TB. If Xpert detects rifampicin resistance in patients considered at risk of MDR-TB, an appropriate MDR-TB regimen should be started while additional sputum specimens are obtained for culture and drug susceptibility testing. Subsequent testing will confirm the presence of rifampicin resistance and enable testing for drug resistance to isoniazid and other first-line drugs and second-line drugs. Although the development of the Xpert MTB/RIF assay is undoubtedly a landmark event, clinical and programmatic effects and cost-effectiveness remain to be defined.

References

1. Hopewell PC, Pai M, Maher D, Uplekar M, Raviglione MC. International standards for tuberculosis care. Lancet Infect Dis. 2006;6:710-25.
2. Heifets LB. Clinical mycobacteriology. Drug susceptibility testing. Clin Lab Med. 1996;16:641-56.

3. Kent PT, Kubica GP. Public Health Mycobacteriology. A guide for the Level III Laboratory. Atlanta, GA: CDC. 1985.
4. Heifets L. Conventional methods for antimicrobial susceptibility testing of *Mycobacterium tuberculosis*. In: Multidrug-resistant Tuberculosis, Ed.: Bastian I, Portaels F. Kluwer Academic Publishers, Dordrecht, The Netherlands 2000.
5. Rüsch-Gerdes S, Pfyffer GE, Casal M, Chadwick M, Siddiqi S. Multicenter laboratory validation of the BACTEC MGIT 960 technique for testing susceptibilities of *Mycobacterium tuberculosis* to classical second-line drugs and newer antimicrobials. J Clin Microbiol. 2006;44:688-92.
6. Wilson SM, l-Suwaidi Z, McNerney R, Porter J, Drobniewski F. Evaluation of a new rapid bacteriophage-based method for the drug susceptibility testing of *Mycobacterium tuberculosis*. Nat Med. 1997;3:465-8.
7. Jacobs WR Jr, Barletta RG, Udani R, et al. Rapid assessment of drug susceptibilities of *Mycobacterium tuberculosis* by means of luciferase reporter phages. Science. 1993;260:819-22.
8. McNerney R. Phage replication technology for diagnosis and susceptibility testing. In: Parish T, Stocker NG, eds. *Mycobacterium tuberculosis* protocols. Methods in Molecular Medicine. Humana Press, Totowa, NY. 2001;145-54.
9. Albert H, Heydenrych A, Brookes R, et al. Performance of a rapid phage-based test, FASTPlaqueTB, to diagnose pulmonary tuberculosis from sputum specimens in South Africa. Int J Tuberc Lung Dis. 2002;6:529-37.
10. Pai M, Kalantri S, Pascopella L, Riley LW, Reingold AL. Bacteriophage-based assays for the rapid detection of rifampicin resistance in *Mycobacterium tuberculosis*: A meta-analysis. J Infect. 2005;51:175-87.
11. Banaiee N, Bobadilla-del-Valle M, Riska PF, et al. Rapid identification and susceptibility testing of *Mycobacterium tuberculosis* from MGIT cultures with luciferase reporter mycobacteriophages. J Med Microbiol. 2003;52:557-6.
12. Hazbon MH. Recent advances in molecular methods for early diagnosis of tuberculosis and drug-resistant tuberculosis. Biomedica. 2004;24:149-62.
13. Palomino JC. Non-conventional and new methods in the diagnosis of tuberculosis: feasibility and applicability in the field. Eur Respir J. 2005;26:1-12.
14. Martin A, Portaels F, Palomino JC. Colorimetric redox-indicator methods for the rapid detection of multidrug resistance in *Mycobacterium tuberculosis*: a systematic review and meta-analysis. J Antimicrob Chemother. 2007;59:175-83.
15. Pai M, Kalantri S, Dheda K. New tools and emerging technologies for the diagnosis of tuberculosis: Part II. Active tuberculosis and drug resistance. Expert Rev Mol Diagn. 2006;6:423-32.
16. Angeby KA, Klintz L, Hoffner SE. Rapid and inexpensive drug susceptibility testing of *Mycobacterium tuberculosis* with a nitrate reductase assay. J Clin Microbiol. 2002;40:553-5.
17. Musa HR, Ambroggi M, Souto A, Angeby KA. Drug susceptibility testing of *Mycobacterium tuberculosis* by a nitrate reductase assay applied directly on microscopy-positive sputum samples. J Clin Microbiol. 2005;43:3159-61.
18. Solis LA, Shin SS, Han LL, Llanos F, Stowell M, Sloutsky A. Validation of a rapid method for detection of *M. tuberculosis* resistance to isoniazid and rifampin in Lima, Peru. Int J Tuberc Lung Dis. 2005;9:760-4.
19. Moore DA, Evans CA, Gilman RH. Microscopic-observation drug-susceptibility assay for the diagnosis of TB. N Engl J Med. 2006;355:1539-50.
20. Caviedes L, Moore DA. Introducing MODS: A low-cost, low-tech tool for high-performance detection of tuberculosis and multidrug-resistant tuberculosis. Ind J Med Microbiol. 2007;25:87-8.

21. Robledo JA, Mejía GI, Morcillo N, et al. Evaluation of a rapid culture method for tuberculosis diagnosis: A Latin-American multi-center study. Int J Tuberc Lung Dis. 2006;10:613-9.
22. Garcia de Viedma D. Rapid detection of resistance in *Mycobacterium tuberculosis*: a review discussing molecular approaches. Clin Microbiol Infect. 2003;9:349-59.
23. Jalava J, Marttila H. Application of molecular genetic methods in macrolide, lincosamide and streptogramin resistance diagnostics and in detection of drug-resistant *Mycobacterium tuberculosis*. APMIS. 2004;112:838-55.
24. Jureen P, Engstrand L, Eriksson S, Alderborn A, Krabbe M, Hoffner SE. Rapid detection of rifampin resistance in *Mycobacterium tuberculosis* by Pyrosequencing technology. J Clin Microbiol. 2006;44:1925-9.
25. Engstrom A, Morcillo N, Imperiale B, Hoffner SE, Jureen P. Detection of First- and Second-Line Drug Resistance in Mycobacterium tuberculosis Clinical Isolates by Pyrosequencing. J. Clin. Microbiol. 2012;50:2026. DOI: 10.1128/JCM.06664-11.
26. De Beenhouwer H, Lhiang Z, Jannes G, et al. Rapid detection of rifampicin resistance in sputum and biopsy specimens from tuberculosis patients by PCR and line probe assay. Tuber Lung Dis. 1995;76:425-30.
27. Morgan M, Kalantri S, Flores L, Pai M. A commercial line probe assay for the rapid detection of rifampicin resistance in *Mycobacterium tuberculosis*: A systematic review and meta-analysis. BMC Infect Dis. 2005;5:62.
28. Hillemann D, Rüsch-Gerdes S, Richter E. Application of the Genotype MTBDR assay directly on sputum specimens. Int J Tuberc Lung Dis. 2006;10:1057-9.
29. Hillemann D, Rüsch-Gerdes S, Richter E. Evaluation of the GenoType MTBDRplus assay for rifampin and isoniazid susceptibility testing of Mycobacterium tuberculosis strains and clinical specimens. J Clin Microbiol. 2007;45:2635-40.
30. Hillemann D, Rüsch-Gerdes S, Richter E. Evaluation of the GenoType MTBDRplus assay for rifampin and isoniazid susceptibility testing of *Mycobacterium tuberculosis* strains and clinical specimens. J Clin Microbiol. 2007;45:2635-40.
31. Brossier F, Veziris N. Detection by GenoType MTBDRsl Test of Complex Mechanisms of Resistance to Second-Line Drugs and Ethambutol in Multidrug-Resistant *Mycobacterium tuberculosis* Complex Isolates. J Clin Microbio. 2010;48:1683-9.
32. Shamputa IC, Rigouts L, Portaels F. Molecular genetic methods for diagnosis and antibiotic resistance detection of mycobacteria from clinical specimens. APMIS. 2004;112:728-52.
33. Espasa M, Gonzalez-Martin J, Alcaide F, et al. Direct detection in clinical samples of multiple gene mutations causing resistance of *Mycobacterium tuberculosis* to isoniazid and rifampicin using fluorogenic probes. J Antimicrob Chemother. 2005;55:860-5.
34. Gryadunov D, Mikhailovich V, Lapa S, et al. Evaluation of hybridisation on oligonucleotide microarrays for analysis of drug-resistant *Mycobacterium tuberculosis*. Clin Microbiol Infect. 2005;11:531-9.
35. Cepheid announces new diagnostic technology in ongoing efforts to halt the spread of TB. Available at: http://www.finddiagnostics.org/export/sitesdefault/media/press/090324.html. Foundation for Innovative New Diagnostics, 2009. Accessed April 2, 2011.
36. Steingart KR, Sohn H, Schiller I, Kloda LA, Boehme CC, Pai M, Dendukuri N. XpertMTB/RIF assay for pulmonary tuberculosis and rifampicin resistance in adults. Cochrane Database of Systematic Reviews 2013, Issue 1. Art. No.: CD009593. DOI: 10.1002/14651858.CD009593.pub2.

Chapter 17

Extensively Drug-resistant Tuberculosis: Management

Introduction

Extensively drug-resistant TB (XDR-TB) is, by definition, resistant to both quinolones and injectable agents, the most potent second-line agents that form the cornerstone of Multidrug-resistant Tuberculosis (MDR-TB) treatment. As a result, treatment of XDR-TB is more difficult and less successful than that of MDR-TB. Effective drugs may not be available for XDR-TB patients, who have had extensive prior TB treatment. However, many principles of the treatment of MDR-TB patients are applicable to XDR-TB patients.[1,2] The treatment can be an individualized regimen or a standardized one, depending on the previous drugs taken by the patient (by constructing a drug-o-gram), the degree of resistance in the community and the financial status of the patient. A drug may be considered likely to be effective if the baseline DST shows susceptibility to that drug; if no DST results are available, a drug may still be considered likely to be effective if the patient has not received the drug for atleast 1 month.[3] This chapter aims to review the management of XDR-TB.

Management Guidelines for Patients with Documented, or Almost Certain, XDR-TB[4]

Hierarchical system of drug groups usage applies in XDR-TB also. Atleast five drugs with proven susceptibility or which are most likely to be effective should be used (Table 17.1). Use any Group 1 agents that may be effective. Use an injectable agent to which the strain is susceptible and consider an extended duration of use (12 months or possibly the whole treatment). If resistant to all injectable agents, it is recommended to use the one which the patient has never used before (strain may be resistant to injectable in vitro, though not necessarily in vivo). Usually capreomycin is preferred. Use a later-generation fluoroquinolone such as moxifloxacin. Use all Group 4 agents that have not been used extensively in a previous regimen or any that are likely to be effective. Use two or more agents from Group 5. Consider high-dose isoniazid treatment if low-level resistance is documented. Consider adjuvant surgery if there is localized disease.

Ensure strong infection control measures. Treat HIV disease if present. Provide comprehensive monitoring and full adherence support.

A standardized regimen for the management of XDR-TB patients consist of seven drugs, with two reserve/substitute drugs. The dosages of the drugs would vary as per the weight of the patient (≤ 45kg or >45kg). All drugs are to be given on a daily basis preferably under supervision. Injection capreomycin is given 6 days/week. The details of the drugs and dosages are as per Table 17.2.

The reserve/substitute drugs would be used in the following conditions:

- If the patient has taken PAS during his previous MDR treatment, PAS will be replaced with one of the reserve drugs used in the management of XDR-TB
- If the patient is unable to tolerate one or more of the drugs
- If the patient is found to be resistant to Capreomycin.

The treatment would be of 24 to 30 months' duration, with 6 to 12 months' Intensive Phase (IP) and 18 months' Continuation Phase (CP). The Intensive Phase

TABLE 17.1: Grouping of antituberculosis drugs

Group 1 First line oral agents	Ethambutol (E); Pyrazinamide (Z); Rifabutin (Rfb)
Group 2 Injectable agents	Kanamycin (Km); Amikacin (Amk); Capreomycin (Cm); Streptomycin (S)
Group3: Fluoroquinolones	Moxifloxacin (Mfx); Levofloxacin (Lfx); Ofloxacin (Ofx)
Group 4 Oral bacteriostatic second-line agents	Ethionamide (Eto); Prothionamide (Pto); Cycloserine (Cs); Terizidone (Trd); Para-aminosalicylic acid (PAS)
Group 5 (drugs with unclear efficacy or unclear role in MDR-TB treatment, not recommended by WHO for routine use in MDR-TB patients)	Clofazimine (Cfz); Linezolid (Lzd); Amoxicillin/clavulanate (Amx/Clv); Thioacetazone (Thz); Imipenem/cilastatin (Ipm/Cln); high-dose isoniazid (high-dose H); Clarithromycin (Clr)

TABLE 17.2: Standardized regimen for the management of XDR-TB (as per body weight)

Drugs	*Dosage/day*	
	≤ 45 kg	*> 45 kg*
Capreomycin (Cm)	750 mg OD	1000 mg OD
Na PAS	10 g OD	12 g OD
Moxifloxacin (Mfx)	400 mg OD	400 mg OD
High dose INH (High dose-H)	600 mg OD	900 mg OD
Clofazimine (Cfz)	200 mg OD	200 mg OD
Linezolid (Lzd)	600 mg OD	600 mg OD
Amoxyclav (Amx/Clv)	875/125 mg BD	875/125 mg BD
Pyridoxine	100 mg OD	100 mg OD
Reserve/Substitute drugs		
Clarithromycin (Clr)	500 mg BD	500 mg BD
Thiacetazone (Thz)	150 mg OD	150 mg OD

will consist of Capreomycin, PAS, Moxifloxacin, High dose-INH (600–900 mg), clofazamine, linezolid, and amoxycillin/clavulanate while the continuation phase will consist of PAS, moxifloxacin, High dose-INH (600–900 mg), clofazamine, linezolid and amoxycillin/clavulanate. Reserve/substitute drugs would be clarithromycin and thiacetazone. The change from IP to CP will be done only after achievement of culture conversion, i.e. two consecutive negative cultures taken at least one month apart. In case of delay in culture conversion, the IP will be extended from 6 months up to a maximum of 12 months.[5] In case of extension, capreomycin injection can be used intermittently (three times/week) for seven to twelve months.

Monitoring of Treatment

No randomized controlled trials have been conducted on XDR-TB, regarding the appropriate duration of treatment or regarding the appropriate monitoring techniques. Therefore, it is largely based on consensus.[5] Essentially the treatment should be given directly observed for a minimum of 6 days/week as treatment success is critical. Ensure strict compliance and prompt identification and management of side effects.

Baseline Evaluation

- Complete Blood Count with platelets
- Thyroid function test
- Liver function test
- Kidney function test
- S electrolytes
- Blood sugar
- Pregnancy test
- All patients would be offered HIV testing after pretest counseling, unless known to be HIV positive
- Chest X-ray
- Surgical evaluation.

Follow-up schedule:

a. Culture monthly during IP starting after 3 months of starting treatment, i.e. 3, 4, 5 and 6, 7 and quarterly during CP, i.e. 9, 12, 15, 18, 21 and 24. In case of extension of IP due to delay in culture conversion, the follow-up schedule will be modified accordingly. The treatment follow-up culture in XDR-TB can be reduced as per Chennai consensus[6](culture examination done at least at 4, 6, 12, 18 and 24 months of treatment).
b. Other tests:
   - Complete Blood Count: Weekly in first month, then monthly to rule out bone marrow suppression, anemia as a side effect of linezolid
   - Renal function tests, serum electrolytes: Monthly during the period that the capreomycin is being administered
   - Liver function tests: Monthly in IP and 3 monthly during CP
   - CXR: 6 monthly
   - Thyroid function tests and other tests when clinically indicated.

Assess side effects due to drugs and manage appropriately. Smear status at 6th month may be used as a surrogate marker for response to treatment and those who remain smear positive at 6 months can be considered for change of treatment.[7]

Role of Surgery

With the emergence of MDR and XDR-TB, the role of surgery has again surfaced due to an inability to ensure complete cure with the available chemotherapy. In XDR-TB patients with localized disease, surgery, as an adjunct to chemotherapy, can improve outcomes provided skilled thoracic surgeons and excellent post-operative care are available. It is adjunct to chemotherapy and should not be considered as last resort. Chemotherapy should be given atleast for two months prior to surgery and continued for 12 to 24 months after resection. It is indicated in patients who remain sputum positive, with resistance to large number of drugs; and localized pulmonary disease.[4] Most common operative procedure in patients with XDR-TB is resection surgery.[8] Resection surgery should be timed to offer the patient the best possible chances of cure with the least morbidity, for example, when the disease is still localized to one lung or one lung lobe. Specialized surgical facilities should include stringent infection control measures, since infectious substances and aerosols are generated in large quantities during surgery and during mechanical ventilation and postoperative pulmonary hygiene maneuvers. Computerized tomography, pulmonary function testing and quantitative lung perfusion/ventilation are recommended as part of the preoperative work-up. It has been shown that overall cure rate was substantially higher (81% v/s 56%) when surgery was more frequently and aggressively applied in cases of resistant pulmonary tuberculosis.[9,10] The same principle can be applied to surgically feasible XDR-TB patients.

Human Immunodeficiency Virus (HIV) and XDR-TB

The treatment of drug-resistant tuberculosis (DR-TB) in patients with HIV is very similar to that in patients without HIV except that antiretroviral treatment (ART) plays a crucial role, as mortality in XDR-TB/HIV patients without the use of ART is extremely high.[4,11] Adverse effects are more common in patients with HIV. The multiple medicines involved in XDR-TB with recognized high toxicity risks, often combined with ART, results in a high incidence of adverse effects. Some toxicities are common to both antituberculosis treatment and ART, which may result in added rates of adverse events. Monitoring needs to be more intense for both response to therapy and adverse effects. The use of Thioacetazone is not recommended for patients with HIV or for routine use in populations with high rates of HIV.[12] Immune Reconstitution Inflammatory Syndrome (IRIS) may complicate therapy.

XDR-TB in Pediatric Patients

Children with DR-TB generally have primary resistance transmitted from an index case with DR-TB. When DST is available, it should be used to guide therapy, although children with paucibacillary TB are often culture negative. Nevertheless, every effort should be made to confirm XDR-TB bacteriologically by the use of drug susceptability testing (DST) and to avoid exposing children unnecessarily to toxic drugs. The treatment of culture-negative children with clinical evidence of active TB disease and contact with a documented case of DR-TB should be guided by the results of DST and the history of the contact's exposure to antituberculosis drugs.[12] There is only limited reported experience with the use of second-line drugs for extended periods in children. The risks and benefits of each drug should be carefully considered in designing a regimen. Frank discussion with family members is critical, especially at the outset of therapy. XDR-TB is life-threatening, and no antituberculosis drugs are absolutely contraindicated in children. Children who have received treatment for DR-TB have generally tolerated the second-line drugs well.[13,14] Experience with the use of fluoroquinolones has not demonstrated side effects in humans. So, it is considered that the benefit of fluoroquinolones in treating XDR-TB in children outweighs any risk.[15,16] Additionally, ethionamide, PAS and cycloserine have been used effectively in children and are well tolerated. In general, antituberculosis drugs should be dosed according to body weight (Table 17.3). Monthly monitoring of body weight is, therefore, especially important in pediatric cases, with adjustment of doses as children gain weight. All drugs, including the fluoroquinolones, should be dosed at the higher end of the recommended ranges whenever possible, except ethambutol. Ethambutol should be dosed at 15 mg/kg, and not at 25 mg/kg as sometimes used in adults with DR-TB, as it is more difficult to monitor for optic neuritis in children. In children who are not culture-positive initially, treatment failure is difficult to assess. Persistent abnormalities on chest radiograph do not necessarily signify a lack of improvement. In children, weight loss or, more commonly, failure to gain weight adequately, is of particular concern and often one of the first or only signs of treatment failure. This is another key reason to monitor weight carefully in children.[4]

TABLE 17.3: Pediatric dosing of second-line antituberculosis drugs

Drug	*Daily dose (mg/kg)*	*Frequency*	*Maximum*
Streptomycin	20–40	Once daily	1 g
Kanamycin	15–30	Once daily	1 g
Amikacin	15–22.5	Once daily	1 g
Capreomycin	15–30	Once daily	1 g
Ofloxacin	15–20	Twice daily	800 mg
Levofloxacin	7.5–10	Once daily	750 mg
Moxifloxacin	7.5–10	Once daily	400 mg
Ethionamide	15–20	Twice daily	1 g
Prothionamide	15–20	Twice daily	1 g
Cycloserine	10–20	Once or twice daily	1 g
P-aminosalicylic acid	150	Twice or thrice daily	12 g

XDR-TB in Pregnancy

All female patients of childbearing age should be tested for pregnancy upon initial evaluation. Pregnancy is not a contraindication for treatment of active XDR-TB, which poses great risks to the lives of both mother and fetus.[4,17,18] However, birth control is strongly recommended for all nonpregnant women receiving therapy for XDR-TB because of the potential consequences for both mother and fetus resulting from frequent and severe adverse drug reactions. The risks and benefits of treatment should be carefully considered, with the primary goal of smear conversion to protect the health of the mother and child, both before and after birth. The following are some general guidelines:

- Start treatment of drug resistance in second trimester or sooner if condition of patient is severe. Since the majority of teratogenic effects occur in the first trimester, therapy may be delayed until the second trimester. The decision to postpone the start of treatment should be agreed by both patient and doctor after analysis of the risks and benefits. It is based primarily on the clinical judgment resulting from the analysis of life-threatening signs/symptoms and severity of the disease. When therapy is started, three or four oral drugs with demonstrated efficacy against the infecting strain should be used and then reinforced with an injectable agent and possibly other drugs immediately postpartum.[19]
- Avoid injectable agents for the most part, aminoglycosides should not be used in the regimens of pregnant patients and can be particularly toxic to the developing fetal ear. Capreomycin may also carry a risk of ototoxicity but is the injectable drug of choice if an injectable agent cannot be avoided
- Avoid ethionamide as it can increase the risk of nausea and vomiting associated with pregnancy, and teratogenic effects have been observed in animal studies. If possible, ethionamide should be avoided in pregnant patients.

Breastfeeding

A woman who is breastfeeding and has active XDR-TB should receive a full course of antituberculosis treatment. Timely and properly applied chemotherapy is the best way to prevent transmission of tubercle bacilli to her baby. In lactating mothers on treatment, most antituberculosis drugs will be found in the breast milk in concentrations that would equal only a small fraction of the therapeutic dose used in an infant. However, any effects on infants of such exposure during the full course of DR-TB treatment have not been established. Therefore, when resources are available, it is recommended to provide infant formula options as an alternative to breastfeeding. However, if the mother is sputum smear-positive, the care of the infant should be left to family members until she becomes sputum smear-negative, if this is feasible. When the mother and infant are together, this common time should be spent in well-ventilated areas or outdoors. In some settings, the mother may be offered the option of using a surgical mask or an N-95 respirator until she becomes sputum smear-negative.

Contraception

There is no contraindication to the use of oral contraceptives with the nonrifamycin-containing regimens. Patients who vomit directly after taking an oral contraceptive can be at risk of decreased absorption of the drug and, therefore, of decreased efficacy. These patients should be advised to take their contraceptives apart from times when they may experience vomiting caused by the antituberculosis treatment. Patients who vomit at any time directly after, or within the first two hours, after taking the contraceptive tablet, should use a barrier method of contraception until a full month of the contraceptive tablets can be tolerated.

WHO Response Strategies for XDR-TB[20]

To combat the threat of XDR-TB, WHO convened a Global Task Force on XDR-TB on 17th October, 2006 and recommended to strengthen basic activities to control TB and HIV/AIDS and to avoid additional emergence of MDR-TB and XDR-TB as well as acceleration of treatment of MDR and XDR-TB cases with universal access to sound management of MDR and XDR-TB by 2015 in all countries and near to universal access in the high burden countries by 2010. The revised plan recommended the treatment of 1.6 million MDR-TB and XDR-TB cases by 2015 instead of 800,000 MDR-TB cases. During this meeting, eight recommendations were put forward to the international TB community, outlining key areas of response, beginning with strengthening of basic TB and HIV/AIDS control and proper management of MDR-TB. The eight recommendations are:

- Strengthening basic activities to control TB and HIV/AIDS, as detailed in the Stop TB Strategy and the Global Plan, to avoid additional emergence of MDR-TB and XDR-TB;
- Scaling-up the programmatic management of MDR-TB and XDR-TB to reach the targets set forth in the Global Plan;
- Strengthening laboratory services for adequate and timely diagnosis of MDR-TB and XDR-TB;
- Expanding surveillance of MDR-TB and XDR-TB to better understand the magnitude and trends of drug resistance and the links with HIV;
- Fostering sound infection-control measures to avoid MDR-TB and XDR-TB transmission to protect patients, health workers, others working in congregate settings and the broader community, especially in high HIV prevalence settings;
- Strengthening advocacy, communication and social mobilization for sustained political commitment and a patient-centered approach to treatment.

Management of Contacts of XDR-TB Patients

There is little evidence available to inform the management of contacts of XDR-TB patients. The United States Centre for Disease Control and Prevention recommends using two drugs to which the isolate is susceptible in treating contacts of MDR-TB.[21,22] However, without the ability to use a quinolone or injectable agents, there are no available bactericidal options for treating latent infection with XDR-TB. One option is to follow infected contacts of XDR-TB for 2 years to detect early progression to active disease, if it occurs. While contact investigation is not routinely performed in low-income, high-TB incidence countries, a recent review found that the pooled yield of active household-contact investigations in low- and middle-income nations is 8.5% for active disease in children under 5 years of age. Targeting this high-risk group of young children for active contact investigations and treatment of latent TB infection could have a large impact on *M. tuberculosis* transmission [23] and is recommended by the International Union Against Tuberculosis and Lung Disease and the WHO.[24]

Treatment Outcome in XDR-TB

Treatment outcomes have been significantly worse for patients with XDR-TB than for patients with tuberculosis that is either drug-susceptible or MDR.[25-27] In the first recognized outbreak of XDR-TB, Gandhi et al.[28] reported that 53 patients in KwaZulu-Natal, South Africa, who were coinfected with XDR-TB and human immunodeficiency virus (HIV) survived for a median of only 16 days, with a mortality of 98%. Although some subsequent studies have reported better outcomes,[29] therapeutic options for XDR-TB are extremely limited because second-line drugs are less effective, more toxic, and more costly than are first-line therapies, and XDR-TB strains are, by definition, resistant to the more potent second-line options. The treatment outcomes of XDR-TB vary greatly between studies, possibly related to variations in method of analysis, definition of treatment success and failure, drug susceptibility testing and clinical follow-up. The outcomes also depend on adverse events due to drugs and their management, as well as supply and availability of the agents for treatment. Prior antituberculosis therapy, extensive in vitro drug resistance, fluoroquinolone resistance or prior fluoroquinolone use, capreomycin resistance, positive sputum smear, radiological cavitation, HIV seropositivity, other immunocompromized states, low body mass index, hypoalbuminemia, older age, male sex, low hematocrit, and early default during one year of treatment constitute important risk factors for poor outcomes. There are many studies reporting on treatment outcome in patients with XDR-TB.[3,11,25 27,-36] Out of these 13 studies, four (31%) used the WHO definition of cure,[11,29,30,35] six (46%) used the Laserson, et al.[37] definition of cure[3,25,28,32,33,36] and two did not specify the definition used.[31,34] Although one study used the WHO definition,[27] its cohort data were re-evaluated using the Laserson, et al.[37]definition in order to improve comparability. In these studies, the overall success rate (cured and completed) ranged from 34%[27] to 67%.[33] Experience from Peru and other countries suggests that strategies to support adherence, as well as psychological, nutritional and even financial interventions, may further contribute to improved outcomes in XDR-TB patients. The promising results obtained from Korea and Peru also suggest that strict and well-defined rules like management of XDR-TB cases in specialized reference centers are essential to improve prognosis. High success rates can also be achieved without hospital care in community DR-TB programs. Indeed, hospital care may be associated with nosocomial transmission of XDR-TB if adequate infection control strategies are not implemented. The lingering question for further study is whether these encouraging results, achieved with significant effort, can be reproduced in the conditions faced by most TB control programs worldwide, and what interventions would be needed to achieve high success rates. Encouraging results from some countries in Asia and Europe have also suggested that management in specialized reference centers could improve outcome, although high success rates could be achieved with treatment in some community settings.[38] Perhaps most importantly, XDR-TB has been shown in the current literature to be a treatable as well as curable condition. While this is an encouraging finding, complacency is not appropriate. XDR-TB patients do more poorly in terms of smear and culture conversion, treatment duration, treatment failure and death. With clear indications that XDR-TB results from mismanaged cases of drug-susceptible and MDR-TB, the first imperative is to treat susceptible TB appropriately to completion and to provide rapid diagnosis and aggressive, appropriate treatment of MDR-TB to avoid the unnecessary development of additional cases of XDR-TB.[39]

Control of XDR-TB

The primary aim in the control of extensively drug-resistant tuberculosis is to prevent its development in the first place. This can be done by Directly Observed Treatment Short Course (DOTS), which is the most cost-effective way of treatment and prevention of MDR-TB. At the same time, since MDR-TB and XDR-TB cases respond poorly to short course chemotherapy, careful introduction of second-line drugs to treat MDR-TB and proper management of MDR-TB cases to prevent XDR-TB cases, should be ensured to reduce further transmission of such strains.[20] Since new drugs for tuberculosis are unlikely to come up in the near future, the key to success remains in prompt and correct diagnosis and effective treatment of infectious patients. Apart from a strong tuberculosis control program, there is also a need for a continuous and periodic survey of drug resistance which will provide information on the type of chemotherapy to be used for the treatment of patients and also serve as a useful parameter in the evaluation of current and past chemotherapy programs. There is a need for revision of guidelines of national programs based on levels of resistance, training of professionals in private sector, strengthening of existing National Tuberculosis Control Program, and by ensuring compliance-enhancing measures like providing free/subsidized anti-tubercular drugs, supervized treatment and health education.

References

1. Mukherjee JS, Rich ML, Socci AR. Programmes and principles in treatment of multidrug-resistant tuberculosis. Lancet. 2004;363:474-81.

2. Treatment of Tuberculosis, American Thoracic Society, Center for Disease Control and Prevention, and Infectious Diseases Society of America. MMWR. 2003;52:RR-11.
3. Mitnick CD. Comprehensive treatment of extensively drug-resistant tuberculosis. N Engl J Med. 2008;359:563-74.
4. Guidelines for the programmatic management of drug-resistant tuberculosis—WHO 2008, 2011.
5. Guidelines on programmatic management of drug-resistant tuberculosis, 2012. India.
6. Multi-drug resistant and Extensively drug resistant TB in India. Consensus statement on the problem, prevention, management and control. www.tbcindia.org/.../Consensus%20statement%20on%20MDR%20XDR%20TB%20-Final. Acessed on May 1, 2011.
7. Thomas A, Ramachandran R, Rehaman F, Jaggarajamma K, Santha T, Narayanan PR, et al. Management of multi-drug resistance tuberculosis in the field: tuberculosis research centre experience. Ind J Tuberc. 2007;54:117-24.
8. Migliori GB, et al. Extensively drug-resistant tuberculosis, Italy and Germany [letter]. In: Emerging Infectious Diseases [serial on the Internet], May2007.
9. Francis RS, Curwen MP. Major surgery for pulmonary tuberculosis: final report. A national survey of 8232 patients operated on from April 1953 to March 1954 and followed up for five years. Tubercle. 1964;5:5-79.
10. Pomerantz M, Madsen LA, Goble M. Iseman MD, Surgical management of resistant mycobacterial pulmonary infection. Ann Thorac Surg. 1991;52:1108-12.
11. Gandhi NR, Moll A, Sturm AW, Pawinski R, Govender T, Lalloo U, et al. Extensively drug-resistant tuberculosis as a cause of death among patient coinfected with tuberculosis and HIV in a rural area in South Africa. Lancet. 2006;368:1575-80.
12. Wells CD. HIV infection and multidrug-resistant tuberculosis: the perfect storm. Journal of Infectious Diseases. 2007;196 Suppl 1:S86-107.
13. Swanson DS, Starke JR. Drug resistant tuberculosis in pediatrics. Pediatric Clinics of North America. 1995;42:553-81.
14. Mukherjee JS. Clinical and programmatic considerations in the treatment of MDR-TB in children: a series of 16 patients from Lima, Peru. Int J Tuber Lung Dis. 2003;7:637-44.
15. Warren RW. Rheumatologic aspects of pediatric cystic fibrosis patients treated with fluoroquinolones. Ped Infectious Dis J. 1997;16:118-22.
16. Hampel B, Hullmann R, Schmidt H. Ciprofloxacin in pediatrics: worldwide clinical experience based on compassionate use—safety report. Ped Infectious Dis J. 1997;16:127-9.
17. Figueroa-Damián R, Arredondo-García JL. Neonatal outcome of children born to women with tuberculosis. Archives of Medical Research. 2001;32:66-9.
18. Brost BC, Newman RB. The maternal and fetal effects of tuberculosis therapy. Obstetrics and Gynecology Clinics of North America. 1997;24:659-73.
19. Duff P. Antibiotic selection in obstetric patients. Infectious Disease Clinics of North America. 1997;11:1-12.
20. The Global MDR-TB and XDR-TB Response Plan 2007–2008. Geneva, World Health Organization, 2007 (WHO/HTM/TB/2007.387).
21. Peloquin C. Therapeutic drug monitoring in the treatment of tuberculosis. Drugs. 2002;62:2169-83.
22. Center for Disease Control and Prevention.Targeted tuberculin testing and treatment of latent tuberculosis infection. MMWR. 2000;49:1-54.
23. Villarino ME, Dooley SW, Geiter LJ, Castro KG, Snider DE. Management of persons exposed to multidrug-resistant tuberculosis. MMWR. 1992;41:59-71.

24. Morrison J, Pai M, Hopewell PC. Tuberculosis and latent tuberculosis infection in close contacts of people with pulmonary tuberculosis in low-income and middle-income countries: a systematic review and meta-analysis. Lancet Infect. Dis. 2008;8:359-68.
25. Kim HR, Hwang SS, Kim HJ. Impact of extensive drug resistance on treatment outcomes in non-HIV-infected patients with multi-drug-resistant tuberculosis. Clin Infect Dis. 2007;45:1290-5.
26. Andrews JR, Gandhi NR, Moll AP. High mortality among patients with multidrug and extensively drug-resistant tuberculosis in rural South Africa [abstract PS72041-12]. In: Program and abstracts of the 38th Union World Conference Lung Health (Cape Town, South Africa) 2007.
27. Migliori GB, Besozzi G, Girardi E. Clinical and operational value of the extensively drug-resistant tuberculosis definition. Eur Respir J. 2007;30:623-6.
28. Keshavjee S, Gelmanova IY, Farmer PE, et al. Treatment of extensively drug-resistant tuberculosis in Tomsk, Russia: a retrospective cohort study. Lancet. 2008;372:1403-9.
29. Banerjee R, Allen J, Westenhouse J, et al. Extensively drug-resistant tuberculosis in California, 1993–2006. Clin Infect Dis. 2008;47:450-7.
30. Migliori GB, Ortmann J, Girardi E, et al. Extensively drug-resistant tuberculosis, Italy and Germany. Emerg Infect Dis. 2007;13:780-2.
31. Chan ED, Strand MJ, Iseman MD. Treatment outcomes in extensively resistant tuberculosis. N Engl J Med. 2008;359:657-9.
32. Eker B, Ortmann J, Migliori GB, et al. Multidrug- and extensively drug-resistant tuberculosis, Germany. Emerg Infect Dis. 2008;14:1700-6.
33. Kwon YS, Kim YH, Suh GY, et al. Treatment outcomes for HIV uninfected patients with multidrug-resistant and extensively drug-resistant tuberculosis. Clin Infect Dis. 2008;47:496-502.
34. Lai CC, Tan CK, Huang YT, et al. Extensively drug-resistant *Mycobacterium tuberculosis* during a trend of decreasing drug resistance from 2000 through 2006 at a Medical Center in Taiwan. Clin Infect Dis. 2008;47:e57-63.
35. Bonilla CA, Crossa A, Jave HO, et al. Management of extensively drug-resistant tuberculosis in Peru: cure is possible. PLoS ONE. 2008;3:e2957.
36. Kim DH, Kim HJ, Park SK, et al. Treatment outcomes and long-term survival in patients with extensively drug-resistant tuberculosis. Am J Respir Crit Care Med. 2008;178:1075-82.
37. Laserson KF, Thorpe LE, Leimane V, et al. Speaking the same language: treatment outcome definitions for multidrug-resistant tuberculosis. Int J Tuberc Lung Dis. 2005;9:640-5.
38. Sotgiu G, Ferrara G, Matteelli MD, et al. Epidemiology and clinical management of XDR-TB: a systematic review by TBNET. Eur Respir J. 2009;33:871-81.
39. Raviglione MC, Uplekar MW. WHO's new Stop TB Strategy. Lancet. 2006;367:952-5.

Chapter 18

Extensively Drug-resistant Tuberculosis Failure: Management

Introduction

This chapter aims to describe the clinical approach in suspected extensively drug-resistant tuberculosis (XDR-TB) treatment failure, discuss indications for suspending treatment for patients in whom an XDR-TB treatment has failed and to outline the supportive care options for such patients.

Assessment of Patients at Risk for Treatment Failure

Patients who do not show signs of improvement after four months of treatment are at risk of treatment failure. All patients who show clinical, radiographical or bacteriological evidence of progressive active disease, or reappearance of disease after four months of treatment, should be considered as being at high risk for treatment failure. The following steps are recommended in such patients:

- The treatment should be reviewed to confirm that the patient has adhered to the treatment
- The treatment regimen should be reviewed in relation to medical history, contacts and all drug susceptibility test reports. If the regimen is deemed inadequate, a new regimen should be designed
- The bacteriological data should be reviewed. Often the smear and culture data are the strongest evidence that a patient is not responding to therapy. One single positive culture in the presence of an otherwise good clinical response can be caused by a laboratory contaminant or error. In this case, subsequent cultures that are negative, or in which the number of colonies is decreasing, may help prove that the apparently positive result did not reflect treatment failure. Positive smears with negative cultures may be caused by the presence of dead bacilli and, therefore, may not indicate treatment failure. Repeated culture and smear negative results in a patient with clinical and radiographical deterioration may indicate that the patient has a disease other than XDR-TB

- It should be confirmed that the patient has taken all the prescribed medicines
- Other illnesses that may decrease absorption of medicines (e.g. chronic diarrhea) or may result in immune suppression (e.g. HIV infection) should be excluded
- If surgical resection is feasible, it should be considered.

If no response is seen, reassessment of the regimen and treatment plan and formulation of a new plan of action are necessary. Patients who have persistent positive smears or cultures at fourth month but who are doing well clinically and radiographically may not require a regimen change. Whenever a regimen change is indicated because of treatment failure, a new regimen is started (with at least seven effective drugs) and options for adjunctive treatment like surgery can be considered. Adding one or two drugs to a failing regimen should be avoided. Changes in treatment can be made as early as 4 to 6 months if conversion is not seen and if there is clinical deterioration.

Indications for Suspending Treatment

It takes 3 to 4 months to evaluate whether a change in treatment plan has been effective. If the patient continues to deteriorate despite the measures described in the previous section, treatment failure should be considered. There is no single indicator to determine whether a treatment regimen is failing. Although there is no simple definition for treatment failure, there often comes a point during the treatment when it becomes clear that the patient is not going to improve. Signs indicating treatment failure include:

- Persistent positive smears or cultures past 8 to 10 months of treatment
- Progressive, extensive and bilateral lung disease on chest X-ray, with no option for surgery
- High-grade resistance with no option to add two additional agents
- Overall deteriorating clinical condition that usually includes weight loss and respiratory insufficiency.

It is not necessary for all of these signs to be present to identify failure of the treatment regimen. However, a cure is highly unlikely when they are all present. The epidemiological definition of treatment failure for recording outcomes is often different from that used in the process of suspending therapy in a patient when the therapy is failing. The epidemiological definition is an outcome to account for the patient in a treatment cohort analysis, while the clinical decision to suspend therapy is made after the clinical search for all other options has been exhausted and cure of the patient is considered to be highly unlikely.

Suspending Therapy

Treatment can be considered to have failed and suspension of therapy is recommended in cases where the medical personnel involved are confident that all the drugs have been ingested and there is no possibility of adding other drugs or carrying out surgery. There are two important considerations in suspending therapy or changing it to a supportive care regimen. The first is the patient's quality of life; the drugs used in XDR-TB treatment have significant adverse effects, and continuing them while the treatment is failing may cause additional suffering. The second is the public health concern; continuing a treatment that is failing can amplify resistance in the patient's strain, resulting in highly resistant strains such as extreme drug resistance (XXDR-TB) or total drug resistance (TDR-TB) that may cause subsequent infection to others.

Approach to Suspending Therapy

The approach to suspending therapy should start with discussions among the clinical team involved in the patient's care. Once the clinical team decides that treatment should be suspended, a clear plan should be prepared for approaching the patient and the family. Home visits during the process offer an excellent opportunity to talk with family members and the patient in a familiar environment. It is not recommended to suspend therapy before the patient understands and accepts the reasons to do so, and agrees with the supportive care offered.

Supportive Care for Patients in Whom all the Possibilities of XDR-TB Treatment have Failed

A number of supportive measures can be used once the therapy has been suspended. It is very important that medical visits continue and that the patient is not abandoned. The supportive measures are described in detail in the Integrated Management of Adolescent and Adult Illness guidelines produced by WHO in a booklet titled *Palliative care: Symptom management and end-of-life care.*[1] The supportive measures are summarized below:

- *Pain control and symptom relief:* Paracetamol, or codeine with paracetamol, gives relief from moderate pain. Codeine also helps control cough. Other cough suppressants can be added. If possible, stronger analgesics, including morphine, should be used, when appropriate, to keep the patient adequately comfortable.
- *Relief of respiratory insufficiency:* Oxygen can be used to alleviate shortness of breath. Morphine also provides significant relief from respiratory insufficiency and should be offered if available.
- *Nutritional support:* Small and frequent meals are often best for a person at the end of life. It should be accepted that the intake will reduce as the patient's condition deteriorates and during end-of-life care. Nausea and vomiting or any other conditions that interfere with nutritional support should be treated.
- *Regular medical visits:* When therapy stops, regular visits by the treating physician and support team should not be discontinued.
- *Continuation of ancillary medicines:* All necessary ancillary medications should be continued as needed. Depression and anxiety, if present, should be addressed.
- *Hospitalization, hospice care or nursing home care:* Having a patient die at home can be difficult for the family. Hospice-like care should be offered to families who want to keep the patient at home. Inpatient end-of-life care should be available to those for whom home care is not available.

- *Preventive measures:* Oral care, prevention of bedsores, bathing and prevention of muscle contractures are indicated in all patients. Regular scheduled movement of the bedridden patient is very important.
- *Infection control measures:* The patient, who is taken off anti-tuberculosis treatment because of failure, often remains infectious for long periods of time. Infection control measures should be continued.

Conclusion

Suspension of therapy should be considered only after all other options for treatment have been explored. Suspending therapy in a patient who has failed XDR-TB treatment is a delicate situation and difficult for family members and caregivers; but it is especially difficult for the patient as treatment is often viewed as his or her only hope. Strong support, care and sympathy must be given to the patient and family.

Reference

1. Palliative care: symptom management and end-of-life care. Geneva, World Health Organization, 2004 (WHO/CDS/IMAI/2004.4).

Chapter 19

Drug Resistance in Extrapulmonary Tuberculosis

Introduction

Tuberculosis is one of the major public health problems especially in developing countries such as India.[1] India had 2.2 million new cases of tuberculosis in 2012. Furthermore, India accounted for an estimated 64,000 patients out of 3,10,000 cases of drug-resistant tuberculosis estimated to have occurred among the notified cases of TB across the globe in a year. Extrapulmonary tuberculosis is a significant health problem in both developing and developed countries. The importance of extrapulmonary tuberculosis, especially the drug-resistant forms among all forms of tuberculosis has not yet been ascertained yet. Drug resistant extrapulmonary tuberculosis is difficult to diagnose because of difficulty in obtaining adequate sample from extrapulmonary sites and also because of paucibacillary nature of disease.[2] The current chapter aims at describing the epidemiology, diagnostic and management issues in drug-resistant extrapulmonary tuberculosis.

Epidemiology

The exact prevalence of drug resistance in extrapulmonary tuberculosis is not known. Data regarding drug resistance in extrapulmonary tuberculosis is very sparse.

Global

An eurosurveillance data from 2002–2011 found that multi-drug-resistant tuberculosis (MDR-TB) is less frequent among extrapulmonary tuberculosis cases than among pulmonary tuberculosis cases with an incidence of 1.3% in extrapulmonary tuberculosis cases.[3] MDR-TB was found in 1.9% of pleural, 1% of extrathoracic lymphatics, 1.7% of intrathoracic lymphatics, 0.9% of genitourinary, 3% of spinal, 2.1% of bone, 2.8% of meningeal, 1.2% of gastrointestinal, 1.5% of disseminated and 1.2 % of tuberculosis involving other sites.[3] In a study of epidemiology of extrapulmonary tuberculosis in the

United States from 1993–2006, extrapulmonary tuberculosis was found to be negatively associated with multi-drug resistance. 0.9% of extrapulmonary cases versus 1.6% of pulmonary tuberculosis cases were found to be MDR-TB giving an odds ratio of 0.6. The proportion of MDR-TB cases varied little between extrapulmonary tuberculosis disease sites.[4] A Korean study of 168 extrapulmonary tuberculosis cases found that out of a total of 168 cases, resistance to at least one antituberculosis drug was found in 15 cases (8.9%), and MDR-TB was found in three cases (1.8%). Of the extrapulmonary drug-resistant cases, any drug resistance was found in lymph node (33%), intra-abdominal (27%), central nervous system (20%), milliary nodules in the lung (20%), genitourinary (13%), musculoskeletal (7%), pleura (7%).[5] In a review on 194 extrapulmonary cases diagnosed between 2005 and 2007 in a tertiary hospital in Pakistan, drug resistance was found in 17% cases. The dominant site of disease in the drug-resistant cases was lymph nodes (54%) followed by musculoskeletal (15%) and spine (12%) cases.[6] A 10-year health data on laboratory-confirmed cases of MDR-TB for the period 1998–2007 found 31 cases of MDR-TB. Pulmonary involvement alone was found in 17 cases, extrapulmonary in 14 (lymph node-7, pleura-3, peritoneum, genitourinary, lymph node plus bone/joint, pleura plus bone/joint involvement-1 case each).[7] A study from Taiwan found that rates of drug resistance were significantly higher amongst mycobacterial tuberculosis isolates recovered from respiratory specimens than amongst those from nonrespiratory specimens to isoniazid (15.3% vs 9.4%), rifampicin (5.5% vs 3.3%), ethambutol (7.3% vs 3.8%), and both isoniazid and rifampicin (4.8% vs 2.5%).[8] On the other hand, a study from Turkey found no significantly different drug resistance between pulmonary tuberculosis (29.9%) and extrapulmonary tuberculosis (25.25%) cases.[9]

India

In a study, 20 extrapulmonary drug-resistant cases were identified out of 350 clinically suspected cases of extrapulmonary tuberculosis. Among *M. tuberculosis* isolates, both initial and acquired resistance was highest for streptomycin followed by isoniazid, rifampicin and ethambutol. No strain showed resistance to pyrazinamide. Two strains were found to be multidrug resistant.[10] A study of 419 samples from suspected extrapulmonary tuberculosis cases found mycobacterial tuberculosis culture positive in 125 (29.8%) samples. Drug susceptibility testing showed that 15 (12%) isolates had MDR-TB, 26 (20.8%) were resistant for any one drug while 84 (67.2%) isolates were pansensitive.[11] Another study found that incidence of MDR-TB in extrapulmonary tuberculosis cases was 13.5%.[12] The study observed that 39.9% were resistant to any first-line antitubercular drug. The overall resistance to first-line agent isoniazid, rifampicin, ethambutol and streptomycin was found in 30.3%, 16.3%, 15.7% and 16.3% respectively. In new cases, resistance to first-line agent isoniazid, rifampicin, ethambutol and streptomycin was found in 27.6%, 14.6%, 14.6% and 13.8% cases respectively. The resistance rate was higher in previously treated patients: isoniazid (30.3%), rifampicin (16.3%), ethambutol (15.7%) and streptomycin (16.3%).

Diagnosis of Drug Resistance in Extrapulmonary Tuberculosis

A patient with extrapulmonary tuberculosis may have general symptoms, like weight loss, fever with evening rise and night sweats. Other symptoms depend on the organs affected like swelling of a lymph node in tuberculosis lymphadenitis, pain and swelling of a joint in tuberculous arthritis, neck stiffness and disorientation in a case of tuberculous meningitis. The diagnosis depends on taking adequate sample from representative tissue and performing the various culture and genotypic based tests on these specimens. Traditionally, Lowenstein-Jensen (LJ) culture has been used for drug sensitivity testing using absolute concentration method, the resistance ratio method and the proportions method. With the conventional methods, 6–8 weeks' time is required before sensitivity results are known.[13] BACTEC and mycobacterial growth indicator tube reduced the time required to detect resistance. More recently, Xpert MTB/RIF has been introduced, which correctly identifies rifampicin resistance in more than 98% of smear positive MDR-TB cases. However, its role in smear negative and extrapulmonary tuberculosis remains to be established. In a study on application of Gen/Xpert to extrapulmonary specimens, it was shown that it correctly identified 98% of phenotypic rifampin resistant cases and 94% of phenotypic rifampicin-susceptible cases.[14]

Management of Drug Resistance in Extrapulmonary Tuberculosis

As per programmatic management of drug-resistant tuberculosis (PMDT), bacteriologically confirmed extrapulmonary MDR-TB patients are treated as per regimen and schedule for pulmonary MDR-TB. Patients are registered in the PMDT Register.

Monitoring of Drug Resistance in Extrapulmonary Tuberculosis

Monitoring and follow-up can be done clinically based on weight gain, decrease or increase in symptoms, increase or regression in size of lymph nodes, appearance of new nodes, in chest symptomatic, monthly sputum for AFB. Monitoring with radiological investigations like X ray, ultrasound, CT scan and MRI are important tools to monitor response to therapy. Bacteriological monitoring, although important, is usually not possible because of difficulties in obtaining adequate specimens from extrapulmonary sites. Monitoring for adverse drug reactions should also be done.

Role of Surgery in Drug-resistant Extrapulmonary Tuberculosis

Some forms of extrapulmonary tuberculosis might benefit from surgical debridement or resection in order to decrease the burden of disease. Surgery may be acceptable for obtaining samples for study and treating some situations, such as constrictive pericarditis, vertebral abscesses compressing the spinal cord or superficial and accessible abscesses in cases of osteoarticular tuberculosis. Surgery is not a replacement for full medical treatment of tuberculosis, but may offer a greater likelihood of success and may give the patient some symptomatic relief while the disease is being treated medically.

Treatment Success in Drug-resistant Extrapulmonary Cases

There is a paucity of follow-up studies in management of extrapulmonary MDR-TB cases. A recent eurosurveillance survey found a high treatment success of 81.4%.[2] Thus, inspite of all the complicating issues regarding diagnosis and management, the success achieved in extrapulmonary MDR-TB cases may be actually better than pulmonary MDR-TB cases.

Problems in Management of Drug Resistance in Extrapulmonary Tuberculosis

Some forms of extrapulmonary tuberculosis (meningitis/pericarditis) are treated with adjunctive corticosteroid treatment in conjunction with an optimal anti-tuberculosis regimen. Use of corticosteroids for patients not receiving adequate antitubercular therapy could be problematic. Studies showing efficacy of corticosteroid therapy are reported for drug-susceptible cases. The indication for corticosteroids in patients with drug-resistant tuberculosis is not clear. Some forms of tuberculosis (particularly lymphadenopathy) are known to worsen as the tuberculosis is being successfully treated. This is due to immune reconstitution as the organism is being eliminated and is particularly common in HIV-infected individuals. This phenomenon is known as immune reconstitution inflammatory syndrome (IRIS). However, if the clinical worsening is actually due to microbiologic failure associated with unrecognized drug resistance, it may inappropriately be attributed to a paradoxical reaction. In this case, the correct diagnosis of drug resistance and treatment failure will be delayed. Also the introduction of steroids in such cases in the belief of suppressing IRIS may prove disastrous. Drug regimens and durations of treatment for drug-susceptible extrapulmonary tuberculosis are based on known penetration of first-line antituberculosis drugs into tissues, years of experience, and some clinical trials. Unfortunately, much less is known regarding the penetration of second-line drugs into tissues. This is compounded by the increased rates of malabsorption and drug interactions experienced by individuals at risk for drug-resistant tuberculosis. Another problem is that serial cultures are often not available. In pulmonary MDR-TB, follow-up cultures are essential periodically but in extrapulmonary MDR-TB, no such cultures are usually available for follow-up. Computed tomography is often useful in following treatment progress in these patients.

Drug-resistant Central Nervous System Tuberculosis

MDR-TB meningitis is especially challenging to treat due to limited CNS penetration of several second line antituberculosis drugs. Nonspecific clinical presentation, especially in young children, poor diagnostics, and delays in instituting appropriate antituberculosis therapy, as drug susceptibility testing may require up to 10 weeks, further increase the risk of mortality or the onset of severe, irreversible neurological damage. Several reports detail poor outcomes of drug-resistant tuberculosis meningitis.[15,16] Most of the patients in these series were HIV-infected and many developed meningitis while already receiving treatment for MDR-TB.[17] The majority of patients were HIV-infected. Any degree of drug resistance will hinder the treatment of tuberculosis meningitis or other central nervous system (CNS) tuberculosis because isoniazid (INH) is the most important drug in the treatment of tuberculous meningitis.

Tuberculosis Drugs and their CNS Penetration

INH is the most important drug in the treatment of tubercular meningitis. INH readily diffuses into the cerebrospinal fluid independent of meningeal inflammation due to its small size and lipophilic nature. Levels approach those in serum. Because of this, some experts recommend the use of INH in MDR-TB meningitis, especially in the setting of low-level INH resistance. Pyrazinamide also crosses freely into the CSF. Ethionamide and cycloserine also have good CNS penetration approaching that in serum. The fluoroquinolones have variable CSF penetration. Levofloxacin levels in the CSF are about 15% to 30% that of serum. Since higher doses are generally used to treat MDR-TB, CSF levels may be adequate to treat tubercular meningitis (MIC 0.5–1.0). Moxifloxacin has shown good CSF penetration in several animal studies (CSF levels approximately 50% of serum). On the other hand, rifampin, rifabutin, ethambutol, para-aminosalicylic acid, and the aminoglycosides penetrate poorly into the CSF with noninflamed meninges, but better with inflamed meninges. For rifampicin, 10% to 20% of the serum level reaches the CSF in the setting of inflamed meninges.

Conclusion

The extrapulmonary forms of tuberculosis are usually paucibacillary. Thus, the chances of resistance are comparatively less than pulmonary tuberculosis. In many situations, nonresponse in extrapulmonary tuberculosis may be due to nonpenetration of drug or due to endarteritis rather than drug resistance. Diagnosis although difficult can be accomplished by high suspicion and appropriate sample collection. Treatment is similar to pulmonary tuberculosis drug-resistant cases. Surgery may play an important role in the management of drug-resistant extrapulmonary tuberculosis. Surgical resection and drainage may decrease bacterial burden and improve outcome.

References

1. TB India 2013. RNTCP Status Report. Central TB Division, Directorate General of Health Services, Ministry of Health and Family Welfare, Nirman Bhawan, New Delhi.
2. Chakravorty S, Sen MK, Tyagi JS. Diagnosis of extrapulmonary tuberculosis by smear, culture, and PCR using universal sample processing technology. J Clin Microbiol. 2005;43:4357-62.
3. Sandgren A, Hollo V, van der Werf MJ. Extrapulmonary tuberculosis in the European Union and European Economic Area, 2002 to 2011. Euro Surveill. 2013;18:pii=20431. Available online: http://www.eurosurveillance.org/ViewArticle.aspx?ArticleId=20431.
4. Peto HM, Pratt RH, Harrington TA, LoBue PA, Armstrong LR. Epidemiology of extrapulmonary tuberculosis in the United States, 1993-2006.Clin Infect Dis. 2009;49:1350-7.
5. Cho OH, Park KH, Park SY, Moon SM, Chong YP, Kim MN, et al. Drug-resistant Extrapulmonary Tuberculosis. Infect Chemother. 2011;43:258-61.
6. Chandir S, Hussain H, Salahuddin N, Amir M, Ali F, Lotia I, et al. Extrapulmonary Tuberculosis: A retrospective review of 194 cases at a tertiary care hospital in Karachi, Pakistan. J Pak Med Assoc. 2010;60:105-9.
7. Lavender CJ, Brown LK, Johnson PD. Multi-drug-resistant tuberculosis in Victoria: a 10-year review. Med J Aust. 2009;191:315-8.
8. Lai CC, Liu WL, Tan CK, Huang YC, Chung KP, Lee MR, et al. Differences in drug resistance profiles of Mycobacterium tuberculosis isolates causing pulmonary and extrapulmonary tuberculosis in a medical centre in Taiwan, 2000–2010. Int J Antimicrob Agents. 2011;38:125-9.
9. Gunal S, Yang Z, Agarwal M, Koroglu M, Kazgan Z, Durmaz R: Demographic and microbial characteristics of extrapulmonary tuberculosis cases diagnosed in Malatya, Turkey, 2001–2007. BMC Publ Health. 2011;11:154.
10. Sachdeva R, Gadre DV, Talwar V. Characterisation and drug susceptibility patterns of extrapulmonary mycobacterial isolates. Indian J Med Res. 2002;115:102-7.
11. Sankar MM, Singh J, Diana SC, Singh S. Molecular characterization of Mycobacterium tuberculosis isolates from North Indian patients with extrapulmonary tuberculosis. Tuberculosis. 2013;93:75-83.
12. Maurya AK, Kant S, Nag VL, Kushwaha R, Dhole TN. Trends of anti-tuberculosis drug resistance pattern in new cases and previously treated cases of extrapulmonary tuberculosis cases in referral hospitals in northern India. J Postgrad Med. 2012;58:185-9.
13. Revised National Tuberculosis Control Program. DOTS-Plus Guidelines 2010. Central TB Division, Directorate General of Health Services, Ministry of Health and Family Welfare, Nirman Bhawan, New Delhi.
14. Vadwai V, et al. Xpert MTB/RIF: a new pillar in diagnosis of extrapulmonary tuberculosis. J. Clin. Microbiol. 2011;49:2540-5.
15. Guidelines on Programmatic Management of Drug Resistant TB (PMDT) in India. Central TB Division, Directorate General of Health Services, Ministry of Health and Family Welfare, Nirman Bhavan, New Delhi.
16. De Vincenzo JP, Berning SE, Peloquin CA, Husson RN. Multidrug-resistant tuberculosis meningitis: clinical problems and concentrations of second-line antituberculous medications. Ann Pharmacother. 1999;33:1184-8.
17. Patel VB, Padayatchi, Bhigjee NA, Allen J, Bhagwan B, Moodley AA, et al. Multidrug-Resistant Tuberculous Meningitis in Kwa Zulu-Natal, South Africa. Clinical Infectious Diseases. 2004;38:851-6.

Chapter 20

Fluoroquinolone Resistance in Tuberculosis

Introduction

Fluoroquinolones are an important class of drugs used in the treatment of drug-resistant tuberculosis. They are almost certainly effective in the treatment of MDR-TB, and outcomes are uniformly worse in patients in whom they cannot be used. Several studies show that quinolone use in multi-drug-resistant tuberculosis correlates with survival.[1,2] Newer members of this class, such as levofloxacin, moxifloxacin, and gatifloxacin are very active in vitro and in animal models of tuberculosis.[3,4] These drugs have potent sterilizing activity.[5,6,7] In addition, they may prevent resistance to other agents in a multi-drug regimen. Although formal studies with prolonged dosing are lacking, the fluoroquinolones appear to be well tolerated,[8] even when administered for 12 months as part of treatment of multi-drug-resistant tuberculosis.[1] The fluoroquinolone resistance has increased from 0% in 1995 to 8% in 1998 and then to 35% in 2004. The aim of this chapter is to discuss the fluoroquinolone resistance in tuberculosis.

Prevalence of Fluoroquinolone Resistance

Fluoroquinolone resistance was first reported in 1995.[9] Sullivan, et al. first identified 22 patients in New York City with fluoroquinolone-resistant tuberculosis from 1991 to 1993.[10] Fluoroquinolone resistance has now been found to be a global phenomenon with studies showing fluoroquinolone resistance to range from 0.7% to 43%.[11-16] In the United States and Canada, the fluoroquinolone resistance among Mycobacterium tuberculosis isolates between 1996 and 2000 was 1.8%.[12] A study in Baltimore, Maryland reported fluoroquinolone resistance in 4%.[16] In other recent studies, rate of fluoroquinolone resistance has been found to be 3.6% in India, 1.8% in Thailand, 6.1% in Spain and 18% in Phillipines.[16] Among the patients who have received prior tuberculosis treatment, rates of fluoroquinolone resistance are higher—as high as 43% in the study from Phillipines.[16] In another study, fluoroquinolone resistance was found to be 19% in multi-drug-resistant tuberculosis.[17] In HIV-infected patients, fluoroquinolone resistance was reported in 1%.[11,12] In India, a study done by Hemvani N, et al. at Indore in 2001 showed

Fluoroquinolone resistance to be. 3.6%[18] Another study done by Agrawal et al at Mumbai in 2004 reported the total fluoroquinolone resistance to be 35%.[19] Recent state-wide surveillance of drug-resistant tuberculosis in the state of Gujarat has reported resistance to fluoroquinolones (FQ) in 24% cases (19% among new and 25% among previously treated TB cases).[20]

Mechanism of Resistance to Fluoroquinolones

Mutations in the *gyrA* gene were the most common mechanism of fluoroquinolone resistance in Mycobacterium Tuberculosis.[9,11,21] Isolates with *gyrA* mutations in this study had single mutations, which generally confer a 2–8-fold increase in the mean inhibitory concentration.[22] Isolates with 2 mutations in *gyrA,* which confer high-level fluoroquinolone resistance, have been selected in laboratory experiments[22] but were not identified in these clinical isolates. As has been documented in previous studies,[9,21] a minority of fluoroquinolone-resistant Mycobacterium tuberculosis isolates do not have recognized mutations in the *gyrA* gene. The mechanism of fluoroquinolone resistance among isolates having wild-type *gyrA* has yet to be identified, but it may include a mutation in *gyrB* gene, altered cell permeability, an efflux pump that decreases intracellular concentrations of the drug, or intracellular inactivation of the fluoroquinolone.[23] The increasing use of fluoroquinolones has led to increasing resistance to these antimicrobials.[24] When used for treatment of nontuberculous conditions, fluoroquinolones can lead to delayed diagnosis of tuberculosis in undiagnosed tuberculosis cases.[25,26] Previous monotherapy with fluoroquinolones for bacterial infections can lead to selection of fluoroquinolone-resistant mutants against Mycobacterium tuberculosis. Even a short 13-day course of quinolones can lead to subsequent resistance when used for tuberculosis.[27]

Cross Resistance amongst Fluoroquinolones

Increase of fluoroquinolone resistance correlates well with the very widespread use of fluoroquinolones in lower-respiratory, gastrointestinal, genitourinary infections[20] and in tuberculosis. The prevalence of fluoroquinolone resistance in tuberculosis is increasing.[28,29] All 32 isolates that contained *gyrA* mutations exhibited cross-resistance to other fluoroquinolones, although moxifloxacin, gatifloxacin and sitafloxacin (MIC for 90% of strains < 4 mg/L) were apparently more active than ofloxacin, levofloxacin and sparfloxacin (MIC for 90% of strains > 16 mg/liter). On the other hand, 23 isolates without discernible *gyrA* mutations were also classified as resistant with a breakpoint of ≥2 mg/L for ofloxacin.[30] The cross resistance among the fluoroquinolones is such that reduced susceptibility to one quinolone is likely to confer reduced susceptibility to all fluoroquinolones[23] but in some other studies, fluoroquinolones are believed to have variable cross resistance between each other, with in vitro data showing that some later-generation fluoroquinolones remain susceptible when earlier generation fluoroquinolones are resistant.[24, 31-33] Given its clinical effectiveness and superior *in vitro* potency against Mycobacterium tuberculosis compared with other fluoroquinolones,[3] moxifloxacin might be considered the preferred fluoroquinolone for treating multi-drug-resistant (MDR) and extensively drug resistant (XDR) tuberculosis. Gatifloxacin may be as active but is associated with a risk of dysglycemia when used for community-acquired pneumonia in the elderly.[34] The OFLOTUB study, carried out at several sites in South Africa, compared several fluoroquinolones to ethambutol and found that moxifloxacin and gatifloxacin resulted in higher culture conversion rates on solid media after eight weeks, whereas ofloxacin did not.[35]

Minimum Inhibitory Concentration of Fluoroquinolones

Representative values for minimum inhibitory concentration (MIC) of fluoroquinolones for Mycobacterium tuberculosis in communities with a low prevalence of primary fluoroquinolone resistance are shown in Table 20.1. The threshold MIC for declaring ofloxacin-resistance is normally taken to be 2µg/mL. Of greater importance than MIC is the relation of peak serum concentration with usual doses (Cmax) to MIC, also shown. For comparison, usual values for isoniazid MIC for isoniazid-sensitive strains are also given.[23,36]

It appears from these data that the fluoroquinolones most closely approximating the values seen with isoniazid, at the doses currently used, are levofloxacin and gatifloxacin. It should be noted, however, that the dose of ofloxacin represented in this data is much lower than that of levofloxacin. Gatifloxacin and moxifloxacin were found to kill rifampicin-tolerant bacteria much more effectively than levofloxacin or ofloxacin suggesting they may possess greater sterilizing activity.[37]

Early Bactericidal Activity

Early bactericidal activity (EBA) is conventionally but arbitrarily defined as the decline in colony-forming units in sputum over the first two days of treatment.[38-43] It is thought that this reflects rapid killing of metabolically active organisms, and that this is an important factor in interrupting transmission. EBA over the period of 2–5 days (extended EBA) has been proposed as an index of a drug's ability to kill more slowly metabolizing organisms.

TABLE 20.1: MIC90 and C_{max} for fluoroquinolones and isoniazid

	MIC_{90}, µg/mL	C_{max}, µg/mL	C_{max}/MIC
Ciprofloxacin 500 mg	0.5–1.0	3.0	3–6
Ofloxacin 400 mg	0.5–1.3	4.6	3–9
Levofloxacin 750 mg	0.5–1.0	8.6	8–15
Sparfloxacin 400 mg	0.25–0.5	1.3	3–6
Gatifloxacin 400 mg	0.25–0.5	4.2	8–15
Moxifloxacin 400 mg	0.25–0.5	3.2	6
Isoniazid 300 mg	0.01–0.06	3-5	20–50

It appears that ciprofloxacin has lower EBA than the other fluoroquinolones. Data for extended EBA are very sparse, but it does not appear likely that there are any important differences among the fluoroquinolones tested Tables 20.2 and 20.3.

Development of Resistance During Treatment

Acquisition of fluoroquinolone resistance during treatment has been observed frequently.[23,44] This is of concern because it results in early relapse and often involves resistance to other fluoroquinolones.[45] In vitro resistance to fluoroquinolones does not exclude effective treatment[46] but previous use of fluoroquinolones in a patient's treatment decreases the chances of successful treatment of MDR-TB.[47] Fluoroquinolone-resistant strains of Mycobacterium tuberculosis in patients with MDR-TB is related, in most communities, to previous tuberculosis treatment of those patients with fluoroquinolones. Fluoroquinolone-resistant MDR-TB in patients not previously treated for Mycobacterium tuberculosis with fluoroquinolones is increasing and has become common in many areas.[48] This has been attributed to use of fluoroquinolones in patients who have unsuspected tuberculosis. A recent study has shown resistance to ofloxacin among 26.3% cases, with 36.2% resistance in MDR and 20.7% in non-MDR isolates in those who had received ofloxacin for more than 4 weeks previously.[49] There are reports of the acquisition of fluoroquinolone resistance by Mycobacterium tuberculosis after as little as 23 and 13 days of fluoroquinolone treatment.[23,36] It has been suggested that a mutant prevention concentration (MPC) of an antibiotic for a particular organism can be defined, at which the selection of resistant mutants

TABLE 20.2: EBA (days 0–2) for fluoroquinolones

	EBA (days 0–2) (log CFU/mL/d)				
	Ciprofloxacin varying doses	*Ofloxacin 800 mg*	*Levofloxacin 1000 mg*	*Gatifloxacin 400 mg*	*Moxifloxacin 400 mg*
Johnson, et al. 2006[39]	-	-	0.45	0.35	0.33
Gosling, et al. 2003[40]	-	-	-	-	0.53
Sirgel, et al. 1997[41]	0.09 (500 mg), 0.205 (1500 mg)	-	-	-	-
Sirgel, et al. 2000[42]	-	0.17	-	-	-
Ginsburg, et al. 2003[27]	0.09 (500 mg)	0.39	-	-	-

TABLE 20.3: Extended EBA (days 2–5) for fluoroquinolones

	Extended EBA (days 2-5) (logCFU/mL/d)				
	Ciprofloxacin 750 mg	*Ofloxacin 800 mg*	*Levofloxacin 1000 mg*	*Gatifloxacin 400 mg*	*Moxifloxacin 400 mg*
Johnson, et al. 2006[39]	-	-	0.18	0.17	0.17
Sirgel, et al. 2000[42]	-	0.20	-	-	-
Kennedy et al, 1995[43]	0.20	-	-	-	-

during treatment is suppressed. For Mycobacterium tuberculosis, the MPC90 (MPC for 90% of strains) for fluoroquinolones have been reported to be 2, 1.8, 1.0 and 1.2 µg/mL for ciprofloxacin, levofloxacin, gatifloxacin and moxifloxacin respectively.[50] The Cmax/MPC ratios for these drugs would then be 1.5, 4.8, 4.2 and 2.7 respectively, and all except ciprofloxacin would seem likely to be roughly equivalent. It has been suggested that gatifloxacin and moxifloxacin are less likely to provoke the development of resistance,[23,39] but there are no clinical data supporting this suggestion.

Treatment Outcome in Fluoroquinolone-resistant Tuberculosis Patients

MDR-TB and resistance to any fluoroquinolone plus one second-line injectable drug was, in fact, the only combination of drug resistance significantly associated with an increased risk of death or failure. Successful treatment outcome is reported in 46% MDR TB patients with fluoroquinolone susceptibility in comparison to 34% in MDR TB patients with fluoroquinolone resistance.[51] In another study, an MDR TB patient with resistance to one second-line injectable drug and any fluoroquinolone is associated with successful treatment outcome in 45.8% cases.[52] The patients with MDR TB resistant to fluoroquinolone and streptomycin but susceptible to second-line injectable had significantly better long-term treatment outcomes than did the patients with XDR TB. Long-term treatment outcome in MDR-TB patients was 83% in comparison to 75% in MDR TB patients with resistance to fluoroquinolone and streptomycin but susceptible to second-line injectable and 20% in extensively drug-resistant (XDR) TB patients.[53] Under the programatic management of drug-resistant tuberculosis (PMDT), baseline ofloxacin monoresistance is treated by substitution of levofloxacin from MDR regimen by a combination of Moxifloxacin and PAS.[54]

References

1. Yew WW, Chan CK, Chau CH. Outcomes of patients with multidrug-resistant pulmonary tuberculosis treated with ofloxacin/levofloxacin-containing regimens. Chest 2000;117:744-51.
2. Chan ED, Laurel V, Strand MJ. Treatment and outcome analysis of 205 patients with multidrug resistant tuberculosis. Am J Respir Crit Care Med 2004;169:1103-9.
3. Ji B, Lounis N, Maslo C, Truffot-Pernot C, Bonnafous P, Grosset J. In vitro and in vivo activities of moxifloxacin and clinafloxacin against Mycobacterium tuberculosis. Antimicrob Agents Chemother 1998;42:2066-9.
4. Miyazaki E, Miyazaki M, Chen JM, Chaisson RE, Bishai WR. Moxifloxacin (BAY12-8039), a new 8-methoxyquinolone, is active in a mouse model of tuberculosis. Antimicrob Agents Chemother 1999; 43:85-9.
5. Lounis N, Bentoucha A, Truffot-Pernot C. Effectiveness of once weekly rifapentine and moxifloxacin regimens against Mycobacterium tuberculosis in mice. Antimicrob Agents Chemother 2001; 45:3482-6.
6. Tuberculosis Research Centre, Chennai. Shortening short course chemotherapy: a randomized clinical trial for treatment of smear-positive pulmonary tuberculosis with regimens using ofloxacin in the intensive phase. Indian J Tuberc 2002; 49:27-38.

7. Nuermberger EL, Yoshimatsu T, Tyagi S. Moxifloxacin-containing regimen greatly reduces time to culture conversion in murine tuberculosis. Am J Respir Crit Care Med. 2004;169:421-6.
8. El-Sadr W, Perlman DC, Matts JP. Evaluation of an intensive intermittent-induction regimen and short course duration of treatment for HIV-related pulmonary tuberculosis. Clin Infect Dis 1998; 26:1148-58.
9. Sullivan EA, Kreiswirth BN, Palumbo L. Emergence of fluoroquinolone-resistant tuberculosis in New York City. Lancet 1995;345:1148-50.
10. Udwadia ZF, Jain S, Rodrigues C, Mehta A. XDR tuberculosis in India: what's in a name? Lancet Infect Dis 2007;7:441-2.
11. Perlman DC, El Sadr WM, Heifets LB. Susceptibility to Levofloxacin of Mycobacterium tuberculosis isolates from patients with HIV-related tuberculosis and characterization of a strain with levofloxacin monoresistance. Community Programs for Clinical Research on AIDS 019 and the AIDS Clinical Trials Group 222 Protocol Team. AIDS 1997;11:1473-8.
12. Bozeman L, Burman W, Metchock B, Welch L, Weiner M, Tuberculosis Trials Consortium. Fluoroquinolone susceptibility among Mycobacterium tuberculosis isolates from the United States and Canada. Clin Infect Dis 2005;40:386-91.
13. Riantawan P, Punnotok J, Chaisuksuwan R, Pransujarit V. Resistance of M. tuberculosis to anti-tuberculosis drugs in the central region of Thailand, 1996. Int J Tuberc Lung Dis 1998;2:616-20.
14. Casal M, Ruiz P, Herreras A. Study of the in vitro susceptibility of M. tuberculosis to ofloxacin in Spain. Spanish Study Group of M. tuberculosis Resistance. Int J Tuberc Lung Dis 2000;4:588-91.
15. Huang TS, Kunin CM, Shin-Jung Lee S, Chen YS, Tu HZ, Liu YC. Trends in fluoroquinolone resistance of Mycobacterium tuberculosis complex in a Taiwanese medical centre: 1995–2003. J Antimicrob Chemother 2005;56:1058-62.
16. Grimaldo ER, Tupasi TE, Rivera AB. Increased resistance to ciprofloxacin and ofloxacin in multidrug-resistant tuberculosis isolates from patients seen at a tertiary care hospital in the Philippines. Int J Tuberc Lung Dis 2001;5:546-50.
17. Jann-Yuan Wang, Li-Na Lee, Hsin-Chih Lai. Fluoroquinolone resistance in Mycobacterium tuberculosis isolates: associated genetic mutations and relationship to antimicrobial exposure. J Antimicrob Chemother. 2007;59:860-5.
18. Hemvani N, Chitris DS, Bhatia GC, Sharma N, Drug resistance among tubercle bacilli from pulmonary tuberculosis in control India. Indian J Medical Sci. 2001;55:382-92.
19. Agrawal D, Udwadia ZF, Rodriguez C, Mehta A; Increasing incidence of fluoroquinolone-resistant Mycobacterium tuberculosis in Mumbai, India. Int J tuberc lung dis 2009;13:79-83.
20. Ramachandran R, Nalini S, Chandrasekar V, Dave PV, Sanghvi AS, Wares F. Surveillance of drug-resistant tuberculosis in the state of Gujarat, India. Int J Tuberc Lung Dis 2009;13:1154-60.
21. Yew WW, Chan ED, Chan CY, Cheng AF. Genotypic and phenotypic resistance of Mycobacterium tuberculosis to rifamycins and fluoroquinolones. Int J Tuberc Lung Dis 2002; 6:936-7.
22. Kocagoz T, Hackbarth CJ, Unsal I, Rosenberg EY, Nikaido H, Chambers HF. Gyrase mutations in laboratory-selected, fluoroquinolone resistant-mutants of Mycobacterium tuberculosis H37Ra. Antimicrob Agents Chemother 1996;40:1768-74.
23. Ginsburg AS, Grosset JH, Bishai WR. Fluoroquinolones, tuberculosis and resistance. Lancet Infect Dis 2003; 3:432-42.

24. Jacoby GA. Mechanisms of resistance to quinolones. Clin Infect Dis 2005; 41: S120-S126.
25. Yoon YS, Lee HJ, Yoon HI. Impact of fluoroquinolones on the diagnosis of pulmonary tuberculosis initially treated as bacterial pneumonia. Int J Tuberc Lung Dis 2005;9:1215-9.
26. Singh A. Quinolones to treat acute bacterial exacerbation of chronic bronchitis in TB endemic areas: a word of caution. Eur Respir J 2007;30:1233-5.
27. Ginsburg AS, Woolwine SC, Hooper N. The rapid development of fluoroquinolone resistance in M. tuberculosis. N Engl J Med 2003;349:1977-8.
28. Xu P, Li X, Zhao M, Gui X, DeRiemer K, Gagneux S. Prevalence of fluoroquinolone resistance among tuberculosis patients in Shanghai, China. Antimicrob Agents Chemother 2009;53:3170-2.
29. Devasia RA, Blackman A, Gebretsadik T, Griffin M, Shintani A, May C. Fluoroquinolone resistance in Mycobacterium tuberculosis: the effect of duration and timing of fluoroquinolone exposure. Am J Respir Crit Care Med 2009;180:365-70.
30. Canetti G, Wallace F, Khomenko A, Mahler H, Menon N, Mitchison D, Rist N, and Smelev N. Advances in techniques of testing mycobacterial drug sensitivity and the use of sensitivity tests in tuberculosis control programmes. Bull, WHO. 1969;41:21-43.
31. Zhao BY. Fluoroquinolone action against clinical isolates of Mycobacterium tuberculosis: effects of a C-8 methoxyl group on survival in liquid media and in human macrophages. Antimicrobial agents and Chemotherapy, 1999;43:661-6.
32. Dong Y. Fluoroquinolone action against mycobacteria: effects of C-8 substituents on growth, survival and resistance. Antimicrobial Agents and Chemotherapy, 1998, 42:2978 84.
33. Lounis N. Which aminoglycoside or fluoroquinolone is more active against Mycobacterium tuberculosis in mice? Antimicrobial Agents and Chemotherapy, 1997, 41:607-10.
34. Park-Wyllie LY, Juurlink DN, Kopp A, Shah BR, Stukel TA, Stumpo C. Outpatient gatifloxacin therapy and dysglycemia in older adults. N Engl J Med 2006;354:1352-61.
35. Rustomjee R, Lienhardt C, Kanyok T, Davies GR, Levin J, Mthiyane T. A Phase II study of the sterilising activities of ofloxacin, gatifloxacin and moxifloxacin in pulmonary tuberculosis. Int J Tuberc Lung Dis 2008;12:128-38.
36. Hooper DC. Fluoroquinolones. UptoDate, Rose BD, Waltham MA, 2006, Issue 3.
37. Hu Y, Coates AR, Mitchison DA: Sterilizing activities of fluoroquinolones against rifampin-tolerant populations of Mycobacterium tuberculosis. Antimicrob Agents Chemother 2003;47:653-7.
38. O'Brien RJ. Studies of the early bactericidal activity of new drugs for tuberculosis: a help or a hindrance to anti-tuberculosis drug development. Am J Respir Crit Care Med. 2002;166:3-4.
39. Johnson JL, Hadad DJ, Boom WH. Early and extended bactericidal activity of levofloxacin, gatifloxacin and moxifloxacin in pulmonary tuberculosis. Int J Tuberc Lung Dis 2006;10:605-12.
40. Gosling RD, Uiso LO, Sam NE, Bongard E, Kanduma EG, Nyindo M, et al. The bactericidal activity of moxifloxacin in patients with pulmonary tuberculosis. Am J Respir Crit Care Med. 2003;168:1342-5.
41. Sirgel F, Botha FJ, Parkin DP, Van de Wal BW, Donald PR, Mitchison D. The early bactericidal activity of ciprofloxacin in patients with pulmonary tuberculosis. Am J Respir Crit Care Med 1997;156:901-5.
42. Sirgel FA, Donald PR, Odhiambo J. EBA Collaborative Study Group A multicentre study of the early bactericidal activity of anti-tuberculosis drugs. J Antimicrob Chemother. 2000;45:859-70.

43. Kennedy N, Fox R, Kisyombe GM, Saruni AO, Uiso LO. Early bactericidal and sterilizing activities of ciprofloxacin in pulmonary tuberculosis. The American review of respiratory disease. 1993;Dec;148(61):1547-51.
44. Tsukamura M, Nakamura E, Yoshii S, Amano H. Therapeutic effect of a new antibacterial substance, ofloxacin (DL8280) on pulmonary tuberculosis. Am Rev Respir Dis 1985;131:352-356.
45. Marra F, Marra CA, Moadebi S. Levofloxacin treatment of active tuberculosis and the risk of adverse events. Chest 2005;128:1406-13.
46. Burman WJ, Goldberg S, Johnson JL. Moxifloxacin versus ethambutol for the first 2 months of treatment for pulmonary tuberculosis. Am J Respir Crit Care Med 2006; 174:331-8.
47. Yew WW, Chan CK, Leung CC. Comparative roles of levofloxacin and ofloxacin in the treatment of multidrug-resistant tuberculosis: Preliminary results of a retrospective study from Hong Kong. Chest 2003;124:1476-81.
48. Suarez PG, Floyd K, Portocarrero J. Feasibility and cost-effectiveness of standardised second-line drug treatment for chronic tuberculosis patients: A national cohort study in Peru. Lancet 2002; 359:1980-9.
49. Jain A, Dixit P, Prasad R. Pre-XDR & XDR in MDR and Ofloxacin and Kanamycin resistance in non-MDR Mycobacterium tuberculosis isolates. Tuberculosis 2012; 92: 404-6.
50. Rodriguez JC, Cebrián L, López L. Mutant prevention concentration: comparison of fluoroquinolones and linezolid with Mycobacterium tuberculosis. J Antimicrob Chemother 2004;53:441-4.
51. Migliori GB. Fluoroquinolones: are they essential to treat multidrug resistant tuberculosis. Eur Respir J 2008;31:904-10.
52. Migliori GB, Lange C, Centis R. Resistance to second-line injectables and treatment outcomes in multidrug-resistant and extensively drug-resistant tuberculosis cases. Eur Respir J 2008;31:1155-9.
53. Chan ED, Strand MJ, Iseman MD. Multidrug-resistant Tuberculosis (TB) Resistant to Fluoroquinolones and Streptomycin but Susceptible to Second-Line Injection Therapy Has a Better Prognosis than Extensively Drug-Resistant TB. Clin Infect Dis. 2009;48:50-2.
54. Guidelines on Programmatic Management of Drug Resistant TB (PMDT) in India. Central TB Division, Directorate General of Health Services, Ministry of Health and Family Welfare, Nirman Bhavan, New Delhi.

Chapter 21

Multi-drug-resistant and Extensively Drug-resistant Tuberculosis and HIV

Introduction

HIV coinfection is a significant challenge for the prevention, diagnosis and treatment of drug-resistant tuberculosis (DR-TB), especially in the case of multi-drug-resistant tuberculosis (MDR-TB) and extensively drug-resistant tuberculosis (XDR-TB). Reports have shown high mortality rates among HIV-infected patients with MDR-TB[1,2] and alarming mortality rates in patients coinfected with XDR-TB and HIV.[3] Early diagnosis of multi-drug-resistant and extensively drug-resistant tuberculosis (M/XDR-TB) and HIV, prompt treatment with adequate regimens, sound patient support and strong infection control measures are all essential components in the management of M/XDR-TB in HIV-infected people. HIV is a powerful risk factor for all forms of TB, and DR-TB outbreaks, including MDR and XDR-TB outbreaks.[3-7] The use of Antiretroviral treatment (ART) in addition to treatment of M/XDR-TB has been reported to improve outcomes of M/XDR-TB in HIV-infected people.[8,9] The chapter addresses relationship between HIV and M/XDR-TB, collaborative TB/HIV activities, diagnostic and clinical guidelines for management of M/XDR-TB in HIV-infected patients, potential drug interactions, toxicities and monitoring requirements in the concomitant treatment of M/XDR-TB and HIV and infection control implications in the context of HIV and M/XDR-TB.

Relationship HIV AND M/XDR-TB

There are several reasons why drug-resistant TB may be associated with HIV. Firstly, people living with HIV in Eastern Europe, particularly those infected earlier in the epidemic and whose weakened immune systems have since left them vulnerable to TB, frequently come from socially vulnerable populations, including injecting drug users. Sociobehavioral problems and/or lack of access to proper care may make these populations, as TB patients, vulnerable to developing drug resistance as a result of poor adherence to treatment or suboptimal treatment. Furthermore, people living with HIV may also be more likely to be exposed to M/XDR-TB patients, due either to increased hospitalizations in settings with poor infection control or association with peers who may have M/XDR-TB. Secondly, acquisition of rifampicin resistance among people living with HIV under treatment for TB may also be the result of anti-TB drug malabsorption, which has been documented in patient cohorts in settings of high HIV prevalence. Outbreaks of drug-resistant forms of tuberculosis among HIV-infected patients have been widely documented in nosocomial and other congregate settings[10,11] but little information is available about the association of HIV and drug-resistant TB on a population level.[12,13] The primary reason for the lack of information is that HIV and anti-TB drug susceptibility testing have not been sufficiently accessible for joint surveys under routine conditions. The accelerating and amplifying influence of HIV infection and the delay in recognition and diagnosis of tuberculosis were found to contribute to outbreaks of MDR-TB among HIV-infected patients in USA.[10,14-16] Shafer et al[17] studied temporal trends and transmission patterns in New York City using restriction fragment length polymorphism (RFLP) and found clustering of MDR-TB cases, particularly among HIV-infected persons, who suffered disproportionately from drug-resistant disease, findings consistent with the above scenario. A subsequent survey of 167 consecutive cases of tuberculosis seen at five New York hospitals during 1992 and 1993 demonstrated that HIV-infected persons were significantly more likely to have been recently infected with MDR-TB; indeed, 79% of the drug-resistant cases were shown by RFLP to be clustered with the clear implication of recent transmission.[17] In the Fourth WHO/IUATLD global drug surveillance report,[18] eight settings in seven countries reported data on drug resistance stratified by HIV status: Cuba, Honduras, Latvia, The Russian Federation (Tomsk Oblast), Spain (Barcelona and Galicia), Ukraine (Donetsk Oblast) and Uruguay. In addition, preliminary results of a survey conducted in Mozambique in 2007 have also found a significant association. Four countries were not able to discriminate between negative and unknown HIV status. The data reported from the majority of countries were not strong enough to examine an association between HIV and drug resistance. However, the data available from Donetsk Oblast, Ukraine and Latvia indicated a significant association between HIV and MDR-TB. Additional information on risk factors including history of hospitalization or imprisonment were not available for this analysis. So the specific reasons for the association are not known. Both the countries have a high underlying prevalence of MDR-TB, as well as an emerging HIV epidemic, that initially was concentrated among risk groups, but has now become more generalized. However, several studies in India and other South-East Asian countries, having high prevalence of HIV seropositivity, have reported very low prevalence of MDR-TB in HIV-seropositive patients contrary to western literature. HIV-infected TB cases are more likely to be smear negative, and delayed diagnosis of drug resistance as well as unavailability of treatment have led to high death rates in people living with HIV. Both these factors may suggest a lower rate of transmission. However, HIV-infected cases progress rapidly to disease, and in settings where MDR-TB is prevalent, this may lead to rapid development of a pool of drug-resistant TB patients, or an outbreak. Despite some of the weakness in these data and subsequent analysis, the association between HIV and MDR-TB is concerning particularly given the implications for the clinical management of these patients. Rapid progression to death in HIV-infected M/XDR-TB patients in both outbreaks and treatment cohorts has been widely documented.[3,10,19] Antiretroviral treatment for HIV does appear to benefit coinfected MDR-TB patients; however, comanagement of treatment for both diseases is very complicated. Currently, most TB control programs in high-burden countries do not have the diagnostic infrastructure to either detect an outbreak nor the programmatic capacity to manage an outbreak. Given the impact on mortality, outbreaks should be avoided at all costs. The development of infection control measures in congregate settings as well as diagnostic screening tools to rapidly identify drug-resistant TB are a priority, for all countries, but particularly for those with high prevalence of HIV or MDR-TB. From a global perspective, routine diagnosis of both HIV and drug-resistant TB should be scaled up for the patient's benefit. Better surveillance data may help in developing an understanding of the relationship between HIV and M/XDR-TB.

Collaborative TB/HIV Activities

WHO recommends that certain collaborative activities are carried out to decrease the joint burden of TB and HIV. These activities are the backbone of the TB/HIV collaborative strategy that, along with the implementation of effective DOTS programs, will strengthen and increase the success of M/XDR-TB/HIV control and treatment activities. The activities described below are based on TB/HIV activities and are adapted to be specifically applicable to M/XDR-TB.

Perform provider initiated HIV testing and counseling in all TB suspects: As there are high levels of HIV and TB coinfection in many settings, provider-initiated HIV counseling and testing is recommended for all TB suspects.[20,21] Provider-initiated testing can be done at the same time the sputum is sent for smear microscopy or culture. This is more efficient and more likely to be successful than referring patients elsewhere for HIV testing and counseling.[22]

Use standard algorithms to diagnose pulmonary and extrapulmonary TB: New recommendations for improving the diagnosis and treatment of smear-negative pulmonary and extrapulmonary TB by WHO[23] must be used. Mycobacterial cultures of sputum or other fluids and tissues are recommended to help in the diagnosis of sputum smear negative and extrapulmonary TB.[23] The heavy reliance on smear microscopy has significant limitations and is insufficient to reliably diagnose a significant proportion of HIV-coinfected patients, especially as the degree of immunosuppression advances.[24] Rapid methods such as liquid culture or molecular techniques should be considered.[25] Drug Susceptibility Test (DST) should be performed at the start of antituberculosis therapy as unrecognized M/XDR-TB carries a high risk of mortality in patients with HIV.[26] Prompt initiation of appropriate antituberculosis treatment and subsequent initiation of Antiretroviral treatment can reduce mortality among HIV-infected patients infected with M/XDR-TB.[27,28] While performing DST for all TB/HIV co-infected patients is the standard of care for many areas, but this may be difficult or impossible in many resource-limited settings. Programs ideally should determine the extent of the overlap of the M/XDR-TB and HIV epidemics.[29]

Introduce Antiretroviral treatment (ART) promptly in M/XDR-TB/HIV patients: Guidelines recommend the prompt initiation of ART in HIV-infected patients with M/XDR-TB according to WHO guidelines.[30]

Consider empirical therapy with second-line antituberculosis drugs: Patients with a very high risk of M/XDR-TB can be empirically started on Category IV regimens. This strategy can be applied to all patients regardless of HIV status but is especially important in those with HIV.

Provide Cotrimoxazole prevention therapy (CPT) for patients with active TB and HIV: CPT should be provided to all patients with HIV according to WHO recommendations.[31] This therapy is not known to interact significantly with any of the second-line antituberculosis agents. There are overlapping toxicities between ART, antitubercular therapy and CPT, and vigilance in terms of monitoring adverse effects is required.

Arrange treatment follow-up by a specialized team: The team of care providers should be familiar with the treatment of both M/XDR-TB and HIV, with close monitoring of potential additive adverse effects and nutritional status as well as periodic assessments of therapeutic response for both infections.

Implement additional nutritional and socioeconomic support: Patients with M/XDR-TB and HIV may suffer from severe wasting, diarrheal diseases, and malabsorption syndromes. Coinfected patients often come from socially marginalized groups or from families with low economic resources. Additionally, M/XDR-TB therapy with second-line antituberculosis medications may result in adverse effects that affect treatment adherence and require more frequent visits to health facilities. Wherever possible, patients with M/XDR-TB/HIV and limited means should be offered socioeconomic and nutritional support.[32]

Ensure effective infection control: Infection control procedures can reduce the risk of *M. tuberculosis* transmission in HIV/AIDS care facilities. Infection control measures should be ensured as per WHO guidelines.[33]

Involve key stakeholders in M/XDR-TB/HIV activities: The local/national TB/HIV-coordinating bodies, community groups and key stakeholders should be involved in the planning and monitoring of M/XDR-TB/HIV activities and programs.

Clinical Features and Diagnosis of M/XDR-TB in HIV-infected Patients

The diagnosis of TB including MDR-TB and XDR-TB in HIV-infected people is more difficult and may be confused with other pulmonary or systemic infections. The presentation is more likely to be extrapulmonary or sputum smear negative than in HIV-uninfected TB patients, especially as immunosuppression advances.[34] This can result in misdiagnosis or delays in diagnosis, and, in turn, higher morbidity and mortality. Algorithms have recently been published by the WHO with the aim of improving the diagnosis of smear-negative pulmonary and extrapulmonary TB.[23] The new algorithms emphasize the use of clinical criteria first and, if needed, the use of additional laboratory data (culture) and radiography to diagnose TB. Clinical criteria have been shown to have an 89 to 96% positive predictive value of smear-negative and extrapulmonary TB when compared with culture.[21] For patients with advanced HIV disease, mycobacterial culture of other fluids (e.g. blood, pleural fluid, ascitic fluid, cerebrospinal fluid and bone-marrow aspirates) and histopathology (e.g. lymph node biopsies) may be helpful in diagnosis. In many programs and areas, all HIV patients with TB are screened for drug resistance with DST. Rapid drug-resistance testing is the DST technique of choice since this allows prompt diagnosis of M/XDR-TB, decreasing the time the patient may be on an inadequate regimen and the period during which the patient may be spreading M/XDR-TB. Programs without facilities or resources to screen all HIV-infected patients for M/XDR-TB should put significant efforts into obtaining them, especially if M/XDR-TB rates are moderate or high. Some programs may adopt a strategy of targeted DST for patients with increased risk of M/XDR-TB such as those in whom treatment has failed or who are contacts of M/XDR-TB cases. Programs may also choose to use targeted DST for those with lower CD4 counts (e.g. less than 200 cells/mm) since these patients are at a very high risk of death due to unrecognized M/XDR-TB.

Concomitant Treatment of M/XDR-TB and HIV

The treatment of M/XDR-TB in patients with HIV is very similar to that in patients without HIV, with the following exceptions:

1. Antiretroviral Treatment (ART) plays a crucial role as mortality in M/XDR-TB/HIV patients without the use of ART is extremely high.
2. Adverse effects are more common in patients with HIV. The multiple medicines involved in M/XDR-TB with recognized high toxicity risks, often combined with ART, result in a high incidence of adverse effects. Some toxicities are common to both antituberculosis treatment and ART, which may result in added rates of adverse events.
3. Monitoring needs to be more intense for both response to therapy and adverse effects.
4. The use of thioacetazone is not recommended for patients with HIV[35] or for routine use in populations with high rates of HIV.
5. Immune reconstitution inflammatory syndrome (IRIS) may complicate the therapy.

Initiating ART Treatment in Patients with M/XDR-TB

The use of ART in HIV-infected patients with TB improves survival for both drug-resistant and susceptible disease.[9,23,36] However, the likelihood of adverse effects could compromise the treatment of either HIV or M/XDR-TB if both the treatments are started simultaneously. On the other hand, undue delay in the start of ART could result in significant risk of HIV-related death among patients with advanced disease.[37] The optimal timing for the introduction of ART in patients receiving TB treatment is unknown. The Timing of ART [30] in the ART-naive patient starting antituberculosis therapy for M/XDR-TB is as below:

1. ART should be started in all TB patients, including those with drug-resistant TB, irrespective of the CD4 count.
2. Antituberculosis treatment should be initiated first, followed by ART as soon as possible within the first eight weeks of treatment.
3. The HIV-positive TB patients with profound immunosuppression (such as CD4 counts less than 50 cells/mm^3) should receive ART immediately within the first two weeks of initiating TB treatment.

4. ART should be started in any child with active TB disease as soon as possible and within eight weeks following the initiation of antituberculosis treatment, irrespective of the CD4 count and clinical stage.
5. Efavirenz should be used as the preferred NNRTI in patients starting ART while on antituberculosis treatment.

M/XDR-TB in Patients Already Receiving ART

There are two issues to consider in patients who are diagnosed with M/XDR-TB while on ART. The first is whether modification of ART is needed due to drug-drug-interactions or to decrease the potential of overlapping toxicities.The second issue is whether the presentation of active M/XDR-TB in a patient on ART constitutes ART failure.

Drug-drug Interactions in the Treatment of HIV and M/XDR-TB

Currently, little is known about drug-drug interactions between second-line antituberculosis agents and antiretroviral therapy. While rifampicin derivatives are not routinely used in M/XDR-TB treatment, they are used in the treatment of rifampicin-sensitive poly- and mono-resistant TB. Buffered didanosine contains an aluminum-magnesium-based antacid and, if given jointly with fluoroquinolones, may result in decreased fluoroquinolone absorption; it should be avoided, but if it is necessary, it should be given six hours before or two hours after fluoroquinolone administration. The enteric-coated (EC) formulation of didanosine can be used concomitantly without this precaution. Ethionamide/prothionamide is thought to be metabolized by the CYP450 system, although it is not known which of the CYP enzymes are responsible. Whether doses of ethionamide/prothionamide and/or certain antiretroviral drugs should be modified during the concomitant treatment of M/XDR-TB and HIV is completely unknown.[38] Clarithromycin is a substrate and inhibitor of CYP3A and has multiple drug interactions with protease inhibitors and non-nucleoside reverse transcriptase inhibitors (NNRTIs). If possible, the use of clarithromycin should be avoided in patients coinfected with M/XDR-TB and HIV because of both its weak efficacy against M/XDR-TB and multiple drug interactions.

Potential Drug Toxicity in the Treatment of HIV and M/XDR-TB

HIV patients have a higher rate of adverse drug reactions to both TB and non-TB medications, and the risk of adverse drug reactions increases with the degree of immunosuppression.[34,39-41] Identifying the source of adverse effects in patients receiving concomitant therapy for M/XDR-TB and HIV is difficult. Many of the medications used to treat M/XDR-TB and HIV have overlapping, or in some cases additive, toxicities. Often it may not be possible to link adverse effects to a single drug, as the risk of resistance for ART therapy precludes the typical medical challenge of stopping all medications and starting them one by one.[42] Adverse effects that are common to both antiretroviral and antitubercular drugs are listed in Table 21.1. It should be noted that relatively very little is known about the rates of adverse effects in the concomitant treatment of

TABLE 21.1: Adverse effects of antiretroviral and antitubercular drugs

Toxicity	*Antiretroviral agent*	*Antituberculosis agent*	*Comments*
Peripheral neuropathy	D4T, ddI, ddC	Lzd, Cs, H, Sm, Km, Am, Eto/ Pto, E	• Avoid use of D4T, ddI and ddC in combination with Cs or Lzd because of increased peripheral neuropathy • If these agents must be used and peripheral neuropathy develops, replace the ARV agent with a less neurotoxic agent
Central nervous system toxicity (CNS)	EFV	Cs, H, Eto /Pto, Ofx, Lfx, Mfx	Efavirenz has a high rate of CNS adverse effects (confusion, impaired concentration, depersonalization, abnormal dreams, insomnia and dizziness) in the first 2 to 3 weeks, which typically resolve on their own. If these effects do not resolve on their own, consider substitution of the agent
Depression	EFV	Cs, Ofx, Lfx, Mfx, H, Eto/Pto	Severe depression can be seen in 2.4% of patients receiving EFV. Consider substituting for EFV if severe depression develops
Headache	AZT, EFV	Cs	• Rule out more serious causes of headache such as bacterial meningitis, cryptococcal meningitis, CNS toxoplasmosis, etc. • Use of analgesics (ibuprofen, paracetamol) and good hydration may help. • Headache secondary to AZT, EFV and Cs is usually self-limited
Nausea and vomiting	RTV, D4T, NVP	Eto/Pto, PAS, H, E&Z	• Nausea and vomiting are common adverse effects and can be managed. • Persistent vomiting and abdominal pain may be a result of developing lactic acidosis and/or hepatitis secondary to medications
Abdominal pain	All ART treatments have been associated with abdominal pain	Cfz, Eto/Pto, PAS	Abdominal pain is a common adverse effect and often benign; however, abdominal pain may be an early symptom of severe adverse effects, such as pancreatitis, hepatitis or lactic acidosis

Contd...

Contd...

Toxicity	*Antiretroviral agent*	*Antituberculosis agent*	*Comments*
Pancreatitis	D4T, ddl, ddC	Lzd	• Avoid use of these agents together. If an agent causes pancreatitis, suspend it permanently and do not use any of the pancreatitis-producing anti-HIV medications (D4T, ddl, or ddC) in the future. • Also consider gallstones or alcohol as a potential cause of pancreatitis
Diarrhea	All protease inhibitors, ddl (buffered formula)	Eto/Pto, PAS, Ofx, Lfx, Mfx	• Diarrhea is a common adverse effect. • Also consider opportunistic infections as a cause of diarrhea, or clostridium difficile (a cause of pseudomembranous colitis).
Hepatotoxicity	NVP, EFV, all protease inhibitors and all NRTIs	H, R, E, Z, PAS, Eto/Pto, Ofx, Lfx, Mfx	• Also consider TMP/SMX as a cause of hepatotoxicity if the patient is receiving this medication • Also rule out viral etiologies such as cause of hepatitis (Hepatitis A, B, C and CMV)
Skin rash	ABC, NVP, EFV, D4T	H, R, Z, PAS, Ofx, Lfx, Mfx	• Do not rechallenge with ABC (can result in life-threatening anaphylaxis) • Do not rechallenge with an agent that causes Stevens-Johnson syndrome • Also consider TMP/SMX as a cause of skin rash if the patient is receiving this medication. Thioacetazone is contraindicated in HIV because of life-threatening rash.
Lactic acidosis	D4T, ddl, AZT, 3TC	Lzd	If an agent causes lactic acidosis, replace it with an agent less likely to cause lactic acidosis
Renal toxicity	TDF	Sm, Km, Am, Cm	• TDF may cause renal injury with the characteristic features of Fanconi syndrome, hypophosphatemia, hypouricemia, proteinuria, normoglycemic glycosuria and, in some cases, acute renal failure • Use TDF with caution in patients receiving aminoglycosides or Cm. • Frequent creatinine and electrolyte monitoring every 1 to 3 weeks is recommended

Contd...

Contd...

Toxicity	*Antiretroviral agent*	*Antituberculosis agent*	*Comments*
Nephrolithiasis	IDV	None	• No overlapping toxicities regarding nephrolithiasis have been documented between ART and antituberculosis medications • Adequate hydration prevents nephrolithiasis in patients taking IDV. • If nephrolithiasis develops while on IDV, substitute with another protease inhibitor if possible
Electrolyte disturbances	TDF	Cm, Sm, Km, Am	• Diarrhea and/or vomiting can contribute to electrolyte disturbances • Even without the concurrent use of TDF, HIV-infected patients have an increased risk of both renal toxicity and electrolyte disturbances secondary to aminoglycosides and Cm
Bone marrow suppression	AZT	Lzd, R, Rfb, H	• Monitor blood counts regularly. Replace AZT if bone marrow suppression develops. Consider suspension of Lzd. • Also consider TMP/SMX as a cause if the patient is receiving this medication • Consider adding folinic acid supplements, especially if receiving TMP/SMX
Optic neuritis	ddI	E, Eto/Pto (rare)	Suspend agent responsible for optic neuritis permanently and replace with an agent that does not cause optic neuritis
Hyperlipidemia	Protease inhibitors, EFV	None	No overlapping toxicities regarding hyperlipidemia have been documented between ART and antituberculosis medications
Lipodystrophy	NRTIs (especially D4T and ddI)	None	No overlapping toxicities regarding lipodystrophy have been documented between ART and antituberculosis medications
Dysglycemia (disturbed blood sugar regulation)	Protease inhibitors	Gfx, Eto/Pto	• Protease inhibitors tend to cause insulin resistance and hyperglycemia • Eto/Pto tend to make insulin control in diabetics more difficult, and can result in hypoglycemia and poor glucose regulation

Contd...

Contd...

Toxicity	*Antiretroviral agent*	*Antituberculosis agent*	*Comments*
Hypothyroidism	D4T	Eto/Pto, PAS	There is potential for overlying toxicity, but evidence is mixed. Several studies show subclinical hypothyroidism associated with HAART, particularly stavudine. PAS and Eto/Pto, especially in combination, can commonly cause hypothyroidism

Abbreviations:
Antiretroviral agents: Stavudine (D4T), Didanosine (ddl), Zalcitabine (ddC), Ritonavir (RTV), Nevirapine (NVP), Nucleoside reverse transcriptase inhibitors (NRTIs), Abacavir (ABC), Lamivudine (3TC), Tenofovir (TDF), Indinavir (IDV).
Antitubercular agents: Isoniazid (H), Rifampicin (R), Ethambutol (E), Pyrazinamide (Z), Rifabutin (Rfb), Streptomycin (S), Kanamycin (Km), Amikacin (Am), Capreomycin (Cm), Ofloxacin (Ofx), Levofloxacin (Lfx), Moxifloxacin (Mfx), Gatifloxacin, Ethionamide (Eto), Protionamide (Pto), P-aminosalicylic acid (PAS), Cycloserine (Cs), Clofazimine (Cfz), Linezolid (Lzd).

M/XDR-TB and HIV. Often, however, the benefit of using drugs that have overlying toxicities outweighs the risk. Therefore, if two drugs with overlapping toxicities are determined to be essential in a patient's regimen, increased monitoring of adverse effects rather than disallowing a certain combination is recommended.

Potential Overlying and Additive Toxicities of ART and Antituberculosis Therapy

Monitoring of M/XDR-TB and HIV Therapy in Coinfected Patients

HIV treatment must be taken daily without exception to prevent the evolution of drug resistance. Since DOT is an important component of M/XDR-TB therapy, programs would be advised to explore the provision of TB medications and Antiretrovirals (ARVs) through concomitant DOT or other methods of adherence support. This is particularly important in the setting of second-line antituberculosis therapy, since it can result in a large pill burden and numerous adverse effects that make taking ART more difficult. The complexity of antiretroviral regimens and second-line antituberculosis treatment, each with its own toxicity profiles and some of which may be potentiated by concomitant therapy, demands rigorous clinical monitoring.[43] Given that the regimens together are particularly difficult to take, the stigma of both the diseases can result in serious discrimination, and the risk of mortality is very high. Patients with HIV-associated M/XDR-TB may require special socioeconomic, nutritional and psychosocial support in order to successfully complete the treatment.

Immune Reconstitution Inflammatory Syndrome (IRIS)

IRIS has emerged as an important complication of ART. It is relatively common, reported in up to one-third of patients, in mild to moderate forms in patients with TB started on ART;[44,45] however, it is relatively rare in its severe forms. This syndrome can present as a paradoxical worsening of the patient's clinical status, often due to a previously subclinical and unrecognized opportunistic infection.[30,46] These reactions may present as fever, enlarging lymph nodes, worsening pulmonary infiltrates, respiratory distress or exacerbation of inflammatory changes at other sites. It generally presents within three months of the initiation of ART and is more common with CD4 cell count < 50 cells/mm^3.[23,46] It is important to note that IRIS is a diagnosis of exclusion. Patients with advanced AIDS may show clinical deterioration for a number of other reasons. New opportunistic infections or previously subclinical infections may be unmasked following immune reconstitution and cause clinical worsening.[30] IRIS can also be confused with TB treatment failure, and coinfected patients may be demonstrating progression of TB disease due to drug resistance. The management of IRIS is complex and depends on the clinical status of the patient and the site and extent of involvement. Various treatment modalities have been employed, including nonsteroidal anti-inflammatory drugs in mild disease and corticosteroids in moderate to severe disease. Most patients can be treated without interruption of ART.

XDR-TB and HIV

XDR-TB has been described in a number of countries, including settings with a high prevalence of HIV. An algorithm to help diagnose XDR-TB in HIV-infected individuals and Treatment strategies for XDR-TB are outlined in Chapters 16 and 17.

Implications of HIV for M/XDR-TB Infection Control

Delay in recognition of M/XDR-TB, prolonged periods of infectiousness, crowded wards, and mixing TB and HIV patients, all contribute to nosocomial transmission. These practices have contributed to M/XDR-TB outbreaks that affect both HIV-infected and noninfected patients. Implementation of adequate infection control precautions at health facilities significantly reduces nosocomial transmission.[47] Some community-based treatment programs have used home-based measures such as separate living quarters, personal respiratory protection for visitors and adequate ventilation.[48] Infection control measures for M/XDR-TB, including in the setting of high HIV prevalence, are described in Chapter 26.

Conclusion

M/XDR-TB in HIV-infected patients is highly lethal and a growing problem in many parts of the world. Improved case detection, timely and appropriate therapy, close clinical monitoring, management of adverse effects and infection control measures are the essential components of a successful management. TB and HIV control programs will contain the epidemic of HIV-associated M/XDR-TB.

References

1. Park MM, Davis AL, Schluger NW, Cohen H, Rom WN. Outcome of MDR-TB patients, 1983-1993. Prolonged survival with appropriate therapy. Am J Resp Criti Care Med. 1996;153:317-24.

2. Finlay AF, Van der Walt M, Holtz TH, Thorpe LE, Wells CD, Weyer K. Treatment outcomes of patients with multidrug resistant tuberculosis in South Africa using a standardized regimen, 1999–2000 (Poster session 58, N_ 2101). In: Infectious Disease Society of America, Boston, MA, September 2004.
3. Gandhi NR, Moll A, Sturm AW, Pawinski R, Govender T, Lalloo U, et al. Extensively drug-resistant tuberculosis as a cause of death in patients coinfected with tuberculosis and HIV in a rural area of South Africa. Lancet. 2006;368:1575-80.
4. Anti-tuberculosis drug resistance in the world. Fourth global report. The WHO/IUATLD global project on anti-tuberculosis drug resistance surveillance, 2002–2007. Geneva, World Health Organization, 2008 (WHO/HTM/TB/2008.394).
5. Shah NS, Wright A, Bai GH, Barrera L, Boulahbal F, Martín-Casabona N, et al. Worldwide emergence of extensively drug-resistant tuberculosis. Emerging Infectious Diseases. 2007;13:380-7.
6. Masjedi MR, Farnia P, Sorooch S, Pooramiri MV, Mansoori SD, Zarifi AZ, et al. Extensively drug-resistant tuberculosis: 2 years of surveillance in Iran. Clinical Infectious Diseases. 2006;43:841-7.
7. Wells CD, Cegielski JP, Nelson LJ, Laserson KF, Holtz TH, Finlay A, et al. HIV infection and multidrug-resistant tuberculosis: the perfect storm. J Infec Dis. 2007;196:86-107.
8. Burgos, M, Gonzales, LC, Paz, EA, et al. Treatment of multidrug-resistant tuberculosis in San Francisco: an outpatient-based approach. Clinical Infectious Diseases. 2005;40:968-75.
9. Waisman JL, Palmero DJ, Alberti FA, Güemes JL G, Francos JL, Negroni R. [Improved prognosis in HIV/AIDS related multi-drug-resistant tuberculosis patients treated with highly active antiretroviral therapy] Medicina (B Aires). 2001;61:810-4.
10. Edlin BR, Tokars, JI, Grieco MH, et al. An outbreak of multidrug-resistant tuberculosis among hospitalized patients with the acquired immunodeficiency syndrome. N Engl J Med. 1992;326:1514-21.
11. Moro, ML, Gori A, Errante I, Infuso A, Franzetti F, Sodano L, Iemoli E. An outbreak of multidrug resistant tuberculosis involving HIV infected patients of two hospitals in Milan, Italy. AIDS. 1998;12:1095-102.
12. Kenyon TA, Mwasekaga MJ, Huebner R, Rumisha D, Binkin N. Low levels of drug resistance amidst rapidly increasing tuberculosis and human immunodeficiency virus co-epidemics in Botswana. Int J Tuberc Lung Dis. 1999;3:4-11.
13. Chum HJ, O'Brien RJ, Chonde TM, Graf P, Rieder HLI. An epidemiological study of tuberculosis and HIV infection in Tanzania, 1991-1993. AIDS. 1996;10:299-309.
14. Frieden TR, Sterling T, Pablos-Mendez A, Kilburn JO, Cauthen GM, Dooley SW. The emergence of drug-resistant tuberculosis in New York City. N Engl J med. 1993;328:521-6.
15. Coronado VG, Beck-Sague CM, Hutton MD. Transmission of multidrug-resistant *Mycobacterium tuberculosis* among persons with human immunodeficiency virus infection in an urban hospital: epidemiologic and restriction fragment length polymorphism analysis. J Infect Dis. 1993;168:1052-5.
16. Busillo C, Lessnau K-D, Sanjana V. Multidrug-resistant *Mycobacterium tuberculosis* in patients with human immunodeficiency virus infection. Chest. 1992;102:797-801.
17. Shafer RW, Small PM, Larkin C, et al. Temporal trends and transmission patterns during the emergence of multidrug-resistant tuberculosis in New York City: a molecular epidemiologic assessment. J Infect Dis. 1995;152:171-6.
18. Anti-tuberculosis drug resistance in the world: Fourth global report. The WHO/IUATLD Global Project on Anti-Tuberculosis Drug Resistance Surveillance 2002-2007. Geneva: World Health Organization;2008. Available from: http://www.who.int/tb/publications/2008/drs_report4_26feb08.pdf.

19. Mac-Arthur A, Gloyd S, Perdigao P, Noya A, Sacarlal J. Characteristics of drug resistance and HIV among tuberculosis patients in Mozambique. Int J Tuberc Lung Dis. 2001;5:894-902.
20. UNAIDS/WHO policy statement on HIV testing. Geneva, World Health Organization and Joint United Nations Programme on HIV/AIDS 2004 (available at http://www.who.int/hiv/pub/vct/en hivtestingpolicy04.pdf).
21. Guidance on provider-initiated HIV testing and counseling in health facilities. Geneva, World Health Organization, 2007.
22. Tuberculosis care with TB-HIV co-management. Geneva, World Health Organization, 2007 (WHO/HTM/HIV/2007.01).
23. Improving the diagnosis and treatment of smear-negative pulmonary and extrapulmonary tuberculosis among adults and adolescents: Recommendations for HIV-prevalent and resource-constrained settings. Geneva, World Health Organization, 2007 (WHO/HTM/TB/2007.379; WHO/HIV/2007.01).
24. Wilson D, Nachega J, Morroni C, Chaisson R, Maartens G. Diagnosing smear-negative tuberculosis using case definitions and treatment response in HIV-infected adults. Int J Tuberc Lung Dis. 2006;10:31-8.
25. Moore David AJ, Evans Carlton AW, Gilman RH, Caviedes L, Coronel J, Vivar A, et al. Microscopic-observation drug susceptibility assay for the diagnosis of TB. New England Journal of Medicine. 2006;355:1539-50.
26. Fischl Margaret A, Daikos George L, Uttamchandani Raj B, Poblete Rita B, Moreno Jose N, Reyes Ricardo R, et al. Clinical presentation and outcome of patients with HIV infection and tuberculosis caused by multiple-drug-resistant bacilli. Annals of Internal Medicine. 1992;117:184-90.
27. Nunn P, Kibuga D, Gathua S, Brindle R, Imalingat A, Wasunna K, et al. Cutaneous hypersensitivity reactions due to thiacetazone in HIV-1 seropositive patients treated for tuberculosis. Lancet. 1991;337:627-30.
28. Turett GS, Telzak EE, Torian LV, Blum S, Alland D, Weisfuse I, et al. Improved outcomes for patients with multidrug-resistant tuberculosis. Clinical Infectious Diseases. 1995;21(5):1238-44.
29. Guidelines for surveillance of drug resistance in tuberculosis. Geneva, World Health Organization, 2003 (WHO/CDS/TB/2003.312).
30. Antiretroviral therapy for HIV infection in adults and adolescents: recommendations for a public health approach. Geneva, World Health Organization, 2006, 2010, 2013 (available at http: //www. who.int/entity/hiv/pub/guidelines/adult/en/index.html).
31. World Health Organization, 2012. WHO policy on collaborative TB/HIV activities guidelines for national programmes and other stakeholders. WHO/HTM/TB/2012; WHO/HIV/2012.1.
32. The PIH guide to the community-based treatment of HIV in resource-poor settings, 2nd edn.
33. Tuberculosis infection control in the era of expanding HIV care and treament. Addendum to WHO guidelines for the prevention of tuberculosis in healthcare facilities in resource-limited settings, 1999. Geneva, World Health Organization, 2007. TB/HIV: a clinical manual. Geneva, World Health Organization, 2007.
34. TB/HIV: a clinical manual. Geneva, World Health Organization, 2004 (WHO/HTM/TB/2004.329).
35. Nunn P, Kibuga D, Gathua S, Brindle R, Imalingat A, Wasunna K, et al. Cutaneous hypersensitivity reactions due to thiacetazone in HIV-1 seropositive patients treated for tuberculosis. Lancet. 1991;337:627-30.

36. Whalen C, Horsburgh CR, Hom D, Lahart C, Simberkoff M, Ellner J. Accelerated course of human immunodeficiency virus infection after tuberculosis. American Journal of Respiratory and Critical Care Medicine. 1995;151:129-35.
37. Menzies D, Gardam M. Tuberculosis control within Institutions. In: Long R, Ellis E, editors. Canadian tuberculosis standards. 6th ed. Ottawa (ON): Public Health Agency of Canada; 2007;320–47. Available: www.phac-aspc.gc.ca/tbpc-latb/pubs/pdf/tbstand07_e.pdf.
38. Centers for Disease Control and Prevention (CDC). Managing drug interactions in the treatment of HIV-related tuberculosis [online]. 2007 (available at http://www.cdc.gov/ tb/TB_ HIV_ Drugs/ default.htm).
39. Hoffmann CJ, Christopher J Charalambous S, Thio CL, Martin DJ, Pemba L, et al. Hepatotoxicity in an African antiretroviral therapy cohort: the effect of tuberculosis and hepatitis B. AIDS. 2007;21:1301-8.
40. Dean GL, Edwards SG, Ives NJ, Matthews G, Fox EF, Navaratne L, et al. Treatment of tuberculosis in HIV-infected persons in the era of highly active antiretroviral therapy. AIDS. 2002;16:75-83.
41. McIlleron H, Meintjes G, Burman WJ, Maartens G. Complications of antiretroviral therapy in patients with tuberculosis: drug interactions, toxicity and immune reconstitution inflammatory syndrome. J Infec Dis. 2007;196:63-75.
42. Dia-Jeanette T. Mycobacterial Disease in HIV positive patients. J Pharm Practice. 2006;19:10-6.
43. Guidelines for using antiretroviral agents among HIV-infected adults and adolescents. Morbidity and Mortality Weekly Report. 2002;51(RR07).
44. Navas E, Martín-Dávila P, Moreno L, Pintado V, Casado JL, Fortún J, et al. Paradoxical reactions of tuberculosis in patients with the acquired immunodeficiency syndrome who are treated with highly active antiretroviral therapy. Archives of Internal Medicine. 2002;162:97-9.
45. Narita M, Ashkin D, Hollender ES, Pitchenik AE. Paradoxical worsening of tuberculosis following antiretroviral therapy in patients with AIDS. Am J Resp Criti Care Med. 1998;158:157-61.
46. Lawn SD, Myer L, Bekker LG, Wood R. Tuberculosis-associated immune reconstitution disease: incidence, risk factors and impact in an antiretroviral treatment service in South Africa. AIDS. 2007;21:335-41.
47. Basu S, Andrews JR, Poolman EM. Prevention of nosocomial transmission of extensively drug-resistant tuberculosis in rural South African district hospitals: an epidemiological modelling study. Lancet. 2007;370:1500-7.
48. Shin S, Furin J, Bayona J, Mate K, Kim JY, Farmer P. Community-based treatment of multidrug-resistant tuberculosis in Lima, Peru: 7 years of experience. Soc Sci Med. 2004;59:1529-39.

Chapter 22

Interaction between Antitubercular and Antiretroviral Drugs

Introduction

Worldwide, tuberculosis (TB) is one of the most important infectious diseases in subjects with Human Immunodeficiency Virus (HIV) infection. Rifamycin-based anti-tuberculosis therapy can cure HIV-related TB and, where available, the introduction of highly active antiretroviral therapy (HAART) has markedly reduced the incidence of Acquired Immunodeficency Syndrome (AIDS) and death. Although effective therapy is available for both conditions, there are major problems in the concurrent treatment of HIV and TB coinfection. This chapter aims to describe antiretroviral therapy for the treatment of HIV- infection, pharmacokinetic issues in the treatment of HIV-related tuberculosis and interactions between antitubercular and antiretroviral drugs.

Antiretroviral Therapy for the Treatment of HIV Infection

Rapid progress in developing antiretroviral therapy (ART) led in 1996 the introduction of highly active antiretroviral therapy (HAART). HAART is a combination of at least three antiretroviral (ARV) drugs. HAART is the global standard of care in the treatment of HIV infection. Although not a cure for HIV infection, HAART usually results in near-complete suppression of HIV replication. Treatment has to be life-long. ART results in dramatic reductions in morbidity and mortality in HIV-infected people. There are several requirements for successful use of ART. These include considerable efforts to maintain adherence to life-long treatment and to monitor response to treatment, drug toxicities and drug interactions.[1]

Antiretroviral (ARV) Drugs

ARV drugs belong to the following classes:

- Reverse transcriptase inhibitors (RTIs)
- Protease inhibitors (PIs)
- Fusion or Entry Inhibitors, and
- Integrase Inhibitors.

RTIs are further divided into three groups:

i. Nucleoside reverse transcriptase inhibitors (NsRTIs);
ii. Non-nucleoside reverse transcriptase inhibitors (NNRTIs) and
iii. Nucleotide reverse transcriptase inhibitors (NtRTIs).

Nucleoside Reverse Transcriptase Inhibitors (NsRTIs)

NsRTIs inhibit reverse transcription by being incorporated into the newly synthesized viral DNA and preventing its further elongation. Drugs available with their toxicities from this group are tabulated in Table 22.1.

TABLE 22.1: Nucleoside reverse transcriptase inhibitors with their toxicities

Drugs	*Abbreviation*	*Toxicity*	*Food restriction*
Zidovudine	(AZT, ZDV)	Anemia, granulocytopenia, myopathy, lactic acidosis, hepatomegaly with steatosis, headache and nausea	Taken with or without food
Didanosine	(ddl)	Pancreatitis, peripheral neuropathy, abnormalities in liver function tests, lactic acidosis, hepatomegaly with steatosis	Taken on an empty stomach 30 mins before, or 2 hours after a meal
Stavudine	(d4T)	Peripheral neuropathy, pancreatitis, lactic acidosis, hepatomegaly with steatosis, ascending neuromuscular weakness and lipodystrophy	Taken with or without food
Lamivudine	(3TC)	Headache and dry mouth	Taken with or without food
Zalcitabine	(ddC)	Peripheral neuropathy, pancreatitis, lactic acidosis, hepatomegaly with steatosis and oral ulcers	Taken with or without food
Emtricitabine	(FTC)	Headache, nausea, insomnia, hypertrophy of palms and soles	Taken with or without food
Abacavir	(ABC)	Hypersensitivity reaction (can be fatal); fever, rash, nausea, vomiting, malaise or fatigue, and loss of appetite	Taken with or without food

Nucleotide Reverse Transcriptase Inhibitors (NtRTIs)

Mechanism of action is similar to NsRTIs. It undergoes diester hydrolysis to form the Nucleoside monophosphate Tenofovir. Drugs available with their toxicities from this group are tabulated in Table 22.2.

TABLE 22.2: Nucleotide reverse transcriptase inhibitors with their toxicities

Drug	*Abbreviation*	*Toxicity*	*Food restriction*
Tenofovir	(TDF)	Potential for renal toxicity	Taken with or without food

Non-nucleoside Reverse Transcriptase Inhibitors (NNRTIs)

*NNRTIs i*nhibit reverse transcriptase directly by binding to the enzyme and interfering with its function. Drugs available with their toxicities from this group are tabulated in Table 22.3.

TABLE 22.3: Non-nucleoside reverse transcriptase inhibitors with their toxicities			
Drug	*Abbreviation*	*Toxicity*	*Food restriction*
Delavirdine	(DLV)	Skin rash, abnormalities in liver function tests	Taken with or without food
Efavirenz	(EFV)	Rash, dysphoria, elevated liver function tests, drowsiness, abnormal dreams, depression	Taken on empty stomach
Nevirapine	(NVP)	Skin rash, hepatotoxicity	Taken with or without food
Etravirine	(ETR)	Elevation in Liver function tests	Taken following a meal

Protease Inhibitors (PIs)

PIs target viral assembly by inhibiting the activity of protease, an enzyme used by HIV to cleave nascent proteins for final assembly of new virions. Drugs available with their toxicities from this group are tabulated in Table 22.4.

TABLE 22.4: Protease inhibitors with their toxicities			
Drug	*Abbreviation*	*Toxicity*	*Food restriction*
Amprenavir	(APV)	Nausea, vomiting, diarrhea, rash, oral paresthesias, elevated liver function tests, hyperglycemia, fat redistribution, lipid abnormalities	Taken with or without food; avoid high fat meals
Fosamprenavir	(FOS-APV)	Vomiting, elevated liver function tests, hyperglycemia, fat redistribution	Taken with or without food
Atazanavir	(ATV)	Hyperbilirubinemia, PR prolongation, nausea, vomiting, hyperglycemia, fat maldistribution	Taken with food
Darunavir	(DRV)	Diarrhea, nausea, headache	Taken with food
Indinavir	(IDV)	Nephrolithiasis, hyperglycemia, fat redistribution, lipid abnormalities, indirect hyperbilirubinemia	Taken on an empty stomach 60 minutes before or 2 hours after a meal. Avoid taking within an hour of taking Didanosine
Lopinavir/Ritonavir	(LPV/RTV)	Diarrhea, hyperglycemia, fat redistribution, lipid abnormalities	
Nelfinavir	(NFV)	Diarrhea, loose stools, hyperglycemia, fat redistribution, lipid abnormalities	Taken with food
Ritonavir	(RTV)	Nausea, abdominal pain, hyperglycemia, fat redistribution, lipid abnormalities, may alter levels of many other drugs, including saquinavir	Taken with food
Saquinavir	(SQV)	Diarrhea, nausea, headaches, hyper glycemia, fat redistribution, lipid abnormalities	Taken within two hours of food
Tipranavir	(TPV)	Nausea, vomiting, diarrhea, elevation in liver function tests, increased total cholesterol and triglyceride, rash and intracranial hemorrhage	Taken with or without food

Fusion or Entry Inhibitors

It interfere with binding, fusion and entry of HIV to the host cell by blocking one of several targets. Drugs available with their toxicities from this group are tabulated in Table 22.5.

TABLE 22.5: Fusion or entry inhibitors with their toxicities

Drug	*Abbreviation*	*Toxicity*	*Food restriction*
Maraviroc	MVC	Diarrhea, nausea, fatigueness, cough, headache, joints pain, muscle pain, hepatitis	Must be prepared from a powder and injected into thigh, arm or abdomen
Enfuvirtide	T-20	Local injection reactions, hypersensitivity reactions, increased rate of bacterial pneumonia	Taken with or without food

Integrase Inhibitors

It inhibits the enzyme integrase, which is responsible for integration of viral DNA into the DNA of the infected cell. Drugs available with their toxicities from this group are tabulated in Table 22.6.

TABLE 22.6: Integrase inhibitors with their toxicities

Drug	*Abbreviation*	*Toxicity*	*Food restriction*
Raltegravir	(RAL)	Nausea, diarrhea, elevation in amylases, diziness, pruritus and rash	Taken with or without food

Pharmacokinetic Issues in the Treatment of HIV-related Tuberculosis

Two pharmacokinetic issues complicate the treatment of HIV-related tuberculosis. The possibility of malabsorption of antituberculosis drugs, and the complex drug-drug interactions. There are conflicting data on whether patients with HIV-related tuberculosis are more prone to malabsorption of antituberculosis drugs than are HIV-uninfected patients. It appears that serum drug concentrations, particularly of rifampin, are somewhat lower in tuberculosis patients with HIV- infection and very low CD4 cell count.[2]

Interaction between Antiretroviral and Antitubercular Drugs

Treatment of TB in the presence of HIV infection is complicated by drug-drug interactions between the rifamycin class of antimycobacterial drugs (rifampin, rifabutin and rifapentine), and the PI and the NNRTI classes of drugs used to treat HIV infection.[3,4] Both PIs and NNRTIs are metabolized by hepatic CYP3A, specifically the CYP3A4 isozyme. Rifamycins are inducers of the CYP3A family of enzymes, which includes the CYP3A4 isozyme. This will adversely affect the ability of the antiretroviral regimen to adequately suppress the virus, which is the goal of antiretroviral treatment regimen.

Rifamycins and Nucleoside/Nucleotide Analogues

Rifamycins are inducers of the CYP3A system but rifampin is not metabolized by this system. Of the three available rifamycins, rifampin is the most potent inducer of CYP3A and rifabutin is the least potent, with rifapentine falling somewhere in between. Rifapentine should not be used for the treatment of TB in HIV-infected individuals because of the increased rate of acquired rifamycin resistance. Rifabutin has been used extensively in the developed world as a substitute for rifampin in the treatment of active TB, outcomes are similar with rifampin or rifabutin. Rifabutin is metabolized by the CYP3A system and there are significant interactions when rifabutin is coadministered with PIs and NNRTIs. Rifabutin dosing has to be adjusted according to the choice of the coadministered antiretroviral drug.

Rifamycins and Protease Inhibitors

Protease inhibitors (PIs) and the rifamycins have opposite effects on CYP3A family of enzymes in the liver. This causes the following types of drug-drug interactions when PIs are taken together with rifamycins. PI serum concentrations and overall bioavailability may decrease to subtherapeutic levels because rifamycins accelerate the metabolism of PIs by inducing the CYP3 enzymes. Rifampin levels are not affected since it is not metabolized by the CYP3A and Rifabutin bioavailability may increase to toxic levels because PIs decrease its metabolism. Rifampicin causes a 75 to 95% reduction in serum concentrations of PI other than ritonavir. Such reductions lead to loss of antiretroviral activity of PI-containing regimens and consequently can result in the emergence of resistance to one or more of the other drugs in the HAART regimen. Currently, most patients are given combinations of PI, which includes low-dose ritonavir [usually 100 mg per dose] in order to take advantage of its enzyme-inhibiting properties. In effect, ritonavir boosts the concentrations of the other PI allowing easier and more tolerable dosing. Rifabutin can be used with single (unboosted) PI except saquinavir. However, because of the balance between rifabutin induction and protease inhibition of CYP3A4, when this combination is used, a modification in the dose of the PI may be required and the dose of rifabutin should be decreased by half to 150 mg.

Rifamycins and Non-nucleoside Reverse Transcriptase Inhibitors (NNRTIs)

The NNRTIs are all metabolized by the hepatic CYP3A. Therefore, NNRTI levels are adversely affected by the rifamycins. The effect of NNRTIs on the CYP3A is less uniform; delavirdine inhibits the CYP3A, whereas nevirapine and efavirenz induce the CYP3A. Delavirdine should not be used with either rifampin or rifabutin because both rifamycins greatly diminish the levels of delavirdine.

Rifampin modestly decreases the efavirenz activity. Therefore, it is probably safe to use rifampin concomitantly with efavirenz at a slightly higher dose (800 mg of efavirenz instead of the usual 600 mg). Efavirenz effectiveness is not significantly affected by rifabutin, but efavirenz does decrease rifabutin bioavailability. Therefore, the rifabutin dosage must be increased (from the usual dosage of 300 mg to a daily dose of 450–600 mg) when it is given with efavirenz. Bioavailability of nevirapine is reduced by rifampin. Rifabutin decreases bioavailabilty of nevirapine and nevirapine also slightly decreases rifabutin bioavailability. Therefore, nevirapine can be used with rifabutin, both at their usual doses.

Rifamycins and Nucleoside Reverse Transcriptase Inhibitors (NRTIs)

There is a slight decrease in the level of zidovudine and probably abacavir when coadministered with rifampin. The other NRTIs do not interact significantly with rifamycins. Rifamycins can, therefore, be included in the anti-TB regimen if a PI- or NNRTI-sparing antiretroviral regimen is chosen. The fusion inhibitor enfuvirtide is not known to be a substrate for the CYP450 enzymes or to have any effect on the levels of these enzymes and can be used with all anti-TB drugs.

Isoniazid and Antiretroviral Drug Interactions

Pharmacokinetic or clinical interactions between isoniazid and antiretroviral agents have not been extensively studied. In vitro studies have shown that isoniazid, at clinically relevant concentrations, is a reversible inhibitor of CYP3A4 and CYP2C19, and that it mechanistically inactivates CYP1A2, CYP2A6, CYP2C19 AND CYP3A4 in human liver microsomes.[5] Isoniazid, co-administered with drugs such as PI and NNRTI, which are metabolized by these isoforms, may result in significant drug-drug interactions. These interactions might be significant when isoniazid is given alone to treat latent TB infection in an HIV co-infected patient who is receiving PI or NNRTI.

Drug-drug Interactions in the Treatment of HIV and Drug Resistant-TB (DR-TB)

Currently, little is known about drug-drug interactions between second-line anti-tuberculosis agents and antiretroviral therapy. Buffered didanosine contains an aluminium/magnesium-based antacid and, if given jointly with fluoroquinolones, may result in decreased fluoroquinolone absorption; it should be avoided, but if it is necessary, it should be given six hours before or two hours after fluoroquinolone administration. The enteric coated formulation of didanosine can be used concomitantly without this precaution. Ethionamide/protionamide is thought to be metabolized by the CYP450 system, although it is not known which of the CYP enzymes are responsible. Whether doses of ethionamide/protionamide and/or certain antiretroviral drugs should be modified during the concomitant treatment of DR-TB and HIV is completely unknown.[6] Clarithromycin is a substrate and inhibitor of CYP3A and has multiple drug interactions with protease inhibitors and NNRTIs. If possible, the use of clarithromycin should be avoided in patients co-infected with DR-TB and HIV because of both its weak efficacy against DR-TB and multiple drug interactions.

Conclusion

With nonrifamycin containing regimens, drug-drug interactions might be fewer but a nonrifamycin regimen is inferior to a rifampicin-based regimen for the treatment of HIV-related tuberculosis. These should be only contemplated in patients with serious toxicity to rifamycins, where desensitization/reintroduction has failed, or in those with rifamycin-resistant isolates. The various options to reduce drug-drug interactions are: (i) to postpone antiretroviral therapy; (ii) to use no PI or NNRTI containing antiretroviral combinations; (iii) to use certain PIs and/or NNRTIs with modification in doses; (iv) Efavirenz (EFZ) or Saquinavir with Ritonavir, without the need to adjust the doses; and (v) to use nonrifamycin regimens, e.g. 2SHEZ + 10HE.

References

1. TB/HIV Clinical manual; second edition. WHO/HTM/TB/2004.329.
2. Corbett EL, Watt CJ, Walker N, et al. The growing burden of tuberculosis: global trends and interactions with the HIV epidemic. Arch Intern Med. 2003;163:1009-21.
3. UNIADS/WHO. AIDS epidemic update: December 2003. UNAIDS/WHO 2003. http://www.unaids.org/wad/2003/epiupdate2003.
4. Sahai J, Gallicano K, Swick L, Tailor S, Garber G, Seguin I, et al. Reduced plasma concentrations of antituberculous drugs in patients with HIV infection. Ann Intern Med. 1997;127:289-93.
5. Desta Z, Soukhova NV, Flockhart DA. Inhibition of cytochrome P450 (CYP450) by isoniazid: potent inhibition of CYP2C19 and CYP3A. Antimicrob Agents Chemother. 2001;45:382-92.
6. Centers for Disease Control and Prevention (CDC). Managing drug interactions in the treatment of HIV-related tuberculosis [online]. 2007(available at http://www.cdc. Gov /tb/ TB_ HIV_ Drugs /default.htm.

Chapter 23

Multi-drug-resistant and Extensively Drug-resistant Tuberculosis: Prevention

Introduction

Tuberculosis is a very important aspect of medical diseases throughout the world. It occurs worldwide and remains an important cause of morbidity and mortality in many countries. According to WHO, in 2011, there were an estimated 8.7 million new cases of tuberculosis and an estimated 12 million prevalent cases causing death to 1.4 million people. There were an estimated 2.2 million (25% of the total cases) new cases in India and 0.30 million people are dying every year in our country due to tuberculosis. It is a cause for concern as India stands first in terms of absolute number of cases, closely followed by China.[1] It is a real paradox because pathogenesis, transmission, prevention, diagnosis and specific therapy are all well-known for tuberculosis.

Ideally good chemotherapy should achieve 100% sputum conversion if correct regimens are prescribed and taken. There will be hardly any relapse if duration of treatment has been sufficient and there will be no emergence of drug resistance. Every treatment failure should be regarded as a failure by the doctor. He has either prescribed a bad or unreliable regimen or he has failed to ensure that the patient takes the regimen as prescribed.[2–4] Drug-resistant tuberculosis has been reported since the early days of introduction of anti-TB chemotherapy, but multi-drug-resistant tuberculosis (MDR-TB) and, more recently, extensively drug resistant tuberculosis (XDR-TB) has been an area of growing concern, and is posing threat to global efforts of tuberculosis control. Prevalence of Drug-Resistant TB mirrors the functional state and efficacy of tuberculosis control programmes and realistic attitude of the community towards implementation of such programs.[5] Poor TB control generates MDR-TB and the misuse of second-line drugs generates XDR-TB. Drug resistance in our country is due to inadequate tuberculosis control services, less well-trained doctors in modern chemotherapy, widespread inadequate treatment by private practitioner of various systems of medicine and quacks and inadequate management of already drug-resistant tuberculosis.[6–9] Drug-resistant tuberculosis is one of the important reasons of morbidity and mortality in tuberculosis.

The fourth WHO-IUATLD, global drug resistance surveillance carried out in 2002-2007 in 93 settings in 81 countries, reported median prevalence of primary and acquired multi-drug-resistant tuberculosis (MDR-TB) as 2.9% and 15.3% respectively. It is estimated that 440,000 MDR-TB cases emerged in 2008 globally. Data from nine sites in India show that drug resistance among new cases is relatively low. The estimated prevalence of primary and acquired MDR-TB in India is 2.8% and 17.2% respectively. It is estimated that 99,000 MDR-TB cases emerged in India in 2008, representing over 20% of the global burden. In 2006, XDR-TB was reported in all regions of the world and it has become a serious emerging threat to global public health especially in countries with a high prevalence of Human Immunodeficiency Virus (HIV). Combining data from 46 countries, 5.4% of MDR-TB cases were found to have XDR-TB. Eight countries reported XDR-TB in more than 10% of MDR-TB cases; six of these countries were located in Eastern Europe and Central Asia. To date, a cumulative total of 84 countries have confirmed at least one case of XDR-TB.[10,11] Although isolated reports, both published and unpublished, indicate the existence of XDR-TB in India, it is not possible as yet to estimate its magnitude and distribution from the available data. According to the data reported on XDR-TB from India, it varied from 1.5% to 11% of MDR-TB cases.[12-14] XDR-TB has raised the possibility that the current drug-susceptible TB will be replaced with a form of TB with severely restricted treatment options. This would halt the progress made in recent years to control TB globally. Thus, it is evident that MDR-TB and XDR-TB is a manmade problem and its emergence can be prevented. Management of MDR-TB and XDR-TB is more difficult, complicated, challenging and more costlier and so the saying "Prevention is better than cure" holds strength here. The present write-up gives an overview for the prevention of MDR-TB and XDR-TB.

General Guidelines for the Prevention of MDR and XDR-TB

1. No single drug therapy. Drug resistance usually follows and is permanent. Never add a single drug to a failing regimen. If he is getting worse, his bacilli may be resistant to all drugs being used. Adding one drug is the same as giving one drug alone. The patient will soon develop resistance to the new drug also.[15]
2. All the drugs should be administered in single dose preferably, as serum peak concentration of drug has greater and more prolonged inhibitory effect on tubercle bacilli compared to minimum inhibitory concentration (MIC) in the serum following administration of the same dose in two divided doses.[16,17]
3. Use only standard, time-tested drug regimens recommended by various national and international agencies.
4. Use drugs in adequate doses and for adequate duration.
5. Never use unreliable chemotherapy even for a short time.
6. Always prescribe good quality medicines. If you are prescribing fixed dose combinations, make sure that they are of good quality as supported by frequent bioavailability test.[18–20]

7. Be kind and sympathetic to the patient. He is much more likely to come back and complete his treatment if he has confidence in you and believes that you are his well-wisher.
8. Follow up the patient regularly, motivate and make sure that the patient takes full recommended course of treatment for adequate duration, i.e. 6 to 9 months for short course chemotherapy and 1 to 2 years for long-term treatment. If possible, make sure that someone watches the patient taking every dose (directly observed therapy).
9. Always assess adverse effects due to medications and address them quickly and adequately.[21]
10. Use rifampicin only in tuberculosis or leprosy. Avoid misuse of rifampicin as it is one of the most potent antituberculosis drugs available at present. Development of resistance to rifampicin will lead to multi-drug-resistant tuberculosis (MDR-TB).
11. Relapse after good and adequate treatment is rare. If relapse has occurred after good and adequate treatment or after too short duration of regular treatment, such cases can be treated with previously used drug regimens. Five drug (2SHREZ/1HRZE/5HRE) regimens either daily or thrice weekly would be much effective and safe.[15]
12. In the group of previously treated patients with one or several courses of chemotherapy and who remain sputum positive (by smear and/or culture) three subpopulations can be observed: (a) Patients existing bacilli still sensitive to all drugs; (b) Patients existing bacilli resistant to atleast Isoniazid but sensitive to Rifampicin; and (c) Patients bacilli resistant to atleast Isoniazid and Rifampicin. The respective proportion of the three subpopulations varies according to chemotherapy applied in the community and number of courses of chemotherapy and type of regimens received by the patients.In the patients who have failed after the first course of chemotherapy, the proportion of patients existing bacilli sensitive to all drugs is usually higher than the proportion of two other subpopulations. For such patients, WHO retreatment regimens or Category-II regimens of five drugs (2SHRZE/1HRZE/5HRE) or ($2\,S_3H_3R_3E_3Z_3/1H_3R_3E_3Z_3/5H_3R_3E_3$) or even four drugs regimen (HRZE/HRE) under direct supervision can cure majority of patients having either sensitive bacilli or bacilli resistant to Isoniazid and/or Streptomycin but still sensitive to Rifampicin.[15,22]
13. In patients who have failed after several courses of previous treatment perhaps with bad or unreliable drug regimens or after two or more courses of chemotherapy under National Tuberculosis Control Programme (last being the fully supervised standard WHO retreatment regimen of five drugs), the proportion of patients with MDR-TB can be as much as 50 to 70%. Treatment of such patients requires expertise and must be carried out under a specialist/specialized center as planning of treatment is very complex and a mistake at this stage can be fatal.[22–24]
14. Early suspicion, diagnosis and appropriate treatment of MDR-TB is essential to prevent morbidity, mortality and transmission of MDR-TB. Under RNTCP, an MDR suspect refers to any patient who fails a Category

I or III treatment regimen or any Category II patient who remains smear positive at the end of the fourth month of treatment or later.[25] Ideally every such patient should be subjected to culture and Drug Sensitivity Testing (DST) for *Mycobacterium Tuberculosis* from a quality-accredited laboratory, before starting a retreatment regimen. Subsequently, when the culture and DST report confirms MDR-TB, an appropriate treatment regimen containing atleast four new drugs the patient has not taken previously or to which the bacilli is considered to be sensitive, are given. There are 5 groups of Antituberculosis drugs. Include drugs from group 1-5 in hierarchical order. Use any first line oral agent such as pyrazinamide (Z), ethambutol (E), rifabutin (Rfb) (Group-1) to which isolate is sensitive, use one injectable—kanamycin (Km), capreomycin (Cm), amikacin (Am) (Group-2), one fluroquinolone-levofloxacin (Lfx), moxifloxacin (Mfx), ofloxacin (Ofx) (Group-3) and add as many second-line bacteriostatic agents—ethionamide (Eto), protionamide (Pto), cycloserine (Cs), terizidone (Trd) and para-aminosalicylic acid (PAS) (Group-4) to make up atleast four effective drugs. Group-5 drugs such as clofazimine (Cfz), linezolid (Lzd), amoxicillin/clavulanate (Amx/Clv), thiacetazone (Thz), imipenem/cilastatin (Ipm/Cln), High-dose Isoniazid (High dose-H) and Clarithromycin (Clr) are not recommended for routine use except where an adequate regimen is impossible with Group 1-4. In standardized treatment, Drug Resistance Surveillance (DRS) data from representative patient populations are used to base regimen design in the absence of individual DST. All patients in a defined group or category receive the same regimen. This type of treatment regimen is followed in resource-poor, low-income nations like India. The Government of India has thereby introduced the DOTS Plus/Category IV as standardized treatment for MDR-TB patients which consists of 6 to 9 months of intensive phase comprising of Kanamycin, Levofloxacin, ethionamide, cycloserine, pyrazinamide and ethambutol followed by 18 months of continuation phase comprising of Levofloxacin, Ethionamide, cycloserine and ethambutol. Para-aminosalicylic acid (PAS) is included in the regimen as a substitute drug if any bactericidal drug (kanamycin, levofloxacin, ethionamide and pyrazinamide) or two bacteriostatic drugs (ethambutol and cycloserine) are not tolerated. Till DOTS-Plus gets introduced in the whole country, all care providers must use proper and appropriate regimens in MDR-TB.

15. Avoid widespread misuse of second-line anti-tuberculosis drugs (SLDs) like ethionamide/prothionamide, cycloserine, PAS, kanamycin/capreomycin, flouroquinolones (levofloxacin, ofloxacin, moxifloxacin), clofazimine, macrolides, etc. in suspected resistant cases if you are not well trained to manage such cases as these are the only drugs available at present which have some hope of cure. Inappropriately using these valuable drugs might convert a MDR-TB case into extensively drug-resistant tuberculosis (XDR-TB). A preliminary study by the author among sixty MDR suspect patients showed 88.8% of MDR and 72.2% MDR suspect cases had taken SLDs for more than one month. The most commonly used SLD was flouroquinolone (63.36%), ethionamide (47.72%) and kanamycin (40.9%).[26]

16. Some physicians (especially engaged in management of drug-resistant cases) feel keeping certain drugs in reserve but this is a serious error. It is a prescription for losing one battle after another. Physicians treating such patient should note that the most powerful drugs available should be used initially and in maximum combination so as to ensure that the first battle is won and won permanently.
17. Treatment of tuberculosis benefits both the community and the patient. Thus, any public/private healthcare provider undertaking to treat a patient with TB is assuming an important public health responsibility that includes not only prescribing an appropriate regimen but also ensuring adherence to the treatment until the treatment is completed. Therefore, the responsibility for successful treatment of TB is placed primarily on the provider of program initiating therapy, rather than on the patient.[27,28] All measures should be taken to ensure adherence by persuading and encouraging such patients and their family members not to stop treatment despite all its discomfort as it is the last thing that stands between the patient and death.[23,24]
18. Delay in recognition of MDR-TB, prolonged periods of infectiousness, crowded wards, and mixing TB and HIV patients, all contribute to nosocomial transmission. However, in view of its seriousness, every program or physician attempting to treat MDR-TB should also undertake a systematic review of current practices and ensure that everything possible is done to prevent transmission among patients and to staff by implementation of adequate infection control precautions.[29]
19. Extrapulmonary drug-resistant tuberculosis is treated with the same strategy and duration as pulmonary drug-resistant tuberculosis. If the patient has symptoms suggestive of central nervous system involvement and is infected with drug-resistant tuberculosis, the regimen should use drugs that have adequate penetration into the central nervous system.[30] Rifampicin, isoniazid, pyrazinamide, protionamide/ethionamide and cycloserine have good penetration into the cerebrospinal fluid (CSF); Kanamycin, amikacin and capreomycin do so only in the presence of meningeal inflammation; PAS and ethambutol have poor or no penetration. The fluoroquinolones have variable CSF penetration, with better penetration seen in the later generations.

Conclusion

In conclusion, the emergence of multi-drug-resistant tuberculosis and extensively drug-resistant tuberculosis is a manmade problem and is always due to medical error. If our tuberculosis control program is effectively implemented, all the doctors can prescribe reliable regimens using reliable drugs and if they can ensure (by directly observed treatment and education of the patient and his family) that it is taken as prescribed, virtually all patients should be cured without any relapse and no drug resistance should occur. Laboratory services for adequate and timely diagnosis of MDR-TB and XDR-TB must be strengthened and programmatic management of MDR-TB and XDR-TB must be scaled up as per the target set by global plan. It must be emphasized that optimal treatment of MDR-TB alone will not curb the epidemic. Efforts must be focused on the effective use of first-line drugs in every new patient so as to prevent the ultimate emergence of multi-drug resistance and extensively drug-resistant tuberculosis. The proper use of second-line drugs in every patient of MDR-TB must be ensured to cure existing multi-drug-resistant tuberculosis, to reduce transmission of MDR-TB and to prevent XDR-TB.

References

1. Global tuberculosis control—surveillance, planning, financing: WHO Report 2012. WHO/HTM/TB/2012.6.
2. Crofton J. The prevention and management of drug-resistant tuberculosis. Bull Int Un Tuberc Lung Dis. 1989;62:6.
3. Crofton J, Horne N, Miller F. Clinical Tuberculosis. Macmillan Education Limited, 1992.
4. Editorial. Multidrug resistance in Tuberculosis. Ind J Tub. 1994;41:1.
5. Prasad R. MDR TB: Current Status (Review article). Ind J Tub. 2005;52:121-31.
6. Mahmoudi A, Iseman MD. Pitfalls in the care of patients with Tuberculosis. JAMA. 1993;270:65.
7. Uplekar MW, Shepard DS. Treatment of Tuberculosis by Private General Practitioners in India. Tubercle. 1991;72:284.
8. Prasad R, Nautiyal RG, Ahuja RC, et al. Treatment of new pulmonary tuberculosis patients: What do allopathic doctors do in India? Int J Tuberc Lung Dis. 2002;6:895-902.
9. Performance in Private Sector in Several Parts of World, International Standards for TB Care. Lancet Infect Dis. 2006;6:710-25.
10. WHO/IUATLD Global Project on Anti-Tuberculosis Drug Resistance Surveillance (2002-2007), Fourth Global Report (2008).
11. World Health Organization. Multidrug and extensively drug-resistant TB (M/XDR-TB): 2010 global report on surveillance and response. WHO/HTM/TB/2010.3.
12. Udwadia Z, Jain S, Rodrigues C, Mehta A. XDR-TB in India: What's in a name? The Lancet Infectious diseases. 2007;7:441-2.
13. Mondal R, Jain A. XDR *Mycobacterium tuberculosis* isolates, India (letter). Emerg Infect Dis 2007. Available from http:/www.cdc.gov/EID/content/13/9/ 1429.htm.
14. Thomas A, Ramachandran R, Rehman F, et al. Management of Multi Drug Resistant Tuberculosis in the field: Tuberculosis Research Centre Experience. Ind J Tuberc. 2007;54:117-24.
15. Caminero JA. Management of multidrug resistant tuberculosis and patients in retreatment. Eur Respir J. 2005;25:928-36.
16. Tuberculosis Research Centre, Indian Council of Medical Research. Low rate of emergence of drug resistance in sputum positive patients treated with short course chemotherapy. Int J Tuberc Lung Dis. 2001;5:40-5.
17. Tuberculosis Chemotherapy Centre, Chennai. A concurrent comparison of INH and PAS with 3 regimens of INH alone in the domiciliary treatment of pulmonary tuberculosis in South India. Bull World Health Organisation.1960;23:535-85.
18. Acocella G. Studies of bioavailability in man. Bull Int Un Tuberc Lung Dis. 1989; 64:40.
19. Editorial. Multidrug formulations. Ind J Tub. 1988;35:161.
20. Good manufacturing practices for pharmaceutical products. WHO Expert Committee on Specifications for Pharmaceutical Preparations. Thirty-second report. Geneva,World Health Organization,1992 (WHO Technical Report Series, No..823), Annex 1.

21. Guidelines for the programmatic management of drug-resistant tuberculosis—WHO 2008, 2011.
22. Mitchison DA, Nunn AJ. Influence of initial drug resistance on the response to short course chemotherapy of Pulmonary Tuberculosis. Am Rev Respir Dis. 1986;133:423.
23. Iseman MD, Madsen LA. Treatment of multidrug resistant tub. N Engl J Med. 1993;329:784.
24. Crofton J, Chaulet P, Maher D. Guidelines for the management of drug resistant tuberculosis. WHO Global Tuberculosis Programme, Geneva 1997. W.H.O./TB/96, 210.
25. DOTS-PLUS guidelines, Revised National Tuberculosis Control Programme, Central TB Division Directorate General Health Services, Ministry of Health & Family Welfare, Nirman Bhawan, New Delhi. Sep. 2008, 2012.
26. Anand SC, Prasad R, Garg R, et al. Observational study to assess the use of second line drugs in patients with tuberculosis. Poster session presented at National Conference on Pulmonary Diseases (NAPCON 2008) at Lucknow on 6–9 November, 2008.
27. Centers for Disease Control and Prevention. Treatment of tuberculosis: American Thoracic Society, CDC and Infectious Diseases Society of America. MMWR Morb Mortal Wkly Rep. 2003;52(RR-11):44.
28. Treatment of Tuberculosis. Guidelines for National Programmes. World Health Organisation, Geneva. 1993, 1997, 2003, 2009.
29. Basu S, et al. Prevention of nosocomial transmission of extensively drug resistant tuberculosis in rural South African district hospitals: an epidemiological modelling study. Lancet. 2007;370:1500-7.
30. Holdiness MR. Cerebrospinal fluid pharmokinetics of antituberculosis drugs. Clinical Pharmacokinetics. 1985;10:532-4.

Chapter 24

Drug-resistant Tuberculosis in Children

Introduction

Emergence of drug-resistant tuberculosis is one of the major challenges faced by health community globally. Drug-resistant tuberculosis is an important cause of morbidity and mortality among children but still very scarce information is available. Despite limited data and difficulties in management, drug-resistant tuberculosis can be successfully treated even in resource poor-settings with proper use of existing technologies. A high index of suspicion and early drug susceptibility testing is the key to early diagnosis and good treatment outcome. Difficulties in establishing the diagnosis, drug toxicities and absence of pediatric formulations add challenges to the management of pediatric MDR-TB cases. Therefore, the current chapter aims at defining epidemiology, diagnosis and treatment of drug-resistant tuberculosis in children.

Epidemiology

Information about MDR-TB in children is scarce. It has been reported that Africa, together with the Americas and western and central Europe, reported the lowest prevalence of multi-drug-resistant tuberculosis (MDR-TB).[1] However, sub-Saharan Africa has a high TB incidence and the highest human immunodeficiency virus (HIV) prevalence in the world and because of the high number of TB cases, Africa still presents 14% of the global burden of new MDR-TB cases. Resistance patterns in children have generally been found to be similar to those of adults from the same areas and similar backgrounds.[2,3] A prospective study in the Western Cape province of South Africa evaluated 149 children in contact with 80 adult MDR pulmonary TB cases and revealed that most of the children in contact with adults having MDR-TB are likely to be infected by these MDR source cases.[4] In a report of 306 children under-five, the incidence of Isoniazid (H) resistance was 5.6% and MDR 1%. Clinical features were similar in children with drug-susceptible and drug-resistant TB.[5] In India, the prevalence of resistance to any drug was 32.4%, while that of multi-drug resistance was 13.3% during 1994-1997.[6] Drug-resistance surveillance in childhood TB in South Africa between 2003 and 2005 had shown a similar rate of MDR-TB but a significant increase in Isoniazid resistance, from 6.9% to 12.8%, which reflected the ongoing transmission of drug-resistant TB.[7] In the last two decades, drug-resistant tuberculosis has increased gradually with emergence of MDR-TB and XDR-TB. The rate of drug resistance to any drug varied from 20% to 80% in different geographic regions.[8] Drug-resistant tuberculosis exists in India, mainly due to poor treatment adherence by the patient and poor management by physicians. Initial drug resistance to isoniazid is reported to be in the range of 10% to 15% and for rifampicin, the range is 2% to 3%.[9] These rates are much higher in patients who have taken prior, irregular treatment. A child with TB was recently shown to be as likely as an adult with TB to have MDR-TB.[10] Thus the prevalence estimates of MDR-TB in children may be derived from total MDR prevalence considering that childhood TB represents at least 10–20% of the total cases in areas with poor epidemic control.

Considering a global prevalence of MDR-TB cases of 450,000,[11] calculated estimated 60,000 pediatric cases of MDR-TB arise per year globally. Similarly, XDR-TB represents 9.0% (6.7%–11.2%) of MDR-TB, thus the calculated estimate of 5000 pediatric cases of XDR TB/year. The corresponding estimates for India regarding pediatric MDR cases are 15000 and XDR cases are 1500 per year.

Pathogenesis

Childhood TB is usually paucibacillary, making the acquisition of drug resistance in previously treated patients less likely, since the chance of developing resistance is proportional to the mycobacterial load.[12,13] Instead, the presence of drug-resistant TB in children most likely reflects transmission of a resistant strain from an adult source case with whom the child had contact. The incidence of TB in children can be used as a marker of successful functioning of the TB control program, as child TB cases represent ongoing transmission within the community. Studies have confirmed transmission of MDR-TB from adult source cases to child contacts using both drug-susceptibility profiles and restriction fragment length polymorphism (RFLP) strain typing.[7] Furthermore, rates of infection in household contacts of MDR-TB cases may be high compared to drug-sensitive cases due to poor treatment response that prolongs duration of infectivity. Because of the paucibacillary nature of the disease and difficulties in getting sputum from young children, childhood pulmonary TB is frequently smear- or culture-negative, and bacteriological confirmation of MDR-TB is often not possible. Outcomes of MDR-TB are generally good if diagnosed early, but with delayed diagnosis, particularly if there is disseminated disease, outcome is often poor.[14,15] A mutation in the 81-base pair region of the rpoB gene is responsible for 97% of rifampicin-resistant strains. Mutations in katG and inhA gene account for majority of the isoniazid-resistant strains. Other genes in which mutation for INH can occur are ahpC and KasA. InhA mutations usually confer resistance to ethionamide. Mutations in rpsi and rrs genes are responsible for streptomycin resistance; mutation in embB gene is responsible for ethambutol resistance and pncA gene for pyrazinamide resistance.[16-18]

Diagnosis of DR-TB in Children

DR-TB in children is usually transmitted from close contact with adult pulmonary DR-TB source cases, although some older children with cavitary pulmonary disease may acquire DR-TB through poor treatment management.[19] The diagnosis of DR-TB in children is either confirmed or presumed.[20] Confirmed disease occurs when Mycobacterium tuberculosis is isolated from child with phenotypic or genotypic resistance. The children with TB often have a negative culture because of the paucibacillary nature of primary TB. In studies of children with clinical evidence of disease with MDR-TB, the proportion of culture-confirmed cases is usually only around 25%.[14,15,21-23] This indicates that a significant proportion of children treated for DR-TB should be presumptively diagnosed. A presumptive diagnosis of DR-TB can be made on clinical symptoms or signs of TB and radiology, in combination with risk factors for drug resistance, such as contact with a confirmed or presumed DR-TB source or the failure to respond to a first-line regimen. The definition of failure in children is challenging and includes persistent microbiological positivity, nonresolving symptoms or signs of TB, persistent or deteriorating radiology, and poor weight gain or weight loss. With effective therapy a child should show improvement by two months.[20]

Children with presumed DR-TB should be started on effective therapy as soon as possible to avoid progression to severe disease, worse clinical outcome, and ongoing transmission. However, empiric therapy for DR-TB may needlessly expose child to toxic medications. Extensive efforts should, therefore, be made to confirm the diagnosis with intensive sampling from the child. Dependent on age of the child and healthcare resources, attempts can be made to obtain sputum samples, gastric aspirates, induced sputum samples, biologic fluid samples, nasopharyngeal aspirates, lymph node aspiration biopsy, or tissue biopsy.[24-26] With extensive sampling, the proportion of children with a confirmed diagnosis can rise to greater than 50%.[27] Invasive methods, such as bronchoalveolar lavage, bronchoscopic biopsy, or open lung biopsy, may be in the child's best interest if a confirmed diagnosis can be made.[28] All isolates confirmed as resistant to rifampin should be sent for full second-line DST assessment. In addition, if rifampin and/or isoniazid resistance is determined by a rapid molecular test, the results should be confirmed by phenotypic testing.

Treatmentof DR-TB in Children

Designing an Effective Regimen for MDR-TB in Children

The drugs used in the treatment of DR-TB have been grouped into five groups as tabulated in Table 24.1.[29] The dosages of various drugs as per weight are elaborated in Table 24.2

As in adults, the decision regarding which drugs to include in a DR-TB treatment regimen, should be guided by the DST of the child's isolate. If this is not available, regimen composition should be guided by the DST pattern of the presumed source case. If DR-TB treatment is given for failure of a first-line regimen, the child should be assumed to have TB that is resistant to rifampin

TABLE 24.1: Drugs used to treat drug resistant tuberculosis in children

Group	*Group Name*	*Drugs*	*Dosage (mg/kg)*	*Adverse Drug Reactions*
1	First-line oral agents	Rifabutin	5	Rash, discoloration of body fluids, neutropenia
		Ethambutol	15–25 (DR-TB: 20–25)	Neuropathy (optic neuritis)
		Pyrazinamide	30–40	Nausea, vomiting, hepatotoxicity
2	Injectable agents	Kanamycin	15–30	Renal, auditory, and vestibular toxicities
		Amikacin	15–22.5	
		Capreomycin	15–30	
3	Fluoroquinolones	Ofloxacin	15–20	Gastrointestinal symptoms, insomnia, dizziness, Q-T interval prolongation, tendon rupture
		Levofloxacin	7.5–10	
		Moxifloxacin	7.5–10	
4	Oral bacteriostatic second-line agents	Ethionamide	15–20	Gastrointestinal intolerance, peripheral neuropathy, psychiatric disturbances
		Prothionamide	15–20	Gastrointestinal intolerance, peripheral neuropathy, psychiatric disturbances
		Cycloserine	15–20	Peripheral neuropathy, central nervous system dysfunction
		Terizidone	15–20	Neurologic and psychiatric disturbances
		P-aminosalicylic acid	150	Gastrointestinal intolerance
5	Agents with unclear efficacy	Clofazimine	3–5	Gastrointestinal intolerance, skin pigmentation
		Linezolid	10	Myelosuppression, peripheral neuropathy
		Amoxicillin-clavulanic acid	10–15	Diarrhea, rash
		Imipenem/cilastatin	500–1000/6 h	Seizures
		Thiacetazone	2.5	Cutaneous hypersensitivity
		High dose isoniazid	15–20	Hepatotoxicity, peripheral neuropathy
		Clarithromycin	7.5–15	Gastrointestinal intolerance, Q-T interval prolongation

TABLE 24.2 Drug dosages for DR-TB cases according to the weight in children

	Isoniazid	*Pyrazinamide*	*Ethambutol*	*Levofloxacin*	*Moxifloxacin*	*Terizidone*	*Ethionamide*	*PAS*
Dosing range, mg/kg	15–20	30–40	20–25	7.5–10	7.5–10	15–20	15–20	150
Weight, kg								
3–4.9	50	125	100	31.5	40	62.5	62.5	500
5–6.9	100	250	100	62.5	60	125	125	1000
7–9.9	150	250	200	125	80	187.5	187.5	1500
10–13.9	200	500	300	125	100	250	250	2000
14–19.9	300	500	400	187.5	200	375	375	3000
20–29.9	400	750	600	250	200	500	500	4000
30–39.9	400	1000	800	312.5	300	625	625	6000
>40	400	1500	1200	375	400	750	750	8000

and isoniazid. In cases with confirmed MDR-TB, there is no role for rifampicin. However, if the child is failing first-line therapy or if there are multiple source cases, it is usually appropriate to include rifampicin to treat potential drug-susceptible organisms.

In regimen designing to treat children with MDR-TB, the target should be to use at least four drugs that are likely to have activity against the infecting organism. Firstly, add any number of first-line drugs to which the organism has not been shown to be resistant. Then add a second-line injectable drug from group 2 and a fluoroquinolone from group 3. Other drugs from group 4 are then added to make an effective regimen of at least 4 new drugs. Finally, agents from group 5 can be added if required to make an effective regimen. Drugs from group 5 are described as having relatively weak or uncertain activity against *M. tuberculosis*. However, clofazimine and linezolid have, in recent adult studies, demonstrated promising efficacy and can be considered useful drug options. Increasing use of linezolid has also been seen in children, but the potential for toxicity must be considered.[29] Novel agent bedaquiline has been recently approved for use in adults in specific circumstances.[30] Other novel agents such as delamanid[31] and PA-824[32] are in advanced stages of clinical trials. However, because no child-friendly formulations have been produced and no pediatric pharmacokinetic studies have been conducted, it will take a number of years before these drugs are available for use in children.

In addition to TB drugs, it is recommended that children with TB should be given pyridoxine if they are HIV-infected, malnourished, breastfed, or are being given cycloserine, terizidone or high-dose isoniazid because pyridoxine deficiency is common. Steroids have been demonstrated to improve outcome in children with TBM[33-35] and are additionally advised for airway obstruction and pericardial TB.[36] Nutritional and metabolic requirements should be assessed because these children are commonly malnourished[21,22] and have often been in a catabolic state before the diagnosis of DR-TB.

Other Adjunctive Treatments

In cases of intrathoracic lymph node disease in children, with external pressure on the airways leading to compression and respiratory compromise, assessment by bronchoscopy is advised. In cases of extensive resistance, where the disease is localized to one anatomical lobe or part of the lung, surgical resection may still have a place. If there are extensive destruction and fibrosis, it may be difficult for some drugs to penetrate into lesions with poor vascularization. Enucleation of the nodes may be required bronchoscopically or surgically to relieve the pressure on the airway and debulk the lymph node lesion.[37,38] In children, some conditions, such as draining of pericardial effusion and insertion of ventriculoperitoneal shunt for noncommunicating hydrocephalus, need surgery as for drug-susceptible TB cases. In children, treatment of MDR and XDR-TB patients is often initially administered in hospitals, due to extensive disease or because of daily administration of injections to children. Poor adherence to treatment by the source case, often the mother or caregiver, raises doubts as to whether the child will be taken for treatment. In some places, children are admitted for the duration of treatment with second-line injectable drugs and, if social circumstances and the clinical condition of the child permit, the rest of the treatment is given in ambulatory basis, preferably under supervision. However, in a study from Peru, the majority of the children managed for MDR-TB were not admitted to the hospital but were treated in the community by DOT.[39]

Treatment Duration for MDR-TB in Children

The decision on number of drugs and duration of therapy is dependent on the extent of disease and the degree of drug resistance as well as penetration to different body sites and treatment response. For children with cavitary or widespread disease with resistance to only rifampin and isoniazid, treatment is usually given for 18 months from the time of sampling of the first negative culture. WHO has recommended that adults should be given injectable drugs for 8 months because longer durations are associated with better outcomes[29] but for most children, 4 to 6 months of treatment are likely to be sufficient except for those with extensive disease.[40] For children with limited, paucibacillary disease like isolated intra- or extra-thoracic lymph node involvement and with susceptibility to the second-line drugs, it is likely that the child can be treated for 12 to 15 months in total, although evidence for such shorter regimens is lacking.

There is limited available evidence for the management of TB in children caused by isolates resistant to isoniazid alone. A single study of children with isoniazid mono-resistant TB describes good treatment outcomes using three to four drugs.[41] Guidelines for children suggest treatment for 6 to 12 months with rifampin, pyrazinamide and ethambutol.[42] In cases of extensive disease or for tuberculous meningitis(TBM), a fluoroquinolone and one other drug can be added. If genotypic tests are used to perform DST, most national programs advise treating Rifampicin monoresistance -TB in adults and children with an MDR-TB regimen because these tests do not identify all the mutations conferring isoniazid resistance.[43]

XDR-TB in Children

Children with XDR-TB generally have primary resistance transmitted from an index case with XDR-TB. When DST is available, it should be used to guide therapy, although children with paucibacillary TB are often culture negative. Nevertheless, every effort should be made to confirm XDR-TB bacteriologically by the use of DST and to avoid exposing children unnecessarily to toxic drugs. In designing regimen for XDR-TB in children include drugs from group 1–5 in hierarchical order. Use any first line oral agent to which isolate is sensitive, use one injectable (Group-2), to which strain is susceptible (preferably capreomycin), use one later generation flouroquinolone, preferably moxifloxacin (Group-3), add as many as Group-4 agents which have not been used extensively and use 2 or more drugs from Group-5.The injectables should be used for extended duration, minimum of 12 months or possibly whole of treatment duration. The treatment is to be given for at least 24 to 30 months. The government of India has decided a standardized treatment for the management of XDR-TB patients. The regimen consists of 7 drugs, with 2 reserve/substitute drugs. The dosages of the drugs vary as per the weight of the patient. All drugs are to be given once daily except amoxicillin-clavulanic acid, linezolid and clarithromycin (usually given twice daily) preferably under supervision. Injections of Capreomycin are to be given 6 days/week. The details of the drugs and dosages with their adverse reactions are tabulated in Table 24.3.

Treatment regimen of XDR-TB would be of 24–30 months' duration, with 6–12 months' Intensive Phase (IP) and 18 months' Continuation Phase (CP). The intensive phase will consist of capreomycin, PAS, moxifloxacin, high-dose INH, clofazamine, linezolid and amoxycillin/clavulanate, while the continuation phase will consist of PAS, moxifloxacin, high-dose INH, clofazamine, linezolid, and amoxycillin/clavulanate. Reserve/substitute drugs would be clarithromycin and Thiacetazone. The reserve/substitute drugs should be used if the patient was on PAS during his MDR-TB treatment, or he is unable to tolerate one or more of the drugs or if he is found to be resistant to Capreomycin. The change from IP to CP will be done only after achievement of culture conversion, i.e. two consecutive negative cultures taken atleast one month apart. In case of delay in culture conversion, the IP will be extended from 6 months up to a maximum of 12 months in case of extension. Capreomycin injection can be given intermittently (3 times/week) for 7–12 months. Treatment of XDR-TB is usually with less effective drugs and in reported studies in children with XDR-TB, more number of drugs have been used and treatment has been continued for atleast 24 months.[6,22]

TABLE 24.3: Dosages and adverse drug reactions of drugs used in XDR-TB in children

Drugs	*Daily Dosing (mg/kg)*	*Adverse drug reactions*
Capreomycin (Cm)	15–30	Renal, auditory and vestibular toxicities
Na PAS	150	Gastrointestinal intolerance
Moxifloxacin (Mfx)	7.5–10	Gastrointestinal symptoms, insomnia, dizziness, Q-T interval prolongation, tendon rupture
High-dose INH (High-dose H)	15–20	Hepatotoxicity, peripheral neuropathy
Clofazimine (Cfz)	4–5	Gastrointestinal intolerance, skin pigmentation
Linezolid (Lzd)	10	Myelosuppression, peripheral neuropathy
Amoxyclav (Amx/Clv)	10–15	Diarrhea, rash
Clarithromycin (Clr)	7.5–15	Gastrointestinal intolerance, Q-T interval prolongation
Thiacetazone (Thz)	2–3	Cutaneous hypersensitivity

Management of Comorbid Conditions

Comorbid medical conditions like HIV infection, diabetes and malnutrition can increase the risk of TB in children and affect treatment outcomes. All children diagnosed with TB, whether DR or not, should be offered testing for HIV infection. The cotreatment of pediatric TB and HIV infection is complicated by practical problems including the timing of initiation of ART, Immune Reconstitution Inflammatory Syndrome (IRIS), drug-drug interactions and overlapping toxicities of ART and TB therapy. As in adults, it is recommended to start ART as early as possible after start of ATT and preferably within 2 weeks of initiating TB therapy. Differentiating IRIS from treatment failure can be challenging but decreasing HIV viral load and improving CD4 count is suggestive of IRIS. ATT, specifically rifampin, ethionamide, PAS and fluoroquinolones can disrupt glycemic control and can thus worsen the blood glucose control in diabetes. Thus, more frequent blood glucose monitoring is required.

Treatment Monitoring

Response to therapy includes clinical, microbiological and radiological monitoring. For children with pulmonary disease and ability to expectorate the schedule for sputum monitoring as in adults is followed. Additionally height and weight should be monitored periodically. Regular monitoring with chest radiograph is advised for children with pulmonary disease. In a recent review, it was found that almost 82% of children on MDR-TB treatment achieved treatment success while default and death were reported in 6% each.[40] It is more difficult to assess adverse effects in children than in adults. Child should be monitored frequently for renal, thyroid, auditory, and visual adverse events. In children treated with MDR regimens, toxicity may occur in up to 40% of cases. However, significant toxicity necessitating treatment modification is less common.

References

1. Schaaf HS, Moll AP, Dheda K. Multidrug- and Extensively Drug-resistant Tuberculosis in Africa and South America: Epidemiology, Diagnosis and Management in Adults and Children. Clinics in Chest Medicine 2009;30:667-83.
2. Steiner P, Rao M. Drug-resistant tuberculosis in children. Sem Pediatr Infect Dis. 1993;4:275-82.
3. Dupon M, Texier-Maugein J, Leroy V, et al. Tuberculosis and HIV infection: a cohort study of incidence and susceptibility to antituberculous drugs, Bordeaux, 1985–1993. AIDS. 1995;9:577-83.
4. Schaaf HS, Van Rie A, Gie RP, Beyers N, Victor TC, Van Helden PD, et al. Transmission of multidrug-resistant tuberculosis. Pediatr Infect Dis J. 2000;19:695-99.
5. Schaaf HS, Gie RP, Beyers N, Sirgel FA, de Klerk PJ, Donald PR. Primary drug-resistant tuberculosis in children. Int J Tuberc Lung Dis. 2000;4:1149-55.
6. Swaminathan S. Tuberculosis in HIV-infected children. Paediatr Respir Rev. 2004;5:225-30.

7. Schaaf HS, Marias BJ, Hesseling AC, Gie RP, Beyers N, Donald PR. Childhood drug resistant tuberculosis in the western Cape province of South Africa. Acta Paediatr. 2006;95:523-28.
8. Mukherjee A, Lodha R, Kabra SK. Changing Trends in Childhood Tuberculosis. Indian J Peds. 2010;78:328-33.
9. Swaminathan S. Management of pediatric tuberculosis; In, Tuberculosis control of India, Directorate General of Health Services/Ministry of Health and Family Welfare Nirman Bhawan, Maulana Azad Road, New Delhi. Elsevier Edition 2005:116-23. Accessed from www.tbcindia.org.
10. Zignol M, Sismanidis C, Falzon D, Glaziou P, Dara M, Floyd K. Multidrug-resistant tuberculosis in children: evidence from global surveillance. Eur Respir J. 2013;42:701-07.
11. World Health Organization. Global tuberculosis report 2013. WHO/HTM/TB/2013.11.
12. Schaaf HS. Drug-resistant tuberculosis in children. S Afr Med J. 2007;97:s995-7.
13. Marais BJ, Gie RP, Schaaf HS, Beyers N, Donald PR, Starke JR. Childhood pulmonary tuberculosis: old wisdom, new challenges. Am J Respir Crit Care Med. 2006;173:1078-90.
14. Schaaf HS, Shean K, Donald PR. Culture-confirmed multidrug-resistant tuberculosis: diagnostic delay, clinical features and outcome. Arch Dis Child. 2003;88:1106-11.
15. Padayatchi N, Bamber S, Halima D, Razia B. Multi-drug resistant tuberculosis in children in Durban, South Africa. Pediatr Infect Dis J. 2006;25:147-50.
16. Laurenzo D, Mousa SA. Mechanisms of drug resistance in Mycobacterium tuberculosis and current status of rapid molecular diagnostic testing. Acta Trop. 2011;119:5-10.
17. Vadwai V, Shetty A, Rodrigues C. Multiplex allele specific PCR for rapid detection of extensively drug resistant tuberculosis. Tuberculosis (Edinb). 2012;92:236-42.
18. Ling DI, Zwerling AA, Pai M. GenoType MTBDR assays for the diagnosis of multidrug-resistant tuberculosis: a meta-analysis. Eur Respir J. 2008;32:1165-74.
19. Schaaf HS, Marais BJ, Hesseling AC, Brittle W, Donald PR. Surveillance of antituberculosis drug resistance amongst children from the Western Cape Province of South Africa—an upward trend. Am J Public Health. 2009;99:1486-90.
20. Seddon JA, Furin JJ, Gale M, Castillo BH, Hurtado RM, Amanullah F, Ford N, Starke JR, Schaaf HS. Caring for children with drug-resistant tuberculosis: practice-based recommendations. Am J Respir Crit Care Med. 2012;186:953-64.
21. Fairlie L, Beylis NC, Reubenson G, Moore DP, Madhi SA. High prevalence of childhood multi-drug resistant tuberculosis in Johannesburg, South Africa: a cross-sectional study. BMC Infect Dis. 2011;11:28.
22. Seddon JA, Hesseling AC, Willemse M, Donald PR, Schaaf HS. Culture-confirmed multidrug-resistant tuberculosis in children: clinical features, treatment and outcome. Clin Infect Dis. 2012;54:157-66.
23. Schluger NW, Lawrence RM, McGuiness G, Park M, Rom WN. Multidrug-resistant tuberculosis in children: two cases and a review of the literature. Pediatr Pulmonol. 1996;21:138-42.
24. Nicol MP, Zar HJ. New specimens and laboratory diagnostics for childhood pulmonary TB: progress and prospects. Paediatr Respir Rev. 2011;12:16-21.
25. Zar HJ, Hanslo D, Apolles P, Swingler G, Hussey G. Induced sputum versus gastric lavage for microbiological confirmation of pulmonary tuberculosis in infants and young children: a prospective study. Lancet. 2005;365:130-34.
26. Zar HJ, Workman L, Isaacs W, Munro J, Black F, Eley B, et al. Rapid molecular diagnosis of pulmonary tuberculosis in children using nasopharyngeal specimens. Clin Infect Dis. 2012;55:1088-95.
27. Marais BJ, Hesseling AC, Gie RP, Schaaf HS, Enarson DA, Beyers N. The bacteriologic yield in children with intrathoracic tuberculosis. Clin Infect Dis. 2006;42:e69-71.

28. Goussard P, Gie RP, Kling S, Nel ED, Louw M, Schubert PT, et al. The diagnostic value and safety of transbronchial needle aspiration biopsy in children with mediastinal lymphadenopathy. Pediatr Pulmonol 2010;45:1173-9.
29. World Health Organization. Guidelines for the programmatic management of drug-resistant tuberculosis update 2011. WHO/HTM/TB/2011.6.
30. World Health Organization. The Use of Bedaquiline in the Treatment of Multidrug-Resistant Tuberculosis: Interim Policy Guidance. Geneva: World Health Organization; 2013. 2, Guidance purpose and target audience. WHO/HTM/TB/2013.6. Available at: http://apps.who.int/iris/bitstream/10665/84879/1/9789241505482_eng.pdf.
31. Gler MT, Skripconoka V, Sanchez-Garavito E, Xiao H, Cabrera-Rivero JL, Vargas-Vasquez DE, et al. Delamanid for multidrug-resistant pulmonary tuberculosis. N Engl J Med. 2012;366:2151-60.
32. Diacon AH, Dawson R, du Bois J, Narunsky K, Venter A, Donald PR, et al. Phase II dose-ranging trial of the early bactericidal activity of PA-824. Antimicrob Agents Chemother. 2012;56:3027-31.
33. Thwaites G, Fisher M, Hemingway C, Scott G, Solomon T, Innes J. British infection society guidelines for the diagnosis and treatment of tuberculosis of the central nervous system in adults and children. J Infect. 2009;59:167-87.
34. Prasad K, Singh MB. Corticosteroids for managing tuberculous meningitis. Cochrane Database Syst Rev. 2008;CD002244.
35. Schoeman F, Van Zyl LE, Laubscher JA, Donald PR. Effect of corticosteroids on intracranial pressure, computed tomographic findings, and clinical outcome in young children with tuberculous meningitis. Pediatrics. 1997;99:226-31.
36. American Academy of Pediatrics. Tuberculosis. In: Pickering LK, ed. Red book: report of the committee on infectious diseases. 28th ed. Elk Grove Village, IL: American Academy of Pediatrics. 2009;680-01.
37. du Plessis J, Goussard P, Andronikou S, Gie R, George R. Comparing three-dimensional volume-rendered CT images with fibreoptic tracheobronchoscopy in the evaluation of airway compression caused by tuberculous lymphadenopathy in children. Pediatr Radiol. 2009;39:694-02.
38. Maydell A, Goussard P, Andronikou S, Bezuidenhout F, Ackermann C, Gie R. Radiological changes post-lymph node enucleation for airway obstruction in children with pulmonary tuberculosis. Eur J Cardiothorac Surg. 2010;38:478-83.
39. Drobac P, Mukherjee JS, Joseph JK, et al. Community-based therapy for children with multidrug-resistant tuberculosis. Pediatrics. 2006;117:2022-29.
40. Ettehad D, Schaaf HS, Seddon JA, Cooke GS, Ford N. Treatment outcomes for children with multidrug-resistant tuberculosis: a systematic review and meta-analysis. Lancet Infect Dis. 2012;12:449-56.
41. Steiner P, Rao M, Victoria M, Steiner M. Primary isoniazid-resistant tuberculosis in children: clinical features, strain resistance, treatment, and outcome in 26 children treated at Kings' County Medical Center of Brooklyn between the years 1961 and 1972. Am Rev Respir Dis. 1974;110:306-11.
42. Drug-resistant tuberculosis: a survival guide for clinicians, 2nd ed. San Francisco, CA: Curry International Tuberculosis Center. 2008.
43. Hazbon MH, Brimacombe M, Bobadilla del Valle M, Cavatore M, Guerrero MI, Varma-Basil M, et al. Population genetics study of isoniazid resistance mutations and evolution of multidrug-resistant mycobacterium tuberculosis. Antimicrob Agents Chemother. 2006;50:2640-49.

Chapter 25

Tuberculosis Control in India: DOTS-Plus

Introduction

The first WHO-endorsed DOTS-Plus programs began in 2000. For this purpose, the Green Light Committee (GLC) was established to promote access to high-quality second-line drugs for appropriate use in TB control Programs. DOTS-Plus is an integral component of RNTCP to manage MDR-TB, which is to be implemented through program infrastructure of the DOTS program. The strategy is designed to manage MDR-TB and XDR-TB using second-line anti-TB drugs within the DOTS strategy in low- and middle-income countries like India. Therefore, in every DOTS-implementing unit of the country, DOTS would be prioritized above DOTS-Plus with the view that DOTS reduces the emergence of MDR-TB, and, therefore, the need for DOTS Plus over time. The present chapter aims to describe framework of DOTS-PLUS program, now known as programmatic management of drug resistant tuberculosis (PMDT) as an integral component of Revised National Tuberculosis Control Programme to manage MDR-TB and XDR-TB.

Framework

The DOTS-Plus framework for the management of multidrug-resistant TB is organized around the same five components of the DOTS strategy, as the underlying principles are the same.

1. **Sustained political and administrative commitment:** It consists of a well functioning DOTS program, long-term investment of staff and resources, coordination efforts between community, local governments and international agencies and addressing the factors leading to the emergence of MDR-TB.
2. **Diagnosis of MDR-TB through quality-assured culture and drug susceptibility testing:** It should include proper triage of patients for culture and DST testing and management under DOTS-Plus and co-ordination with National and Supra-National Reference Laboratories.

3. **Appropriate treatment strategies that utilize second-line drugs under proper management conditions:** Emphasis given on rational standardized treatment design (evidence-based), treatment is directly observed therapy (DOT) ensuring long-term adherence, monitoring and management of adverse drug reactions and adequate human resources.
4. **Uninterrupted supply of quality-assured anti-TB drugs:**
5. **Recording and reporting system designed for DOTS-Plus programs:** It enables performance monitoring and evaluation of treatment outcome.

Each of these components involves more complex and costly operations than those for controlling drug-sensitive TB. Accurate and timely diagnosis is the backbone of the DOTS-Plus activities. MDR-TB must be diagnosed correctly before commencement of treatment. Quality-assured culture and DST is thus indispensable. Nonviable cultures, culture contamination, and unreliable DST results have major consequences for both individual patients and the TB control program as a whole. Therefore, internal quality control and external quality assurance will be in place, including a link for proficiency testing with a recognized reference laboratory such as one of the RNTCP National Reference laboratories. The program is in the process of establishing a network of state level quality-assured culture and DST laboratories. The RNTCP aims to have one such laboratory, known as the Intermediate Reference Laboratory (IRL), for culture and DST in each large state by 2009–10.[1]

Case Finding Strategy

The prevalence of multi-drug-resistant TB (MDR-TB), defined as resistance to isoniazid and rifampicin with or without resistance to other drugs, is found to be at a low level in most of the regions. Data from studies conducted by TRC (TB research centre), Chennai and NTI (National TB Institute), Bengaluru, have found MDR-TB levels of less than 1% to 3% in new cases and around 12% in retreatment cases.[2,3] According to the WHO/IUATLD fourth global survey, the estimated prevalence of primary and acquired MDR-TB in India was 2.8% (95%CI, 2.3–3.4%) and 17.2% (95%CI, 15.0–19.7%) respectively.[4] According to the global tuberculosis report 2012, the prevalence of MDR-TB in India among notified pulmonary tuberculosis patients is 5.3% (3.6–6.2%). Among new tuberculosis cases, the prevalence of MDR-TB is 2.1% (1.5–2.7%) and is 15% (13–17%) among retreatment cases. The RNTCP DOTS-Plus strategy strives to identify and initiate adequate treatment for MDR-TB in a timely manner for confirmed cases of MDR-TB. Timely identification and prompt initiation of treatment prevent the patient from spreading the disease to others, developing a resistant strain to more drugs, and progressing to chronic state of permanent lung damage. RNTCP has undertaken state representative DRS surveys in order to obtain data for new and retreatment patients, to further inform program planning and drug procurement. At present, RNTCP does not have sufficient quality-assured laboratory capacity to do culture and DST in all patients. Hence, the program will use a strategy that enrols patients with a very high risk of MDR-TB into RNTCP DOTS-Plus activities and treatment with the RNTCP Category IV regimen.

Patients who are defined as an "MDR-TB suspect" should be identified and investigated further for MDR-TB. RNTCP uses a strategy that screens patients with initially a very high risk of MDR-TB using DST. As laboratory and treatment capacity builds, the program will scale up to achieve universal access to quality-assured DST. During scale-up, the criteria for referral of a specimen for DST will by necessity differ among the districts. The graded criteria for suspecting MDR TB are as follows:

MDR Suspect Criteria

Criteria A—

- All failures of new TB cases
- Smear positive previously treated cases who remain smear positive at 4th month onwards
- *All pulmonary TB cases* who are contacts of known MDR-TB cases

Criteria B—*In addition to Criteria A*

- All smear positive previously treated pulmonary TB cases at diagnosis
- All smear positive follow-up result in new or previously treated cases

Criteria C—*In addition to Criteria B*

- All smear negative previously treated pulmonary TB cases at diagnosis
- HIV TB coinfected cases at diagnosis.

Enrolment into DOTS-Plus Program

Once the MO PHI confirms that the patient is an MDR-TB suspect, he/she should arrange for sending two sputa samples, one of which is an early morning sample and the other a "supervised" spot sample, from the patient to the RNTCP-certified C-DST laboratory along with the RNTCP Culture and DST request form. All attempts must be made to communicate the DST results to the district as soon as available, so that patient treatment decisions can be smoothly managed.

If results may be delayed more than 7 days of sample collection, the patient should be initiated on RNTCP DOTS treatment till the results are available. Such patients are classified according to the following definition:

Confirmed MDR-TB Case

An MDR-TB suspect who is sputum culture positive and whose TB is due to *Mycobacterium tuberculosis* that are resistant *in-vitro* to at least isoniazid and rifampicin (the culture and DST result being from an RNTCP-accredited laboratory).[1] Internal quality control and external quality assurance of the laboratory are required. Mishandling of a specimen or cross-contamination in the laboratory can result in erroneous reports. It is to be noted that rifampicin resistance is quite rare without isoniazid resistance. The great majority of DST results with rifampicin resistance will also be isoniazid resistance, i.e. MDR-TB. Therefore, RNTCP has taken the programmatic decision that patients who have any Rifampicin resistance, should also be managed as if they are an MDR-TB case, even if they do not formally qualify as an MDR-TB case. Therefore, program and clinical actions will be driven primarily by rifampicin DST results. Once a patient has been confirmed as having MDR-TB, his Category II treatment will be stopped and he/she will be placed on an RNTCP Category IV treatment regimen after pretreatment evaluation. These patients will have to be given a treatment outcome under Category II. The treatment outcome will depend on the duration of Category II treatment completed at the time of confirmation as MDR-TB cases. The outcome will be "Failure" if the patient has completed more than 5 months of Category II treatment or "Switched to Category IV" if the patient has completed less than 5 months of Category II treatment.[5] However, some patients may have other outcomes, e.g. died on Category II treatment or defaulted from Category II treatment prior to culture and DST result being available. After the referral or transportation of sputa samples of an MDR-TB suspect to the RNTCP-certified laboratory, the results of the smear, culture and DST/LPA are entered in the Culture and DST Register held at the laboratory. The culture results are communicated to the DTO immediately by e-mail. In case the culture result is positive, this would be followed by the DST result when available. If the patient is confirmed as a case of MDR-TB, the culture and DST or LPA results are also communicated to the respective DRTB Centre. If the culture result shows contamination, the same is informed to the DTO within 24 hours and he/she should arrange to send a repeat sample (one early morning and one spot) to the laboratory within 3 days. If Rifampicin resistance—with or without INH resistance—is confirmed, the DTO will trace the patient, with help of the Medical Officer—TB control (MO-TC) and Senior Treatment Supervisor (STS) and bring them to the DTC, where they will be counseled by the DTO. After counseling, the patient is referred to the concerned DR-TB Center with their DST result and PMDT referral treatment form, for pre-treatment evaluation and initiation of regimen for MDR-TB.

Drug-Resistant TB Center

Treatment is decentralized, but the complicated clinical care needs require a clinical expert resource center. This is the drug-resistant TB center (DR-TB Center). These DR-TB Centers are utilized to initiate treatment, follow-up case management, and manage complications. One DR-TB Center is expected per 10 million populations roughly, and these sites are being scaled up nationwide in a phased manner. Once confirmed, the MDR-TB patient is referred to the DR-TB Center, with their DST result and request for MDR-TB treatment form. The DR-TB Center Committee will review the patient's details, including previous history, DST result and concurrent illnesses, and make a decision in relation to treatment under RNTCP with a Category IV regimen. If the Committee decides on treatment with an RNTCP Category IV regimen, the patient is initially admitted at the designated DR-TB Center, counseled in regard to their treatment, their treatment card is opened and treatment initiated. If the patient is able to tolerate the Category IV drugs, he/she can be discharged one week post-treatment initiation. In case a patient refuses for hospitalization, all efforts should be made to convince him/her. However, if despite all efforts, the patient is still unwilling for hospitalization, treatment should not be denied and alternative local arrangements should be made for pretreatment evaluation and initiation of treatment. The patient and/or the results of the pretreatment evaluation done at the district level are sent to the DR-TB Center Committee. The committee after reviewing the results will decide on starting Category IV treatment. The decision is communicated to the DTO (District TB Officer) who initiates the treatment with the first dose administered at the DTC (District TB Center). DTO will open the treatment card and send a copy of the same to the DR-TB Center for registration. On registration, the DR-TB Center will convey the DOTS-Plus TB number to the DTO. Once the DR-TB Center decides upon RNTCP Category IV treatment for the patient, the patient is counseled, an RNTCP DOTS-Plus treatment card opened, a DOTS-Plus patient Identity Card issued to the patient, and Category IV treatment initiated. Patients admitted at the DR-TB Center, if clinically appropriate, may be discharged 7 days after treatment initiation to their district of residence with a maximum of 7-day supply of drugs and arrangement for injections in transit. This period of admission will allow for all necessary investigations to be undertaken, initiation of the Category IV regimen, monitoring of patient tolerance of the Category IV regimen, motivation, counseling and providing health education to the patient and their families, developing linkages with the services in the respective district where the patient resides (including identification and training of a local DOT provider and family treatment supporter) and contact assessment.

The patient should be discharged to the district that they reside in, with upto a maximum of one week's supply of drugs, arrangements for injections in transit, and a copy of the treatment card and referral form. The respective DTO should be informed by the attending physician of the patient's planned discharge three days prior to the actual date of discharge. The DTO will inform the respective MO-PHI and the identified DOT provider about the expected discharge of the patient. The three-monthly drug box and the patient records will be passed on to the identified DOT Provider from the respective TU. Local arrangements will need to be made for daily injections during the intensive phase. After discharge, the patient goes to DOTS-Plus site (DR-TB Center) facility for management of severe adverse reactions, change of regimen or dosage and at the end of treatment. It is not essential to send the patient to DOTS-Plus site for change from IP (intensive phase) to CP (continuation phase). The respective DTO can switch the patient to CP after obtaining the approval of the DOTS-Plus Site Committee by e mail.

Pretreatment Evaluation

The patient should be hospitalized at the DR-TB Center for pretreatment evaluation and treatment initiation. Pretreatment evaluation should include a thorough clinical evaluation by a physician, chest radiograph, pregnancy test and relevant hematological (complete blood count with platelets) and bio-chemical tests (blood glucose, liver functions, renal functions, TSH, urine). Since the drugs used for the treatment of MDR-TB are known to produce adverse effects, a proper pretreatment evaluation is essential to identify patients who are at increased risk of developing such adverse effects.

Counseling

Patients should receive counseling on the nature and duration of treatment, need for regular treatment and possible side effects of these drugs and the consequences of irregular treatment or premature cessation of treatment. It is advisable to involve close family members during the counseling, since family support is an essential component in the management. Patients should be advised to report if he/she experiences any unusual problem. Female patients should receive special counseling on family planning.

While the MDR-TB case is undergoing pretreatment evaluation, the DTO should ensure an initial home visit to verify the address and meet the family members. A DOT provider (who can either be a healthcare worker, a community worker or a community volunteer), should be identified in consultation with the patient. The DOT center can be either at the subcenter of the health system or in the community. The DOT provider should be given training for drug administration and to identify possible adverse effects during treatment, and the frequency of follow-up.

Monitoring Progress During Treatment

Clinical Monitoring

Patients should be seen by the respective DTO for clinical evaluation at monthly intervals during the IP, after discharge from the state DOTS-Plus site (DR-TB Center), and at 3-monthly intervals during the CP until the end of treatment. The DTO should screen patients for clinical improvement and possible adverse reactions. Body weight should be monitored by the DTO at every visit. The patient may need to be hospitalized during treatment for medical or sociological reasons.

Investigations During Treatment

Chest radiograph will be done during the pretreatment evaluation, at the end of the IP, end of treatment and when clinically indicated.

Serum Creatinine is to be done every month for the first three months and every three months thereafter till the patient is receiving kanamycin injection.

Liver function tests and Thyroid stimulating hormone (TSH) will be done as and when indicated clinically. These investigations can be done at the DOTS-Plus site or district hospitals/medical colleges as per the arrangement. However, patients should not be charged for these investigations.

Smear and Culture Schedule During Treatment

Sputum specimens are to be collected and examined by smear and culture at least 30 days apart from the third to seventh month of treatment (i.e. at the end of the months 3, 4, 5, 6 and 7) and at 3-monthly intervals from the 9th month onwards till the completion of treatment (i.e. at the end of the months 9, 12, 15, 18, 21 and 24). Category IV patients who after 9 months of treatment do not seem to be responding and the last available culture results (7th month culture) are positive are considered treatment failure and DST for second-line drugs would be done at a National Reference Laboratory (NRL). As in 2012, three NRLs (NTI-Bengaluru, NIRT-Chennai and LRS-New Delhi) are performing the second-line DST in solid and liquid culture. Two early morning sputum samples will be collected from such patients and sent for culture and DST for Kanamycin, Capreomycin and Fluoroquinolones to these accredited laboratories. RNTCP has identified eight laboratories that includes few IRLs (Andhra Pradesh, Delhi, Gujarat, Kerala, Maharashtra-Nagpur, Rajasthan) and Medical College (SMS, Jaipur and JJ Hospital, Mumbai) laboratories to initiate proficiency testing for second-line DST.

Methods for Drug Susceptibility Testing

Presently, three technologies are available for diagnosis of MDR-TB, viz. the conventional solid egg-based Lowenstein-Jensen (LJ) media, the liquid culture (MGIT), and the rapid molecular assays such as Line Probe Assay (LPA) and similar Nucleic Acid Amplification Tests like Xpert MTB/Rif. Conventional DST evaluates if *M. tuberculosis* grows in the presence of drug-containing media, and is also known as *phenotypic DST*. Molecular DST evaluates for the presence of genetic mutations that are highly associated with phenotypic resistance, and is also known as *genotypic DST*.

Phenotypic DST is available for more drugs, and is considered very reliable for isoniazid (H), rifampicin (R), and streptomycin (S), and somewhat less reliable for other drugs such as ethambutol (E). Molecular/genotypic DST is highly reliable for rifampicin, but has limited sensitivity for detection of isoniazid resistance.

Molecular/genotypic tests are much faster than phenotypic tests, as molecular tests do not require growth of the organism, and *M. tuberculosis* is notoriously slow growing. The turnaround time for C-DST results by Solid LJ media is around 84 days, by Liquid Culture (MGIT) is around 42 days, by LPA is around 72 hours and by CB-NAAT is around 2 hours.

Organization and Development of the Laboratory Network

RNTCP has a three-tier laboratory network based on the designated microscopy centers (DMCs) covering one lakh populations and providing sputum smear microscopy services, and IRLs (undertaking training, external quality assessment [EQA] of sputum smear microscopy network in the districts and DMCs, and culture and DST for first-line drugs for *M. tuberculosis*), and NRLs (undertaking training, EQA of sputum smear microscopy network in the states allotted to them, and culture and DST for first- and second-line drugs for *M. tuberculosis*).

Category IV Regimen

The RNTCP will be using a standardized treatment regimen (STR), comprising of six drugs (kanamycin, levofloxacin, ethionamide, cycloserine, pyrazinamide and ethambutol) during 6–9 months of the Intensive Phase and 4 drugs (levofloxacin, ethionamide, cycloserine and ethambutol) during the 18 months of the Continuation Phase. *p*-aminosalicylic acid (PAS) is included in the regimen as a substitute drug if any bactericidal drug (Km, Lfx, Z and Eto) or any 2 bacteriostatic (E and Cs) drugs are not tolerated. In case of intolerance/resistance to kanamycin, capreomycin is used. In case of ofloxacin resistance, moxifloxacin with combination of PAS is used.

Drug Dosages and Administration

Drug dosages for MDR-TB cases are decided according to the weight band as shown in Table 25.1.

All drugs should be given in a single daily dosage under directly observed treatment (DOT) by a DOT Provider. All patients will receive drugs under direct observation for six days of the week. On the seventh day (Sunday), the oral drugs will be administered unsupervised whereas injection kanamycin will be omitted. If intolerance occurs to the drugs, ethionamide, cycloserine and PAS may be split into two dosages and the morning dose administered under DOT. The evening dose will be self-administered. The empty blister packs of the self-administered doses will be checked the next morning during DOT. Pyridoxine at a dose of 100 mg should be administered to all patients on an RNTCP Category IV regimen. If a patient gains 5 kg or more weight during treatment and crosses the weight-bands range, the DOTS-Plus Site Committee may consider moving the patient to the higher weight-band drug dosages. Similarly, if a patient loses 5 kgs or more in weight during treatment and crosses the weight band, the DR-TB Center committee may consider moving the patient to the lower weight band. The new dosages are provided whenever the patient is due for the next supply of drugs in the normal course of treatment and not as soon as change of weight is noted. In deciding about the dosages, apart from the considerations mentioned above, it is also necessary to rule out the existence of medical illnesses or organ dysfunctions in the individual by conducting routine hematological investigations like full blood count, random blood sugar, liver and kidney function

TABLE 25.1: Drug dosages for MDR-TB according to weight band

Sl. No.	*Drugs*	*16–25 kg*	*26–45 kg*	*46–70 kg*
1.	Kanamycin	500 mg	500 mg	750 mg
2.	Levofloxacin	250 mg	750 mg	1000 mg
3.	Ethionamide	375 mg	500 mg	750 mg
4.	Ethambutol	400 mg	800 mg	1200 mg
5.	Pyrazinamide	500 mg	1250 mg	1500 mg
6.	Cycloserine	250 mg	500 mg	750 mg
7.	Pyridoxine	50 mg	100 mg	100 mg
	Reserve/Substitute drugs			
	Na PAS (80% weight/vol)*	5 g	10 g	12 g
	Moxifloxacin (Mfx)	200 g	400 g	400 g
	Capreomycin (Cm)	500 g	750 g	1000 mg

*In case of PAS with 60% weight/volume the dose will be increased to 7 g (16-25 kg); 14 g (26-45 kg) and 16 g (> 45 kg)

tests, etc. and of urine microscopy. Other investigations like skiagram, ultrasound, etc. may be appropriately carried out as required in a particular case.

Treatment Duration

The treatment is given in two phases, the Intensive phase (IP) and the Continuation phase (CP). The total duration of treatment for Regimen for MDR-TB is 24–27 months, depending on the IP duration. IP should be given for at least six months. After six months of treatment, the patient will be reviewed and the treatment changed to CP if the 4th or 5th month culture result in solid or liquid culture is negative respectively. If the 4th or 5th month culture result remains positive, the treatment is extended by one month. Extension of IP beyond one month will be decided on the results of sputum culture of 5th or 6th and 6th or 7th months. If the result of the 4th month culture is still awaited after six months of treatment, the IP is extended until the result is available, with further treatment being decided according to the culture result. The IP can be extended up to a maximum of three months after which the patient will be initiated on the CP irrespective of the culture result. The recommended duration for CP is 18 months.

Regimen for XDR-TB

All XDR-TB patients should also be subject to a repeat full pretreatment evaluation, but also including consultation by a thoracic surgeon for consideration of surgery. Identification must be done for the site (tertiary centers) with such surgical facilities. MDR-TB patients diagnosed as XDR-TB would be given an outcome of "Switched to Regimen for XDR-TB". The decision and initiation of Regimen for XDR-TB is to be taken by the concerned DR-TB Center Committee. The Intensive Phase (6–12 months) will consist of 7 drugs—capreomycin (Cm), PAS, moxifloxacin (Mfx), high dose-INH, clofazimine, linezolid and amoxyclav. The Continuation Phase (18 months) will consist of 6 drugs—PAS, moxifloxacin (Mfx), high dose-INH, clofazimine, linezolid and amoxyclav.

The dosage of the drugs would vary as per the weight of the patient (≤ 45 kg or > 45 kg) (Table 25.2). All drugs are to be given on a daily basis. Injections of Capreomycin will be given for 6 days/week (not on Sundays). All morning doses are to be supervised by the DOT Provider except on Sundays. After taking DOT for morning doses on Saturday, next day medicines would be given to the patient to be taken at home on Sunday. Empty blisters of medicines taken unsupervised in evening and on Sundays are to be collected by DOT Provider.

Duration of Regimen for XDR-TB

The Regimen for XDR-TB would be of 24–30 months duration, with 6–12 months Intensive Phase (IP) and 18 months Continuation Phase (CP). The change from IP to CP will be done only after achievement of culture conversion, i.e. two consecutive negative cultures taken at least one month apart. In case of delay in culture conversion, the IP can be extended from 6 months up to a maximum of 12 months. In case of extension, the DR-TR Center Committee, which will be

TABLE 25.2: Drug dosages for XDR-TB according to weight band

Drugs	*Dosage/day*	
	≤ 45 kg	*> 45 kg*
Inj. Capreomycin (Cm)	750 g	1000 g
PAS	10 g	12 g
Moxifloxacin (Mfx)	400 g	400 g
High-dose INH (High dose-H)	600 g	900 g
Clofazimine (CFz)	200 mg	200 mg
Linezolid (Lzd)	600 mg	600 mg
Amoxyclav (Amx/Clv)	875/125 mg BD	875/125 mg BD
Pyridoxine	100 mg	100 mg
Reserve/Substitute drugs*		
Clarithromycin (Clr)	500 mg BD	500 mg BD
Thiacetazone (Thz)#	150 mg	150 mg

* Reserve/Substitute drugs would be used in case tha patient was already on PAS, unable to tolerate one are more of the drugs and is resistant to capreomycin

responsible for initiating and monitoring the Regimen for XDR-TB, can decide on administering Capreomycin injection intermittently (3 times/week) for the months 7 to 12.

Treatment Interruption and Default

All efforts should be made to ensure that Category IV patients do not interrupt treatment or default. Action should be taken to promptly retrieve patient who fail to come for DOT.

The following situations may be seen in case of treatment interruption:

Category IV patients in IP/CP who miss doses: All the missed doses during IP must be completed prior to switching the patient to CP. Similarly, all missed doses during CP must be completely administered prior to ending treatment.

Category IV patients who interrupt treatment for less than 2 months during IP: When the patient returns to resume treatment, the IP will be continued. However, the duration of treatment will be extended to complete IP. The follow-up cultures will be done as per the revised schedule.

Category IV patients who interrupt treatment for less than 2 months during CP: When the patient returns to resume treatment, the CP will be continued, however the duration of treatment will be extended to complete the CP. The period of interruption shall not be included in the duration of treatment. The follow-up cultures will be done as per the revised schedule.

Category IV patients who default and return back for treatment: These patients will be given an outcome of default in the existing cohort and thereafter reregistered for treatment.

Treatment Outcomes

Standardized treatment outcome definitions are to be used following treatment of an MDR-TB case and are as follows:

Cure: An MDR-TB patient who has completed treatment and has been consistently culture negative (with at least 5 consecutive negative results in the last 12 to 15 months). If one follow-up positive culture is reported during the last three quarters, patient will still be considered cured provided this positive culture is followed by at least 3 consecutive negative cultures, taken at least 30 days apart, provided that there is clinical evidence of improvement.

Treatment completed: An MDR-TB patient who has completed treatment according to guidelines but does not meet the definition for cure or treatment failure due to lack of bacteriological results.

Death: An MDR-TB patient who dies for any reason during the course of MDR-TB treatment.

Treatment failure: Treatment will be considered to have failed if two or more of the five cultures recorded in the final 12–15 months are positive, or if any of the final three cultures are positive.

Treatment default: An MDR-TB patient whose MDR-TB treatment was interrupted for two or more consecutive months for any reasons.

Transfer out: An MDR-TB patient who has been transferred to another reporting unit and for whom the treatment outcome is not known.

Treatment stopped due to adverse drug reactions: A patient on MDR-TB treatment who develops severe adverse reactions and could not continue the MDR-TB treatment in spite of the management of the adverse reactions as per the defined protocols and decision has been taken by the DOTS-Plus site committee to stop treatment.

Treatment stopped due to other reasons: A patient on MDR-TB treatment who could not continue the MDR-TB treatment for any other medical reason (than adverse drug reactions), and a decision has been taken by the DOTS-Plus site committee to stop treatment.

Still on treatment: An MDR-TB patient who, for any reason, is still receiving his/her RNTCP Category IV treatment at the time of the submission of the RNTCP DOTS-Plus Treatment Outcome Report.

Providing Patient and Family Counseling

Providing counseling and health education to the MDR-TB patient about the disease and about the necessity of taking regular and adequate treatment is of utmost importance, for they must clearly understand that by taking the drugs irregularly or inadequately, or by defaulting, they fell into a category that was difficult to treat and that required a prolonged therapy. It is vital for them to realize that this is their last chance of treatment. Hence, it is extremely essential to strictly adhere to the prescribed line of treatment as well as to the scheduled follow-up of sputum and other lab investigations. Health education and counseling are provided to all patients and family members at different levels of healthcare, right from one at the periphery to those at the DOTS-Plus site facility. It is started at the initial point of contact and carried on a continuous basis at all visits by the patient to a health facility. The counseling and motivation are required to be done not only of the patient but also of the family members. In addition to the emphasis on regular treatment, health education also attempts to cross-check the manner and the number of drugs/injections being taken, the occurrence of side-effects like yellowish skin and/or eyes, pain and swelling of joints, imbalance, etc., if any, and the frequency of sputa examinations being performed.

Monitoring for Early Detection of Adverse Reactions

Close monitoring of patients is necessary to ensure that the adverse effects of Category IV anti-TB drugs are recognized early by the DOT provider. DOT makes it possible to closely monitor patients. Patients will not be asked any leading question to elicit any adverse reaction.[11] However, if the patient makes any spontaneous complaint, he/she will be interrogated in detail and the necessary action taken. Commonly, patients will volunteer if they experience any adverse effects. The DOT provider should be trained to recognize adverse reactions like nausea, vomiting, diarrhea, skin rash, ototoxicity, peripheral neuropathy, psychiatric symptoms and jaundice.[12–15] Training should also be provided on the management of minor reactions and when the patients should be referred to the medical officer. In addition to clinical monitoring, certain laboratory investigations may be required to detect certain occult adverse effects.

Common Adverse Reactions to the Drugs Used

Kanamycin: Toxicity includes ototoxicity,[6,7] nephrotoxicity, vertigo and electrolyte imbalance.

Ofloxacin/Levofloxacin:[8,9] Gastrointestinal symptoms include diarrhea, vomiting and abdominal pain. Central nervous system (CNS): dizziness and convulsions, phototoxicity and photosensitivity, tendinopathy and tendonitis, nephrotoxicity, skin rash, cardiotoxicity, arthralgia.

Ethambutol: Visual disturbance.

Pyrazinamide: Arthralgia, hyperuricemia, hepatitis and pruritus with or without rash.

Ethionamide: Gastrointestinal—Epigastric discomfort, anorexia, nausea, metallic taste, vomiting, excessive salivation and sulfurous belching. Psychiatric: hallucination and depression, Hepatitis, Hypothyroidism and goiter with prolonged administration, Gynecomastia, menstrual disturbances, impotence, acne, headache, alopecia and peripheral neuropathy.

Cycloserine:[10] CNS: Dizziness, slurred speech, convulsions, headache, tremor, and insomnia, psychiatric: confusion, depression, altered behavior, and suicidal tendency, hypersensitivity reaction.

P-aminosalicylic acid:[11] Gastrointestinal—anorexia, nausea, vomiting, and abdominal discomfort, skin rashes, hepatic dysfunction, hypokalemia, hypothyroidism and goiter with prolonged administration.

Role of DR-TB Committee in the Management of Adverse Reactions

Whenever a patient has serious adverse reactions necessitating hospitalization or reduction/withholding/termination of any drug in the treatment regimen, the DR-TB Committee should meet and arrange for specialist consultation, if required. The committee also should arrange for the drugs to be given for managing these reactions. Timely and intensive monitoring for identifying and management of adverse reactions to Category IV drugs are essential components of the DOTS-Plus program. This will help to improve patient adherence to treatment, reduce mortality and obtain better treatment outcomes. Ancillary drugs for the management of adverse reactions should be made available to the patient free of cost (pyridoxine will be supplied by RNTCP and the other ancillary drugs should be available through the general health system drug supplies). Proper training of staff and support to the patient are other important activities that are required. In most cases, management of the adverse effects can be accomplished using relatively simple and low-cost interventions without compromising the integrity of the MDR-TB treatment regimen.[12]

Adherence

Patients with MDR-TB may be more likely to have had problems with non-adherence in the past.[13] In addition, adherence with MDR-TB therapy is made more difficult by its prolonged treatment regimens, with larger number of drugs that have more serious adverse effect profiles.[14] Thus, MDR-TB patients are at risk of not being able to appropriately adhere with treatment, an essential element to prevent the generation of panresistant strains with the potential for community-wide spread and virtually no chance of cure for the patient.[15] MDR-TB treatment can be successful with high overall rates of adherence when adequate support measures are provided.[16] These measures include enablers and incentives for delivery of DOT to ensure adherence to treatment and may include the following: reimbursement of travel expenses to patient and attendants for visits to DTC and designated State-level DOTS-Plus site indoor facility; emotional support; patient, family and peer's education on MDR-TB treatment; early and effective management of adverse drug reactions; and honorarium to the nonsalaried DOT providers.

Follow-up of the Nonadherent Patient

When a patient fails to attend a DOT appointment, a system should be in place that allows prompt patient retrieval. The DOT provider should visit the patient's home on the same day to find out why the patient has not appeared for his/

her DOT, and ensure that treatment is resumed promptly and effectively. The situation should be addressed in a sympathetic, friendly, and nonjudgmental manner. Every effort should be made to listen to reasons for why the patient missed a dose(s) and to work with patient and family to ensure treatment continuation.

DOTS-Plus Plan

The RNTCP PMDT Vision is to promptly diagnose and effectively treat all TB patients with drug-resistant TB, through decentralized DST and PMDT treatment services integrated into RNTCP. Given the complexity, scale and cost, a phased approach has been developed, focusing first on those most likely to have drug-resistant TB. PMDT has the following specific objective to realize this vision:

- By end 2012, complete nationwide geographical coverage of access to basic MDR-TB diagnostic and treatment services
- By 2012–13, expanded access to MDR-TB diagnosis and treatment for all smear positive retreatment TB cases and new cases who have failed an initial first-line drug treatment
- By 2015, nationwide access to MDR-TB diagnosis and treatment for all smear positive TB (retreatment or new) cases registered under RNTCP before or early during their treatment.
- RNTCP expects to treat about 160,000 MDR-TB and 4100 XDR-TB cases over the next 5 years (2012–2017).

Recent technological advances in laboratory diagnostics have expanded the list of WHO-recommended methods available for DST, and can significantly reduce the delay between detection of TB and diagnosis of first-line and second-line drug resistance. Rapid methods of DST allow for the timely design of appropriate treatment regimens based on patients' drug resistance profiles using diagnostics that can be feasibly implemented in settings worldwide. This increased capacity for DST also translates into increased capacity for surveillance. After comprehensive review, WHO has endorsed certain new DST methodologies, including molecular line probe assays and liquid culture systems. With liquid culture, confirmation of pulmonary TB can be obtained in less than two weeks, and DST results in an additional one to two weeks. Use of liquid culture methods is possible for susceptibility testing for both first-line and second-line drugs. Molecular line probe assays are a genotypic method of DST that are used to detect the most common mutations of *M. tuberculosis* DNA that confer resistance to antituberculosis drugs, especially for isoniazid and rifampicin. Line probe assays have the great advantage of being able to produce results within 24 to 48 hours, thus representing a revolutionary step forward in the ability to rapidly confirm or rule out MDR-TB. GeneXpert MTB/RIF system is another molecular method to determine rifampicin resistance which is considered to be a surrogate marker for MDR-TB. Xpert MTB/RIF system has been found to be highly sensitive (98%) and specific (98%) in detecting TB and rifampicin resistance directly from sputum, in less than two hours.

References

1. DOTS-Plus guidelines, Revised National Tuberculosis Control Programme, Central TB Divison Directorate General Health Services, Ministry of Health and Family Welfare, Nirman Bhawan, New Delhi. Sep 2008;/Revised National Tuberculosis Control Programme. Guidelines on Programmatic Management of Drug Resistant TB (PMDT) in India. Central TB Division, Directorate General of Health Services, Ministry of Health & Family Welfare, Nirman Bhavan, New Delhi. May 2012.
2. Mahadev B, Kumar P, Agarwal SP, Chauhan LS, Srikantaramu N. Surveillance of drug resistance to anti-tuberculosis drugs in districts of Hoogli in West Bengal and Mayurbhanj in Orissa. Indian J Tuberc. 2005:52;5-10.
3. Paramasivan CN, Venkataraman P, Chandrasekaran V, Bhat S, Narayanan PR. Surveillance of drug resistance in tuberculosis in two districts of South India. Int J Tuberc Lung Dis. 2002:6; 479-84.
4. WHO IUALTD Global Project on Anti-Tuberculosis Drug Resistance Surveillance (2002-2007), Fourth Global Report (2008)./World Health Organization (WHO). Global Tuberculosis Report 2012. WHO/HTM/TB/2012.6.
5. World Health Organization (WHO). Treatment of Tuberculosis: Guidelines for National Programmes, 3rd edition. WHO/CDS/TB 2003.313 Geneva, Switzerland: WHO, 2003, 2009.
6. Moore RD, Smith CR, Lietman PS. Risk factors for the development of auditory toxicity in patients receiving aminoglycosides. J Infect Dis. 1984;149:23-30.
7. De Jager P, Van Altena R. Hearing loss and nephrotoxicity in long-term aminoglycoside treatment in patients with tuberculosis. Int J Tuberc Lung Dis. 2002;6:622-7.
8. Arora VK, Tumbanatham A. Severe arthropathy with ofloxacin in two cases of MDR tuberculosis. Int J Tuberc Lung Dis. 1998;2:941-3.
9. Yew WW, Chan CK, Chau CH, et al. Outcomes of patients with multidrug-resistant pulmonary tuberculosis treated with ofloxacin/levofloxacin-containing regimens. Chest 2000;117:744-51.
10. Akula SK, Aruna AS, et al. Cycloserine-induced Stevens-Johnson syndrome in an AIDS patient with multi-drug-resistant tuberculosis. Int J Tuberc Lung Dis. 1997;1:187-90.
11. Vega P, Sweetland A, Acha J, et al. Psychiatric issues in the management of patients with multidrug-resistant tuberculosis. Int J Tuberc Lung Dis. 2004;8:749-58.
12. Furin JJ, Mitnick CD, Shin SS, et al. Occurrence of serious adverse effects in patients receiving community-based therapy for multidrug-resistant tuberculosis. Int J Tuberc Lung Dis. 2001;5:648-55.
13. Mitchison D. How drug resistance emerges as a result of poor compliance during short course chemotherapy for tuberculosis. Int J Tuberc Lung Dis. 1998;2:10-15.
14. Chaulk C, Chaisson R, Lewis J, et al. Treating multidrug-resistant tuberculosis: compliance and side effects. Journal of the American Medical Association 1994;271:103-4.
15. Espinal M, Dye C, Raviglione M, et al. A rational "DOTS-Plus" for the control of MDR-TB. Int J Tuberc Lung Dis. 1999;3:561-3.
16. Mitnick CD, Bayona J, Palacios E, et al. Community-based therapy for multidrug-resistant tuberculosis in Lima, Peru. New England Journal of Medicine 2003; 348:119-28.

Chapter 26

Infection Control in Multi-drug-resistant Tuberculosis

Introduction

Drug-resistant Tuberculosis (DR-TB) is transmitted in the same manner as drug-susceptible TB. Well documented outbreaks of highly drug-resistant strains of TB constitute convincing evidence that DR-TB is transmissible, especially among highly vulnerable populations and in institutional settings. Moreover, because DR-TB patients may respond to treatment slowly and remain sputum smear positive longer than other TB patients, they may infect more contacts. The management of DR-TB does not significantly alter the basic TB infection control strategies. However, in view of its seriousness, every program attempting to treat DR-TB should also undertake a systematic review of current practices and ensure that everything possible is done to prevent transmission among patients and to staff.[1] Since every instance of transmission averted represents one less potential DR-TB case, infection control needs to be a leading programmatic priority. It is equally important to protect health workers in the setting of DR-TB.This chapter aims to review special considerations for reducing transmission of DR-TB through infection control measures.

TB infection control has the following three components: Administrative controls, environmental or engineering controls, and personal respiratory protection. The administrative controls are the most effective and least expensive and, therefore, have highest priority, especially in resource-constrained settings.

Administrative Controls

Administrative controls include policies and procedures intended to promptly identify infectious cases so that additional precautions can be taken. They necessitate the appointment of an incharge of infection control for the institution, and an infection control committee representing key departments of the facility. The initial task of the committee is the formulation of a comprehensive infection control plan for the institution, including a program for the education of all staff on infection control policies and procedures. An important aspect of administrative control measures is the physical separation of patients known or suspected to have TB or DR-TB (especially smear-positive cases) from other patients, especially those who are immunocompromised. In many resource-limited settings, however, isolation rooms are not available and patients are mixed together in open wards. A second, less satisfactory but practical solution is to separate rather than isolate patients. In this approach, patients with TB are grouped together and apart from those with suspected DR-TB, who are grouped together. This separation may be difficult as wards are usually separated by sex, which increases the number of different areas required. The presence of a substantial number of HIV-infected patients further complicates separation as they are not only potentially infectious but also highly vulnerable to intercurrent infection and reinfection from others. Placing HIV-infected patients on wards with known or suspected TB together with other TB or MDR-TB patients should always be avoided.

Infectious patients with XDR-TB, whether infected with HIV or not, should not be placed in general wards. Given the high mortality associated with XDR-TB, isolation until the patient is no longer infectious is recommended. Another administrative issue is the length of time patients spend in the hospital. In many resource-limited countries, patients are traditionally treated for prolonged periods in the hospital, particularly when they come from great distances. However, this practice involves an increased risk of nosocomial transmission. The risk of transmission to patients and healthcare workers decreases when community-based ambulatory treatment is established and hospital stays are reduced. Although most transmission is likely to have occurred before the diagnosis and start of treatment, ambulatory patients should be advised to avoid contact with the general public and with particularly susceptible people, such as young children or individuals with HIV infection. Healthcare workers visiting TB patients at home before treatment is well established should wear properly fitted personal respirator masks. Attention should also be paid to outpatient clinical settings. Because of the risk of severe morbidity and mortality in HIV-infected persons from DR-TB, persons with known DR-TB should receive routine care outside of normal HIV care settings.[2]

Environmental Controls

Environmental (or engineering) controls assume that unsuspected, untreated TB patients will enter hospitals despite all efforts to identify them. In addition, there are certain high-risk settings, such as sputum induction rooms, bronchoscopy rooms and rooms for the evaluation of newly admitted patients who may have untreated TB or DR-TB, where engineering interventions are necessary to reduce risk. Engineering controls attempt to reduce the concentration of infectious droplet nuclei in the air. They include natural and/or mechanical ventilation, ultraviolet germicidal irradiation (UVGI) and high efficiency particulate air filtration. Environmental methods should never replace administrative controls; in fact, they work together. In warm climates, infection control often depends on natural ventilation. The efficacy of natural ventilation has not been studied, but it probably depends heavily on climatic conditions. In warm climates, patients spend much of their time outdoors where transmission is highly unlikely. However, at night, for security and warmth, patients stay indoors with doors and windows usually closed tightly. The use of exhaust fans to improve ventilation in closed rooms through wall vents can be extremely useful. Mechanical ventilation systems are uncommon in resource-poor settings and, when present, are often poorly maintained. However, a little ventilation is better than none, and in facilities with mechanical ventilation systems, efforts should be made to ensure that they function correctly. Clinics in warm climates should be designed without interior hallways, which tend to trap air and with waiting areas that are open on at least three sides. Ventilation can be supplemented with upper-room ultraviolet germicidal irradiation (UVGI). This has long been known to be extremely effective in inactivating infectious particles in the air above people's heads, while not exposing them to skin or eye irritation, which is the only practical safety concern. Normal convection currents or low-velocity ceiling fans usually ensure good room air mixing, thereby decontaminating air in the breathing zone. Upper-room UVGI is intended for use while rooms are occupied, but not to sterilize empty rooms as is commonly done in some parts of the world. It is much more important to decontaminate air while the infectious source and other occupants are present, and upper-room UVGI is designed to do so without significant radiation risks. A growing number of manufacturers of fixtures designed for upper-room use are established in low-income countries and can providc products at relatively low cost. However, there are currently no standards for these products; the buyer should obtain advice from an engineer knowledgeable in the field. In addition to UVGI designed for upper-room use, ultraviolet germicidal is sometimes used in ventilation ducts or in fan-driven air sterilizing devices mounted on ceilings or walls, or portable units that can be moved from room to room. However, the efficacy of these systems is limited by the number of air turnovers they can produce, especially in large spaces. By irradiating large volumes of upper-room air at one time, upper-room systems have a quantitative advantage, especially when combined with low-velocity ceiling fans to ensure room air mixing. Laboratories that process specimens, that may be DR-TB, require particularly strict environmental controls.[3]

Personal Respiratory Protection (Special Masks)

Because administrative and engineering controls cannot provide complete protection, the third line of defence against nosocomial TB transmission is the use of personal respirators. Personal respirators are fundamentally different from, and more expensive than, the more familiar surgical masks which they resemble. Surgical masks are designed to protect the operating field from relatively large respiratory droplets generated by surgeons and surgical nurses. They are relatively loose fitting and made of paper or cloth; they are not adequate for prevention of TB infection. Masks that prevent TB transmission are known as "particulate respirators" or simply "respirators". They are designed to protect the wearer from tiny (1–5 μm) airborne infectious droplets. The filtration media through which air passes must capture these minute particles; most importantly, the respirator must fit tightly on the face, especially around the bridge of the nose. Ideally, respirators should be "fit tested" for individual wearers. In addition to choosing the proper model for each worker, this process serves to educate workers on how to put on their respirators correctly to minimize face-seal leakage. Men with beards cannot be properly fitted with personal respirators. Institutions purchasing respirators are advised to look for models that are specifically designed to protect against TB and that meet international standards of quality.

Because they are visible and relatively expensive, it is sometimes assumed that personal respirators alone will prevent TB transmission. However, they cannot be worn continuously and are likely not to be in use when unsuspected TB cases, or unsuspected DR-TB, are encountered. For these reasons, administrative controls that aim to detect and separate cases, and engineering controls that can reduce the risk even for unsuspected cases, are more important.

Role of Rapid Tests in Infection Control

The use of a rapid test for rifampicin or other drugs is an excellent method of distinguishing those who may have DR-TB from others. Patients who are identified by rapid tests can be properly separated or isolated immediately.

References

1. Guidelines for the prevention of tuberculosis in healthcare facilities in resource limited settings. Geneva, World Health Organization, 1999 (WHO/TB/99.269).
2. Tuberculosis infection control in the era of expanding HIV care and treatment. Geneva, World Health Organization, 2007.
3. Laboratory services in tuberculosis control. Parts I, II and III. Geneva, World Health Organization, 1998 (WHO/TB/98.258).

Chapter 27

Newer Antitubercular Drugs

Introduction

More than a century after discovery of Mycobacterium tuberculosis, and a half-century after the discovery of drugs to treat the disease, TB still remains a major public health problem. Since the discovery of effective anti-TB drugs in the middle of the last century, drug resistance has been one of the major challenges in the fight against TB. Despite a number of measures and strategies to prevent and control drug resistance, drug-resistant TB continues to be a formidable problem. With the vast majority of TB patients concentrated in the world's poorest countries, there has traditionally been little incentive for the private sector to invest in the major research for development of new TB drugs. However, the early 21st century has seen a dramatic increase in TB research activity and development of new drugs and other forms of therapeutic modalities. As a result, multiple drug candidates are in clinical trials and thousands of potential compounds are being screened, synthesized, or optimized in discovery and preclinical studies. This chapter aims to address newer drugs in the development for treatment of tuberculosis, including drug-resistant tuberculosis.

Difficulties in Antitubercular Drug Development

In addition to the lack of interest and commitment in TB Drug research, there are many issues that delay anti-TB drug development. Many of the metabolic pathways and pathogenic mechanisms of Mycobacterium tuberculosis are still not understood. The bacteria has got a remarkable ability to persist in macrophages and cause relapse later. Any newly developed drug has to be tried as part of a multi-drug regimen to prevent the possibility of relapse. This requires large population studies to clearly demonstrate the efficacy of new drug. Also one of the primary end-points of evaluation of newly developed drug will be relapse rate in five-year or longer follow-up. This makes evaluation of new drugs a very time-consuming effort. Another issue is that the drug should be free from pharmacokinetic and pharmacodynamic interaction with existing anti-TB drugs.

Priorities in Developing Antitubercular Drugs

The development of newer drugs must aim at fulfilling some of the long felt needs like shortening of antitubercular chemotherapy , development of drugs with activity on persisters, treatment of HIV-TB coinfection, treatment of drug-resistant tuberculosis and development of intermittent regimens.

Methods to Develop Newer Antitubercular Drugs

Different approaches are utilized for developing newer anti-TB drugs. Many existing drugs are being evaluated for antitubercular activity. Previously unused compounds are also being evaluated. Sometimes currently used antitubercular drugs are modified to improve their pharmacokinetic or pharmacodynamic properties. Another novel approach is identification of targets in the metabolic pathways and structural components of *Mycobacteria* and developing compounds that specifically interfere them.

Emerging Pipeline of New Anti-TB Drugs

According to information from the Working Group on New Drugs, there are over 60 recorded projects in various stages of development, including translational basic research, lead compound discovery, preclinical and clinical studies.[1] Currently, two fluoroquinolones (Moxifloxacin and Gatifloxacin) are in Phase III clinical development for the treatment of drug-susceptible TB. There are three novel compounds (TMC-207, OPC-67683 and PA-824) in Phase II clinical trials for the treatment of both drug-susceptible and drug-resistant tuberculosis. Additional compounds are in the early stages of clinical and preclinical development, such as LL-3858 and SQ-109.[2,3]

Gatifloxacin

Gatifloxacin is an 8-methoxy fluoroquinolone, acting predominantly on the DNA gyrase of *M. tuberculosis*. It has no cross-resistance or antagonism with other antimycobacterial drugs.[2] In view of its good sterilizing activity, a Phase III trial is being conducted currently in multiple African countries for pulmonary TB to evaluate the potential efficacy of Gatifloxacin-containing regimens for shortening the treatment from 6 to 4 months.[4] However, owing to its significant side effects, especially dysglycemia, Gatifloxacin has been withdrawn from the US and Canadian markets.[5,6]

Moxifloxacin

Moxifloxacin is another 8-methoxy fluoroquinolone with no cross-resistance or antagonism with other antimycobacterial drugs. It has a long plasma elimination half-life of approximately 11 hours.[2] It has good bactericidal and sterilizing activity and good results from a number of Early Bactericidal Activity (EBA) studies.[7-10] It also has a track record of safety when used in a large number of patients on a short-term basis.

TABLE 27.1: Fluoroquinolones as first-line tuberculosis therapy			
Study (Ref)	*Control Group*	*Intervention Group*	*Findings*
Tuberculosis Research Center, Chennai (14)	None	3OHRZ 3OHRZ/1HR 2 times/week 3OHRZ/2HR 2 times/week 2OHRZ/2HR 2 times/week	3-month intensive phase and at least 2 month continuation are necessary to avoid > 4% relapse
OFLOTUB, phase II (13)	2EHRZ/4HR	2OHRZ/4HR, 2GHRZ/4HR, 2MHRZ/4HR	Moxifloxacin accelerated early killing; Moxifloxacin>Gatifloxacin > Ofloxacin = Etambutol but differences in sputum conversion not significant at 8 week
Conde, et al. (12)	2EHRZ/4HR	2MHRZ/4HR	Moxifloxacin improved sputum conversion from 1 through 8 week
REMox, phase III (15)	2EHRZ/4HR	2MHRZ/2MHR, 2EMRZ/2MR	Currently underway
OFLOTUB, phase III (16)	2EHRZ/4HR	2GHRZ/2GHR	Currently underway

* O = Ofloxacin, H= Isoniazid, R = Rifampicin, Z = Pyrizinamide, G = Gatifloxacin, M = Moxifloxacin

In the TB Trials Consortium (TBTC) Study 27, a Phase II trial substituting Moxifloxacin for Ethambutol in the first 8 weeks of therapy, there was no difference in 2-month culture negativity rates (71%), but there appeared to be higher activity at an earlier time point for Moxifloxacin.[11] On the other hand, a study with nearly the same design conducted in Brazil showed that patients in the Moxifloxacin arm had improved culture conversion (80%) in the initial phase of treatment compared with the Ethambutol arm (63%).[12] Another similar Phase II clinical study has shown that patients in Moxifloxacin and Gatifloxacin containing arms cleared their sputum bacilli more quickly than conventional therapy or an Ofloxacin-containing regimen.[13, 14]

Based on the rapid sterilization results of Isoniazid sparing regimen in murine models, the TBTC Study 28 was designed as a double-blind, placebo-controlled study to evaluate the 2-month culture conversion rates when substituting Moxifloxacin for Isoniazid in the 2-month intensive phase of treatment of pulmonary TB.[15-17] Again, only a small insignificant increase in week-8 culture negativity was achieved by substitution of Moxifloxacin for Isoniazid during the intensive phase treatment of pulmonary TB.[18]

Moxifloxacin is currently being tested in the Phase III REMox study, which is within the TB Alliance's drug development portfolio. The REMox study will explore whether Moxifloxacin containing regimens, in which Moxifloxacin replaces either Isoniazid or Ethambutol, can shorten the conventional therapy from 6 to 4 months. Moxifloxacin is the first drug in TB Alliance's portfolio to enter a pivotal Phase III trial for TB, and is one of the most advanced among the TB clinical development programs.[2,19]

Rifapentine

Rifapentine was discovered in 1965, soon after the discovery of rifampicin. Rifapentine (RPT) is a long-acting cyclopentyl rifamycin (elimination half-life: 14 h) with potent anti-TB activity. Moxifloxacin and Rifapentine-based regimens are also under investigation for the treatment of TB, as both are very active agents with long half-lives. It should be noted that when given together, Rifapentine may induce enzymes that metabolize Moxifloxacin, resulting in modestly reduced Moxifloxacin concentration.[20] Using a mouse model of TB, bactericidal activity and treatment-shortening potential were evaluated for regimens consisting of Isoniazid or Moxifloxacin plus Rifapentine and Pyrazinamide administered either daily or three-times weekly.[21] The duration of treatment necessary to achieve stable cure was 10 weeks for daily regimens and 12 weeks for three-times weekly regimens, regardless of whether Isoniazid or Moxifloxacin was used with Rifapentine-Pyrazinamide. By contrast, for the 12-week regimen of Rifampicin-Isoniazid-Pyrazinamide, all mice relapsed. These results in the mouse model suggest further studies are indicated to explore whether Rifapentine-based regimens might shorten the duration of treatment needed to cure human TB.[21] A Phase II clinical trial is using Rifapentine plus Moxifloxacin in the intensive phase of the treatment. Smear-positive pulmonary TB patients will be randomized in the initial 2 months to receive either Isoniazid-Rifapentine-Pyrazinamide-Moxifloxacin or Isoniazid-Rifampicin-Pyrazinamide-Ethambutol, followed by the standard nonexperimental regimen in the continuation phase. The efficacy in terms of sputum conversion rates and treatment outcomes, as well as safety and tolerability of the Rifapentine-Moxifloxacin-containing regimens, will thus be evaluated.[22] In this regard, the potential benefits of using fluoroquinolones to shorten first-line regimens should be balanced against the strategy of sparing them for use in second-line regimens for MDR-TB.

TMC-207

TMC-207 is a novel diarylquinoline with unique activity on the mycobacterial ATP synthase.[23]Thus, it has high specificity for mycobacteria. A recent study has also shown that human mitochondrial ATP synthase displayed more than 20,000-fold lower sensitivity for TMC-207 compared with that of mycobacterial ATP synthase, suggesting that TMC-207 may not elicit ATP synthesis-related toxicity in mammalian cells.[24] It is active against both drug-resistant and drug-susceptible *M. tuberculosis*, as well as other mycobacterial species. It has a long half-life in plasma and tissues of nearly 24 hours. Data have also suggested that TMC-207 might kill dormant bacilli as effectively as aerobically grown bacilli with the same target specificity. It was shown that dormant mycobacteria possessed residual ATP synthase enzymatic activity, which could be blocked by nanomolar concentrations of TMC-207, thereby further reducing ATP levels and causing a pronounced bactericidal effect.[22] TMC-207 is metabolized by CYP3A4. Thus, its plasma level may be reduced by half through interaction with Rifampicin. However, data from the mouse model have demonstrated that TMC-207 had significant activity, even when its exposure was reduced by 50% and when it was added to a strong background regimen of Isoniazid-Rifampicin-Pyrazinamide. In killing kinetics, the bactericidal effect of TMC-207 in mice was modest during the first week of treatment but increased in the following 3 weeks, while the bactericidal activity of Isoniazid was limited to the first week of treatment.[25-26] TMC-207 probably acts synergistically with Pyrazinamide to exert sterilization activity. In the mouse model, 2-month treatment regimens containing TMC-207 and Pyrazinamide led to sterilization. Thus, it has the potential to reduce treatment time.[27] In another mouse model study, the triple combination of TMC-207-Rifapentine-Pyrazinamide given once weekly led to satisfactory lung culture negativity at 2 months, and was more active than the current regimen of Rifampicin-Isoniazid-Pyrazinamide given five times per week.[28] The unprecedented activity of this triple combination suggested that it may be feasible to develop a fully intermittent, once-weekly regimen.[29]

In a mouse model to evaluate the use of TMC-207 in MDR-TB, treatment was given five times per week with TMC-207 alone or various combinations of TMC-207 with Pyrazinamide or other second-line drugs.[30] All TMC-207-containing regimens were significantly more active than the non-TMC-207-containing regimens after 1 month of therapy. When given for 2 months, TMC-207 alone was more active than the first-line regimen Rifampicin-Isoniazid-Pyrazinamide. When TMC-207 was combined with second-line drugs, the combinations were more active than currently used regimen of MDR-TB, and culture negativity of both the lungs and spleen was reached after 2 months of treatment in almost every case.[30]

Phase I trials in healthy volunteers did not show any serious adverse effects, while further Phase I trials are being conducted to investigate the pharmacokinetic interaction with antiretrovirals of the protease inhibitor class.[31] A Phase IIa EBA study with ascending doses of TMC-207 has demonstrated that the drug had a delayed onset of bactericidal activity, with significant activity from day 4–7 when given at a daily dose of 400 mg, which was similar in magnitude to those of Isoniazid and Rifampicin over the same period.[32]

A double-blind, randomized Phase II clinical trial with TMC-207 began in 2007 in MDR-TB patients.[33] The study was conducted in two consecutive stages. In the first exploratory stage for safety and dose determination, newly diagnosed sputum smear-positive patients with MDR-TB were randomized to receive either TMC-207 or placebo for 8 weeks on top of a background regimen. The dose regimen for TMC-207 was validated for further testing in the second stage, being 400 mg daily for 2 weeks followed by 200 mg three times weekly. The second stage was planned to be a proof-of-effectiveness stage, during which patients were randomized to receive either TMC-207 or placebo for 24 weeks on top of a background regimen. After finishing 24 weeks of treatment, patients continued to receive MDR-TB treatment as per national treatment guidelines. Study subjects were followed for safety, tolerability, pharmacokinetics and microbiological efficacy for 2 years.[30] Patients receiving bedaquiline in addition to a baseline Regimen during the initial 8 weeks of MDR treatment reached sputum culture negativity in the MGIT system significantly more quickly than patients receiving placebo and were at lower risk of acquisition of additional drug resistance over the whole duration of follow-up.[34]

WHO has issued interim guidance which lists five conditions that must be in place if bedaquiline is used to treat adults with MDR-TB. Firstly, treatment must be closely monitored for effectiveness and safety, using sound treatment and management protocols approved by relevant national authorities. Secondly, special caution is required when bedaquiline is used in people aged 65 and over, and in adults living with HIV. Use in pregnant women and children is not advised. Thirdly, patients must be fully aware of the potential benefits and harms of the new drug, and give documented informed consent before embarking on treatment. Fourthly, all principles, on which WHO-recommended MDR-TB treatment regimens are based, must be followed, particularly the inclusion of four effective second-line drugs. In line with general principles of TB therapeutics, bedaquiline alone should not be introduced into a regimen in which the companion drugs are failing to show effectiveness. Lastly, active pharmacovigilance measures must be in place to ensure early detection and proper management of adverse drug reactions and potential interactions with other drugs. WHO Expert group has given interim recommendation that bedaquiline may be added to a WHO-recommended regimen in MDR-TB adult patients when an effective treatment regimen containing four second-line drugs in addition to pyrazinamide cannot be designed or when there is documented evidence of resistance to any fluoroquinolone in addition to multidrug resistance. It has also received FDA approval on December 28, 2012 to treat MDR-TB in adults as part of combination therapy when other alternatives are not available.[35]

OPC-67683

OPC-67683 is a nitroimidazole with high potency *in vitro* and *in vivo* against *M. tuberculosis*, inclusive of MDR strains. It probably acts through inhibition of cell wall biosynthesis, a mechanism similar to that of PA-824, but is approximately 20 times more potent. OPC-67683 and PA-824 are relatively closely related compounds and appear to share cross-resistance. OPC-67683 has a long half-life at approximately 7–8 hours, with no cross-resistance or antagonistic activity with first-line anti-TB drugs. In the mouse model, its activity was superior to that of conventional drugs. In mice, 2 months of OPC-Rifampicin-Pyrazinamide followed by another 2 months of OPC-Rifampicin led to complete culture negativity, suggesting that OPC-67683 could shorten TB therapy in combination with other existing drugs.[36] In a Bactec system using drug-tolerant *M. tuberculosis* clinical strains, OPC has shown concentration-dependent sterilization activity that, at the highest dose levels tested (1.0 mg/l), was superior to Isoniazid and equal to Rifampicin.[37] In a phase IIa, open-label, active controlled randomized clinical trial to evaluate the safety, efficacy and pharmacokinetics (PK) of four dosages (100, 200, 300 or 400 mg) of delamanid, administered orally once daily for 14 consecutive days, delamanid at all dosages was found to be safe, well tolerated and demonstrated significant exposure-dependent EBA over 14 days.[38]

PA-824

PA-824 is a nitroimidazopyran, a class of novel antibacterial agents. By means of an agreement in 2002, the TB Alliance was granted worldwide exclusive rights to develop PA-824 and its analogues for anti-TB treatment.[2] PA-824 has many attractive characteristics as a potential anti-TB agent. It is active against drug-susceptible and drug-resistant, as well as actively dividing and nonreplicating *M. tuberculosis*.[39] It has a narrow spectrum of activity, with a relatively specific action against tubercle bacilli and no significant activity against many other Gram-positive and Gram-negative bacteria.[2] In addition, there is no evidence of mutagenicity or significant cytochrome P450 interactions. Its mechanism of action is not very well understood, although it may possibly act by inhibiting both protein production and cell wall lipid biosynthesis in *M. tuberculosis*. A recent report has suggested that PA-824 might act on nonreplicating *M. tuberculosis* by intracellular nitric oxide release.[40] From studying CFU counts in the lungs of mice, PA-824 showed bactericidal activity comparable to that of Isoniazid in the first 8 weeks and sterilizing activity comparable to that of Isoniazid-Rifampicin in the continuation phase.[41] In the mouse model, it has shown excellent tissue penetration. Rifampicin-PA-824-Pyrazinamide for 2 months followed by Rifampicin-PA-824 led to higher sterilization activity in mice compared with conventional TB therapy.[42] A follow-up experiment in mice showed advantages in relapse rate with the same combination of drugs when PA-824 was given at a higher dose of 100 mg/kg.[43] With the novel combination of PA-824-Moxifloxacin-Pyrazinamide, mice were cured more rapidly than with the first-line regimen of Rifampicin-Isoniazid-Pyrazinamide, suggesting that this combination might radically shorten the treatment of MDR-TB in humans.[44]

No serious adverse events were reported in Phase I single-dose and multiple-dose trials in healthy volunteers.[2] A Phase IIa extended EBA study was conducted in Cape Town (South Africa), evaluating the efficacy, safety and pharmacokinetics in newly diagnosed sputum smear-positive patients with drug-susceptible TB.[45] Based on findings from the preclinical and Phase I studies, escalating doses of PA-824 were administered for 14 consecutive days to four groups of patients and compared with a fifth cohort receiving standard first-line TB treatment. The study showed substantial and continued EBA over 14 days with equivalent efficacy at all doses from a daily dose of 200–1200 mg. Although higher doses were associated with more potential adverse events, no significant drug-related events were demonstrated. Based on these findings, the TB Alliance plans to explore lower doses of PA-824 to define the minimum effective dose. However, as PA-824 is 94% plasma-bound, it is necessary to ensure that sufficiently high concentrations of the free drug can be reached in cavities of pulmonary TB to exert bactericidal activity.[46] Recently, a dry powder preparation of PA-824 was tested for aerosol inhalation in guinea pigs.[47] This preparation may have the advantage of a lower dose administration for treatment of pulmonary TB compared with the oral route.

LL-3858

LL-3858 is a pyrrole with activity against drug-susceptible and drug-resistant strains of *M. tuberculosis*. It probably has a novel mechanism of action.[48] It shows *in vitro* synergistic activity with Rifampicin. In the mouse model, it was more effective than Isoniazid as monotherapy. In combination with existing anti-

TB drugs, LL-3858 was reported to sterilize the lungs and spleens of infected animals in a shorter timeframe than conventional therapy.[49] In a Phase I trial in healthy adult male volunteers, LL-3858 was found to be better absorbed under fasting conditions. Doses below 600 mg appeared to be safe and well tolerated. Further studies are being planned to evaluate EBA of LL-3858 in sputum-positive TB patients.[50]

SQ-109

Although SQ-109 is a diamine identified from screening of Ethambutol analogues, it is probably a novel antimycobacterial agent, as suggested by its structural dissimilarity and potential difference in target of action.[2] It is active against *M. tuberculosis* strains, inclusive of those with MDR, and has synergistic activity with Rifampicin and Isoniazid, as well as an additive effect with streptomycin.[51] It probably acts through inhibition of cell wall synthesis. In the mouse model, 2 months of Rifampicin-Isoniazid-SQ-109-Pyrazinamide was found to be superior to the conventional regimen and led to sterilization. Thus, SQ-109 appears to be an effective replacement for Ethambutol.[52] A dose-escalation Phase I study has been completed in 62 subjects. The doses administered were well tolerated up to 300 mg with a half-life of 61 hours.[53] An *in vitro* study has been conducted to investigate interactions of SQ-109 and TMC-207 for synergistic, additive or antagonistic activity, using both drug-susceptible and drug-resistant *M. tuberculosis* strains.[54] SQ-109 and TMC-207 in combination were either synergistic or additive in activity regarding various *M. tuberculosis* strains and showed an increased rate of killing and enhanced postantibiotic effect and intracellular killing activity. Results showed that the drug combination was extraordinarily potent, with greater than 90% kill of *M. tuberculosis* as early as 1 day after drug combination exposure. SQ109 completed three phase I studies in the US. Phase II efficacy studies in tuberculosis patients are currently underway. SQ-109 showed activity against both drug-susceptible and Multi-drug-resistant tuberculosis bacteria, including Extensively drug-resistant tuberculosis strains. In preclinical studies, SQ-109 enhanced the activity of antitubercular drugs isoniazid and rifampin and reduced by > 30% the time required to cure mice of experimental TB.[55]

Other New Drugs

Apart from the aforementioned drugs, there are some new compounds in the portfolios of TB Alliance and other enthusiastic workers in various stages of development.[1,2] Examples include nitrofuranylamides,[56] meropenem-clavulanate,[57] pleuromutilins,[2] malate synthase inhibitors[2] and various others. With this flourishing interest and commitment, it appears that there is a chance of having a new drug available soon.

Adjunctive Immunotherapy in MDR-TB and XDR-TB

Apart from the development of antimicrobials in the treatment of TB, there has been active exploration for effective immunotherapy as a form of complementary treatment to speed up disease recovery and reduce relapse.[58,59] In the host's protective immune response against *M. tuberculosis*, the key cells are macrophages, different types of T cells, alongside their elaborated cytokines. New potential immunotherapeutic modalities explored include cytokines and other agents. Studies with cytokines have moved from preclinical to clinical phase, notably for IFN-γ,[60,61] IFN-α,[62,63] IL-2[64] and IL-12.[65] Earlier studies using IFN-γ[66] and the atypical mycobacterial vaccine *Mycobacterium vaccae*[67] have shown rather encouraging results in terms of bacillary load lowering and radiographic improvement. Two recent negative studies from South Korea have, however, tampered the enthusiasm regarding the use of IFN-γ in the treatment of MDR-TB.[68,69] Nevertheless, another recent report has provided a back swing of the pendulum by demonstrating the possible clinical efficacy of IFN-γ in treatment of MDR-TB, alongside favorable immumodulating profiles involving natural killer cells and some lymphocyte types.[70]Another putative protective cytokine in TB, IL-12, while theoretically attractive, has potentially significant toxicity on administration.[71] Preclinical studies in monoclonal antibodies and polyclonal antibody preparations against *M. tuberculosis* have also demonstrated some beneficial effects.[72,73]

The role of other potential immunomodulators, such as vitamin D, apparently requires further delineation, including both for efficacy and tolerance.[74] Lately, much interest regarding intracellular killing of *M. tuberculosis* has been focused on the phenomenon of autophagy, which is an intracellular homeostatic mechanism for clearing aged intracellular organelles and proteins.[75] Rapamycin, an inhibitor of the target of rapamycin proteins, can enhance autophagy. However, this drug is basically rather toxic. It appears that small-molecule enhancers of rapamycin may assume the role better by inducing autophagy independently or in connection with the target of rapamycin protein.[75] It is clear that much more work needs to be done in the area of immunotherapy for MDR-TB and XDR-TB.

References

1. Working Group on New TB Drugs. Global TB Research and Development Projects—Information as of October 2007. www.stoptb.org/wg/new_drugs/projects.asp.
2. The Global Alliance for TB Drug Development www.tballiance.org.
3. Ma Z. Overview of the global TB drug pipeline. Int J Tuberc Lung Dis 2008;12:S13.
4. ClinicalTrials.gov: NCT00216385. A controlled trial of a 4-month quinolone-containing regimen for the treatment of pulmonary tuberculosis. http://clinicaltrials.gov/ct2/show/NCT00216385term=Gatifloxacin+and+tuberculosis&rank=2.
5. Park-Wyllie LY, Juurlink DN, Kopp A, et al. Outpatient gatifloxacin therapy and dysglycemia in older adults. N Engl J Med. 2006;354:1352-61.
6. Spigelman MK. New tuberculosis therapeutics: a growing pipeline. J Infect Dis. 2007; 196;S28-S34.
7. Johnson JL, Hadad DJ, Boom WH, et al. Early and extended early bactericidal activity of levofloxacin, gatifloxacin and moxifloxacin in pulmonary tuberculosis. Int J Tuberc Lung Dis. 2006;10:605-12.
8. Gosling RD, Uiso LO, Sam NE, et al. The bactericidal activity of moxifloxacin in patients with pulmonary tuberculosis. Am J RespirCrit Care Med. 2003;168:1342-5.

9. Pletz MW, De Roux A, Roth A, Neumann KH, Mauch H, Lode H. Early bactericidal activity of moxifloxacin in treatment of pulmonary tuberculosis: a prospective, randomized study. Antimicrob Agents Chemother. 2004;48:780-2.
10. Gillespie SH, Gosling RD, Uiso L, Sam NE, Kanduma EG, McHugh TD. Early bactericidal activity of a moxifloxacin and isoniazid combination in smear-positive pulmonary tuberculosis. J Antimicrob Chemother 2005;56:1169.
11. Burman WJ, Goldberg S, Johnson JL, et al. Moxifloxacin versus ethambutol in the first 2 months of treatment for pulmonary tuberculosis. Am J Respir Crit Care Med. 2006;174:331-8.
12. Conde MB, Efron A, Loredo C, et al. Moxifloxacin versus ethambutol in the initial treatment of tuberculosis: a double-blind, randomised, controlled Phase II trial. Lancet 2009;373:1183-9.
13. Rustomjee R, Lienhardt C, Kanyok T, et al. A Phase II study of the sterilizing activities of ofloxacin, gatifloxacin and moxifloxacin in pulmonary tuberculosis. Int JTuberc Lung Dis 2008;12:128-38.
14. Tuberculosis Research Centre. Shortening short course chemotherapy: a randomized clinical trial for treatment of smear positive pulmonary tuberculosis with regimens using ofloxacin in the intensive phase. Ind J Tub 2002;49:27-38.
15. Global Alliance for TB Drug Development. Controlled Comparison of Two Moxifloxacin Containing Treatment Shortening Regimens in Pulmonary Tuberculosis (REMoxTB). 2012 September 21. Available from: http://clinicaltrials.gov/ct2/show/NCT00864383 (Accessed June 26, 2013).
16. Merle CS, Sismanidis C, Bah Sow O, Gninafon M, Horton J, et al. 2012. A pivotal registration phase III, multicenter, randomized tuberculosis controlled trial: design issues and lessons learnt from the Gatifloxacin for TB (OFLOTUB) project. Trials13: 61.
17. ClinicalTrials.gov: NCT00144417. TBTC Study 28: moxifloxacin versus isoniazid for TB treatment. http://clinicaltrials.gov/ct2/show/NCT00144417?term=moxifloxacin+and+tuberculosis&rank=3.
18. Dorman S, Johnson J, Goldsberg S, et al. Substitution of moxifloxacin for isoniazid during intensive phase treatment of pulmonary tuberculosis. Am J Respir Crit Care Med. 2009;180:273-80.
19. ClinicalTrials.gov: NCT00864383. Controlled comparison of two moxifloxacin containing treatment shortening regimens in pulmonary tuberculosis (REMox TB). http://clinicaltrials.gov/ct2/show/NCT00864383?term=moxifloxacin+and+tuberculosis&rank=3.
20. Dooley K, Flexner C, Hackman J, et al. Repeated administration of high-dose intermittent rifapentine reduces rifapentine and moxifloxacin plasma concenrations. Antimicrob. Agents Chemother 2008;.52:4037-42.
21. Rosenthal IM, Zhang M, Almeida D, Grosset JH, Nuermberger EL. Isoniazid or moxifloxacin in rifapentine-based regimens for experimental tuberculosis? Am J Respir Crit Care Med. 2008;178:989-93.
22. ClinicalTrials.gov: NCT00728507. Rifapentine plus moxifloxacin for treatment of pulmonary tuberculosis. http://clinicaltrials.gov/ct2/show/NCT00728507?term=moxifloxacin+and+tuberculosis&rank=1.
23. Andries K, Verhasselt P, Guillemont J, et al. A diarylquinoline drug active on the ATP synthase of Mycobacterium tuberculosis. Science 2005;307:223-7.
24. Haagsma AC, Abdillahi-Ibrahim R, Wagner MJ, et al. Selectivity of TMC-207 towards mycobacterial ATP synthase compared with that towards the eukaryotic homologue. Antimicrob. Agents Chemother 2009;53:1290-2.

25. Koul A, Vranckx L, Dendouga N, et al. Diarylquinolines are bactericidal for dormant mycobacteria as a result of disturbed ATP homeostasis. J Biol Chem. 2008; 283:25273-80.
26. Lounis N, Gevers T, Van Den Berg J, Andries K. Impact of the interaction of R207910 with rifampin on the treatment of tuberculosis studied in the mouse model. Antimicrob. Agents Chemother 2008;52:3568-72.
27. Ibrahim M, Andries K, Lounis N, et al. Synergistic activity of R207910 combined with pyrazinamide against murine tuberculosis. Antimicrob. Agents Chemother2007; 51:1011-1015.
28. Veziris N, Ibrahim M, Lounis N et al. A once-weekly R207910-containing regimen exceeds activity of the standard daily regimen in murine tuberculosis. Am J Respir Crit Care Med. 2009;179:75-9.
29. Nuermberger E, Mitchison DA. Once-weekly treatment of tuberculosis with the diarylquinoline R207910: a real possibility. Am J Respir Crit Care Med 2009;179:2-3.
30. Lounis N, Veziris N, Chauffour A, Truffot-Pernot C, Andries K, Jarlier V. Combinations of R207910 with drugs used to treat multidrug-resistant tuberculosis have the potential to shorten treatment duration. Antimicrob Agents Chemother 2006;50:3543-7.
31. ClinicalTrials.gov: NCT00828529. TMC207-TiDP13-C110: interaction study in healthy volunteers with lopinavir/ritonavir http://clinicaltrials.gov/ct2/show/study/NCT00828529?term=TMC-207&rank=1 (Accessed March 4 2009).
32. Rustomjee R, Diacon AH, Allen J, et al. Early bactericidal activity and pharmacokinetics of the diarylquinoline TMC-207 in treatment of pulmonary tuberculosis. Antimicrob Agents Chemother 2008;52:2831-5.
33. ClinicalTrials.gov: NCT00449644. TMC207-TiDP13-C208: anti-bacterial activity, safety, and tolerability of TMC-207 in patients with multidrug-resistant Mycobacterium tuberculosishttp://clinicaltrials.gov/ct2/show/NCT00449644?term=tmc207&rank=2.
34. Diacon AH, Donald PR, Pym A, et al. Randomized pilot trial of 8 weeks of bedaquiline (TMC-207) for MDR-TB: long-term outcome, tolerability and effect on emergence of drug resistance. Antimicrob Agents Chemother. 2012;56:3271-6.
35. World Health Organization. The Use of Bedaquiline in the Treatment of Multidrug-Resistant Tuberculosis: Interim Policy Guidance. Geneva: World Health Organization; 2013. 2, Guidance purpose and target audience. WHO/HTM/TB/2013.6. Available at: http://apps.who.int/iris/bitstream/10665/84879/1/9789241505482_eng.pdf.
36. Matsumoto M, Hashizume H, Tomishige T, et al. OPC-67683, a nitro-imidazooxazole derivative with promising action against tuberculosis in vitro and in mice. PLoS Med 2006;3:E466.
37. Saliu OY, Crismale C, Schwander SK, Wallis RS. Bactericidal activity of OPC-67683 against drug-tolerant Mycobacterium tuberculosis. J Antimicrob Chemother. 2007;60:994-8.
38. Diacon AH, Dawson R, Hanekom M, Narunsky K, Venter A, et al (2011). Early bactericidal activity of delamanid (OPC-67683) in smear-positive pulmonary tuberculosis patients. Int J Tuberc Lung Dis. 15: 949-54.
39. Stover CK, Warrener P, Van Devanter DR, et al. A small-molecule nitroimidazopyran drug candidate for the treatment of tuberculosis. Nature 2000;405:962-6.
40. Singh R, Manjunatha U, Boshoff HI, et al. PA-824 kills nonreplicating *Mycobacterium tuberculosis* by intracellular NO release. Science. 2008;322:1337-8.
41. Tyagi S, Nuermberger E, Yoshimatsu T, et al. Bactericidal activity of the nitroimidazopyran PA-824 in a murine model of tuberculosis. Antimicrob Agents Chemother. 2005;49:2289-93.

42. Nuermberger E, Rosenthal I, Tyagi S, et al. Combination chemotherapy with the nitroimidazopyran PA-824 and first-line drugs in a murine model of tuberculosis. Antimicrob Agents Chemother. 2006;50:2621-5.
43. Tasneen R, Tyagi S, Williams K, Grosset J, Nuermberger E. Enhanced bactericidal activity of rifampin and/or pyrazinamide when combined with PA-824 in a murine model of tuberculosis. Antimicrob Agents Chemother 2008;52:3664-8.
44. Nuermberger E, Tyagi S, Tasneen R, et al. Powerful bactericidal and sterilizing activity of a regimen containing PA-824, moxifloxacin, and pyrazinamide in a murine model of tuberculosis. Antimicrob Agents Chemother. 2008;52:1522-4.
45. Diacon A, Dawson R, Venter A, et al. Update on PA-824. Int J Tuberc Lung Dis. 2008;12:S14.
46. Hu Y, Coates AR, Mitchison DA. Comparison of the sterilizing activities of the nitroimidazopyran PA-824 and moxifloxacin against persisting *Mycobacterium tuberculosis*. Int J Tuberc Lung Dis. 2008;12:69-73.
47. Sung JC, Carcia-Contreras L, Verberkmoes JL, et al. Dry powder nitroimidazopyran antibiotic PA-824 aerosol for inhalation. Antimicrob Agents Chemother. 2009;53:1338-43.
48. Deidda D, Lampis G, Fioravanti R, et al. Bactericidal activities of the pyrrole derivative BM-212 against multidrug-resistant and intramacrophagic Mycobacterium tuberculosis strains. Antimicrob Agents Chemother. 1998;42:3035-7.
49. Sinha RK, Arora SK, Sinha N, Modak VM. In vivo activity of LL-3858 against Mycobacterium tuberculosis. Presented at: 44th Interscience Conference on Antimicrobial Agents and Chemotherapy. Washington, DC, USA, 30 October–2 November 2004 (Abstract F-1116).
50. Arora SK, Anuradha K, Avhad AJ. Phase I clinical trial of LL-3858 (Sudoterb), a potential candidate for the treatment of MDR tuberculosis. Int J Tuberc Lung Dis. 2008; 2:S319-S320.
51. Chen P, Gearhart J, Protopopova M, Einck L, Nacy CA. Synergistic interactions of SQ-109, a new ethylene diamine, with front-line antitubercular drugs in vitro. J Antimicrob Chemother. 2006;58:332-7.
52. Nikonenko BV, Protopopova M, Samala R, Einck L, Nacy CA. Drug therapy of experimental tuberculosis: improved outcome by combining SQ-109, a new diamine antibiotic, with existing TB drugs. Antimicrob Agents Chemother. 2007; 51:1563-5.
53. Ginsberg AM. Development of new drugs for TB. IDSA Annual Meeting 4–7 October, 2007, San Diego, CA, USA. www.idsociety.org/WorkArea/downloadasset.aspx?id=7946.
54. Bio-Medicine. Sequella presents data on synergy between investigational new TB drugs SQ-109 and TMC-207 www.bio-medicine.org/medicine-technology-1/Sequella-Presents-Data-on-Synergy-Between-Investigational-New-TB-Drugs-SQ109-and-TMC-207-3357-2/.
55. Bio-Medicine. Sequella commences Phase 1b study for new tuberculosis drug SQ-109 www.bio-medicine.org/biology-technology-1/Sequella-Commences-Phase-1B-Study-for-New-Tuberculosis-Drug-SQ109-11930-1/.
56. Hurdle JG, Lee RB, Budha NR, et al. A microbiological assessment of novel nitrofuranylamides as antituberculosis agents. J Antimicrob Chemother 2008;62:1037-45.
57. Hugonnet JE, Tremblay LW, Boshoff HI, Barry CE, Blanchard JS. Meropenem-clavulanate is effective against extensively drug-resistant *Mycobacterium tuberculosis*. Science. 2009;323:1215-8.
58. Reljic R, Paul MJ, Arias MA. Cytokine therapy of tuberculosis at the crossroads. Expert Rev. Resp. Med. 2009;3:53-66.

59. Achkar JM, Casadevall A, Glatman-Freedman A. Immunological options for the treatment of tuberculosis: evaluation of novel therapeutic approaches. Expert Rev. Anti Infect ther. 2007;5:461-74.
60. Suárez-Méndez R, García-García I, Fernández-Olivera N, et al. Adjuvant interferon gamma in patients with drug-resistant pulmonary tuberculosis: a pilot study. BMC Infect dis. 2004;4:44.
61. Koh WJ, Kwon OJ, Suh GY, et al. Six-month therapy with aerosolized interferon-γ for refractory multidrug-resistant pulmonary tuberculosis. J Korean Med Sci. 2004;19,167-71.
62. Giosuè S, Casarini M, Ameglio F, et al. Aerosolized interferon—a treatment in patients with multidrug-resistant pulmonary tuberculosis. Eur Cytokine Netw. 2000;11:99-104.
63. Kuchtey J, Fulton SA, Reba SM, Harding CV, Boom WH. Interferon-ab mediates partial control of early pulmonary Mycobacterium bovis bacillus Calmette-Guerin infection immunology. 2006;118:39-49.
64. Johnson JL, Ssekasanvu E, OkweraA, et al. Randomised trial of adjunctive interleukin-2 in adults with pulmonary tuberculosis. Am J Respir Crit Care Med. 2003;168:185-91.
65. Ha SJ, Park SH, Kim HJ, et al. Enhanced immunogenicity and protective efficacy with the use of interleukin-12-encapsulated microspheres plus AS01B in tuberculosis subunit vaccination. Infect Immun. 2006;74:4954-9.
66. Condos R, Rom WN, Schluger NW. Treatment of multidrug-resistant pulmonary tuberculosis with interferon-γ via aerosol lancet. 1997;349:1513-5.
67. Stanford JL, Stanford CA, Grange JM, Lan NN, Etemadi A. Does immunotherapy with heat-killed Mycobacterium vaccae offer hope for the treatment of multidrug-resistant pulmonary tuberculosis? Respir Med. 2001;95:444-7.
68. Park SK, Cho S, Lee IH, et al. Subcutaneously administered interferon-γ for the treatment of multidrug-resistant pulmonary tuberculosis. Int J Infect Dis. 2007;11:434-40.
69. Grahmann PR, Braun RK. A new protocol for multiple inhalation of IFN-γ successfully treats MDR-TB: a case study. Int J Tuberc Lung Dis. 2008;12:636-44.
70. Leonard JP, Sherman ML, Fisher GL, et al. Effects of single-dose interleukin-12 exposure on interleukin-12-associated toxicity and interferon-γ production. Blood. 1997;90:2541-8.
71. Williams A, Reljic R, Naylor I, et al. Passive protection with immunoglobulin A antibodies against tuberculous early infection of the lungs immunology. 2004;11:328-33.
72. Guirado E, Amat I, Gil O, et al. Passive serum therapy with polyclonal antibodies against Mycobacterium tuberculosis protects against post-chemotherapy relapse of tuberculosis infection in SCID mice. Microbes Infect. 2006;8:1252-9.
73. Wejse C, Gomes VF, Rabna P, et al. Vitamin D as supplementary treatment for tuberculosis—a double-blind randomized placebo-controlled trial. Am J Respir Crit Care Med. 2009;179:843-50.
74. Gutierrez MG, Master SS, Singh SB, Taylor GA, Colombo MI, Deretic V. Autophagy is a defense mechanism inhibiting BCG and Mycobacterium tuberculosis survival in infected macrophages cell. 2004;119:753-66.
75. Floto RA, Sarkar S, Perlstein EO, Kampmann B, Schreiber SL, Rubinsztein DC. Small molecule enhancers of rapamycin-induced TOR inhibition promote autophagy, reduce toxicity in Hungtington's disease models and enhance killing of mycobacteria by macrophages autophagy. 2007;3:620-2.

Index

Page numbers followed by *t* refer to table.

N

O